CANCER PATIENT CARE

CANCER PATIENT CARE
PSYCHOSOCIAL TREATMENT METHODS

Edited by

Maggie Watson

Published by BPS BOOKS   and   CAMBRIDGE UNIVERSITY PRESS

(The British Psychological Society)

Cambridge
New York   Port Chester
Melbourne   Sydney

First published in 1991 by BPS Books (The British Psychological Society),
St Andrews House, 48 Princess Road East, Leicester LE1 7DR and
the Press Syndicate of the University of Cambridge
The Pitt Building, Trumpington Street, Cambridge CB2 1RP
40 West 20th Street, New York, NY 10011-4211, USA
10 Stamford Road, Oakleigh, Melbourne 3166 Australia.

A catalogue record for this publication is available from the British Library.
Library of Congress Cataloging-in-Publication Data is available.

Printed and bound in Great Britain by BPCC Wheatons Ltd, Exeter.

ISBN 0 521 41632 9 hard covers
ISBN 0 521 42631 6 paperback

CONTENTS

CONTRIBUTORS

Nicole Alby
Department of Haematology
Saint-Louis Hospital
Paris, France

Gary Bell
Department of Psychological
  Medicine
Medical College of St Bartholomew's
  Hospital
London, UK

Peter M. Black
School of Medicine and Dentistry,
  and
School of Education and Human
  Development
University of Rochester
New York, USA

Kerry Bluglass
The Woodbourne Clinic, and
Department of Psychiatry
University of Birmingham
Birmingham, UK

Gerjanne Bos-Branolte
Department of Gynaecology
University Hospital Leiden
Leiden, The Netherlands

Mary V. Burton
Department of Clinical Psychology
Gulson Hospital
Coventry, UK

Sheila Cassidy
St Luke's Hospice
Plymouth, UK

Ann Cull
ICRF Medical Oncology Unit
Western General Hospital
Edinburgh, UK

Ephrem Fernandez
Department of Psychology
University of Queensland
Brisbane, Australia

Ann Goldman
Symptom Care Team
Great Ormond Street Hospital for
  Sick Children
London, UK

Jennifer Hughes
Department of Psychiatry
Royal South Hants Hospital
Southampton, UK

Richard Lansdown
Department of Psychology
Great Ormond Street Hospital for
  Sick Children
London, UK

Stirling Moorey
CRC Psychological Medicine
  Research Group
The Royal Marsden Hospital
London and Sutton, UK

Gary R. Morrow
School of Medicine and Dentistry
University of Rochester
New York, USA

Clare Moynihan
Academic Department of
  Radiotherapy
The Royal Marsden Hospital
London and Sutton, UK

Dennis C. Turk
Department of Psychiatry, and
Pain Evaluation and Treatment
  Institute
University of Pittsburgh School of
  Medicine
Pittsburgh, USA

Maggie Watson
CRC Psychological Medicine
  Research Group
The Royal Marsden Hospital
London and Sutton, UK

FOREWORD

In the new and burgeoning field of psychosocial oncology, much effort has been devoted to monitoring the nature and extent of psychological ill-health and social disability resulting from cancer and from various cancer treatments. This initial phase of research has yielded useful systematic data about the quality of life of patients which is an important consideration in decisions regarding treatment. But the documentation of psychosocial morbidity, though clearly necessary, is not sufficient. The next logical step is to develop methods of psychological therapy which can reduce such morbidity and thereby improve the quality of life of cancer patients.

Until recently, however, it was widely believed that since emotional distress was an understandable and, perhaps, inevitable reaction to the diagnosis of cancer, psychological intervention was not feasible. The present book finally lays that belief to rest. It is encouraging to learn that, in an increasing number of oncology centres, clinical psychologists, psychiatrists, nurses, physicians and other mental health professionals are contributing directly to the care of patients and, where appropriate, their families. The book outlines specific treatments which are being devised to enable patients to cope with a variety of distressing cancer-related symptoms such as pain, anticipatory nausea and vomiting, anxiety and depression. The kinds of psychological treatment described here include cognitive and behavioural psychotherapy, psychotropic medication and supportive counselling. It is essential that these therapeutic procedures should be subjected to randomized, controlled trials.

In view of the currently fashionable craze for alternative nostrums for cancer, it should be stressed that the psychological therapies recommended in this book are an integral part of orthodox medical treatment. Indeed, the inclusion of psychological therapies within oncology should bring closer the ideal to which medicine pays lip service but which is rarely achieved, namely treatment of the whole person.

S. Greer

Director, Cancer Research Campaign
The Royal Marsden Hospital

INTRODUCTION

Cancer is a major disease with high incidence and mortality rates and in the UK accounts for one quarter of all deaths. During 1988 (the most recent year for which UK mortality figures are available) over 160,000 people died from cancer (Cancer Research Campaign, 1989) and in the USA this figure is closer to 400,000. Worldwide it can be said that in general approximately one out of four to five people will develop cancer in their lifetime (Hirayama *et al.*, 1980).

A few cancers tend to predominate, with lung, colorectal, breast and stomach cancers accounting for a substantial proportion of the cases diagnosed each year. In Europe lung cancer is the leading cause of cancer death in men and breast cancer the leading cause in women, and the UK is 'in the unenviable position of leading the world in terms of breast cancer mortality rates' (Cancer Research Campaign, 1988). Some cancers, although less common, are more likely to affect children and young adults and therefore the significance of their impact is in terms of years of life lost. There is no clear indication that, overall, the mortality trends will decline. (While for some cancers, such as Hodgkin's disease and childhood leukaemias, mortality rates are decreasing, others, such as breast cancer, appear to be showing a gradual increase (Cancer Research Campaign, 1988; Mould, 1983).)

As a disease cancer has strong emotional overtones, being likened to a 'ubiquitous plague' (Weisman, 1981) and described as the 'standardised nightmare of our society' (Rosser and Maguire, 1982). Yet, in spite of this gloomy picture, on average 46 per cent of women and 35 per cent of men with cancer in the UK are alive five years after diagnosis.

Cancer treatments have changed dramatically since the end of the nineteenth century when surgical excision of a tumour was the mainstay of treatment. The discovery of x-rays and radium during the last decade of the nineteenth century led to a major change in treatment methods, and the 1920s and 1930s brought new treatment options with the advent of radiotherapy. However, the most dramatic advance has been in the treatment of cancer by chemotherapy and during the last thirty years there have been major innovations and successes in the use of systemic treatment methods. This success in prolonging life has not been without its cost as chemotherapeutic treatments can be aggressive and cause unpleasant side-effects. Thus for many cancer patients the quality of life that is available to them within the context of cancer treatment has become a real issue. Because of the changes in prognosis and treatments indicated above the rehabilitation of patients and maintenance of a good quality of life has become an important issue.

Psychosocial Oncology

Concern that cancer patients have a good quality of life is not new, but psychosocial oncology as a subspecialism of oncology is a recent arrival on the cancer scene. It has grown from research aimed at understanding and alleviating the emotional and social impact of cancer on patients and their families. Where possible psychosocial oncology bases clinical practice on data, but without losing sight of the individual case. Essentially clinical practice in psychosocial oncology covers the detection of psychological, psychiatric and social morbidity, the diagnosis of this morbidity and the provision of treatments designed to alleviate it. Unlike other specialities within medicine, it is not the property of any one group; indeed it is a multidisciplinary area and the skills may be practised by nurses, oncologists, psychologists, psychiatrists, and social workers. This is not a definitive list, as a wide range of professional groups will make use of the techniques available. However, treatment methods in psychosocial oncology do require full knowledge of the relevant techniques and skill in applying them. The 'tea and sympathy' approach in the care of cancer patients is being slowly left to amateurs. This process of professionalization depends on the development of ideas which are based firmly on research and over the last decade there has been an explosion of studies in psychosocial oncology, with a significant increase in published papers compared to the preceding decade. Yet, in Europe at least, the integration of psychosocial services into cancer treatment centres has been slow to develop. Ganz *et al.* (in press) in their survey of European and American research in psychosocial oncology commented:

> In Europe, consultation liaison psychiatry has had only limited development as a subspeciality and very few psychologists have been integrated into medical settings where cancer treatment is provided. In addition, relatively few European cancer centres and hospitals routinely provide the range of psycho-social services which are often available in American cancer treatment centers.

The Historical Context

However, the present situation must be seen within a historical context which helps explain why the overall well-being of the patient became unfashionable in medical practice. Jewson (1976) has described medical cosmology since 1770 as encompassing, in chronological order, three different frameworks which he has called: Bedside Medicine, Hospital Medicine and Laboratory Medicine.

In the late eighteenth and early nineteenth centuries Bedside Medicine prevailed. In this approach it was considered that each individual patient had their own unique pattern of morbid events. These individual morbid forces were located within the context of the total body system rather than any particular organ or tissue. The essence of Bedside Medicine was the idea that psyche and soma were part of the same system of pathology.

However, a dramatic transformation occurred in the Parisian hospital schools during the middle of the nineteenth century with the advent of morbid anatomy. Diagnosis was now based on the observation of organic structures and not just on the symptoms reported by the patient. It was at this time, when Hospital Medicine prevailed, that psyche and soma became clearly differentiated and, indeed, that psychiatry became a specialized area of clinical study separated from other areas of medicine.

Towards the latter half of the nineteenth century Laboratory Medicine was becoming established within the German schools. This had the effect of banishing the patient from medicine in the sense that illness was viewed as a disturbance in cells and laboratory tests began to provide a basis for diagnosis. Thus medicine became concerned with the cell as:

> the fundamental unit of life. . .Life thus became the process of interaction within and between cells, disease a particular form of these physical and chemical processes. (Jewson, 1976).

As a result of this approach to medicine:

> Interest in the unique qualities of the whole person evaporated to be replaced by studies of specific organic lesions and malfunctions. . . the special qualities of the individual case were swallowed up in vast statistical surveys. (Jewson, 1976)

In what seems a cutting analysis of modern medicine Jewson makes the point that the activity of medical investigators is focused primarily upon the advancement of certified knowledge rather than the 'servicing of clients'. What Jewson appears to suggest is that there are no career rewards for caring for the patient as a whole but only for excellence in a narrowly defined area. This has had the effect of limiting the extent to which psychosocial elements were incorporated into clinical practice.

Despite this view of modern medicine as piecemeal and lacking in humanism, there has been an increasing trend, within oncology, towards total patient care and this has helped foster the growth of psychosocial oncology.

Quality of Life

Research on quality of life is a good indicator of this interest. In reviewing the period from 1956 to 1976 Bardelli and Saracci (1978) found less than five per cent of papers published in six major cancer journals attempted any measurement of 'quality of life'. More recently de Haes (1988) pointed out that within *Index Medicus* the concept of quality of life was contained within philosophy and only became a separate subject in 1977. From around 1977 onwards interest in this area has been growing rapidly, and the assessment of quality of life has increasingly been incorporated into cancer research, particularly in treatment trials. By 1988 a search of the literature for the period between 1972 to 1987 (Aaronson *et al.*, 1988), indicated that more than 3,000 publications on this topic had appeared.

Much of the explanation for this recent interest in quality of life is embedded in the modern approach to the clinical management of cancer and this is reflected in Ganz *et al.*'s (in press) observation that the development of quality-of-life research in oncology has paralleled the expanded use of chemotherapy as a treatment for cancer. Although important progress continues to be made in treatment methods, there are circumstances where treatment is achieved only at the cost of adverse reactions and loss of well-being. The aggressive chemotherapy regimens bring side-effects which can lead some patients to think that the treatment is worse than the disease. However, most patients are undoubtedly prepared to tolerate great discomfort in order to achieve a remission or cure and this was highlighted in a recent study (Slevin *et al.*, 1989). But, where no significant survival advantage can be observed between treatments, other aspects of treatment become important to consider, such as the effects on quality of life. Within the context of cancer clinical trials an assessment of quality of life is being included in order to quantify the impact of treatment side-effects on psychosocial functioning. The issue is now about the cost at which cancer treatment is achieved in terms of damage to quality of life. Medicine is a pragmatic science and its approach to quality of life issues is no exception. Yet through this chink in the high-technology armour of modern oncology has slipped a more human and humane approach to care.

Patients and their families have also contributed to the development of psychosocial services by demanding that physicians pay attention to their emotional needs. Cassileth (1987) describes this very aptly when she talks about the typically American approach to illness, with people now saying:

> We want attention to ourselves, our souls and our emotions, as well as to our disease. We want a concern for us as people, and we want the inclusion of healing methods such as nutritional attention and spiritual and emotional support, that display such concern.

The self-help movement.   It could also be argued that the burgeoning self-help movement is an attempt, by patients, to fulfil these other needs that the medical system does not address.

In the US the self-help movement has made significant advances over the last 20 years and has become a well-established source of emotional and social support for patients and their families. Other countries have been slower to follow but the American example has had a ripple effect. A UK survey of cancer support and self-help groups (Alderson, 1988) showed that prior to 1979 five groups were founded. There was, however, an upsurge during 1982–84 and at the time of the survey some 300 British groups existed. These groups are based primarily in the community and only 38 per cent had been instituted by a 'professional'. The benefits or otherwise of self-help groups are not the issue here, rather they reflect a growing demand by patients and their families for resources directed at their emotional and social needs.

PSYCHOLOGICAL MORBIDITY AND PROBLEMS

From this background the relatively new subspeciality of psycho-social oncology has emerged. It is becoming more widely accepted that attention to psychological problems is essential to good clinical practice and much of this change, in Europe, has ridden on the back of the quality-of-life interests. In the United States a more pragmatic approach has been adopted in psychosocial oncology, with a concentration on the psychological and psychiatric sequelae of cancer. The last decade in particular has provided an expanding data base relating to levels of psychological morbidity, variety of presenting problems and methods of psychosocial intervention.

One of the most widely quoted studies, by Derogatis *et al.* (1983) in the United States, indicated that the prevalence of psychiatric disorders, as defined by DSM III criteria, was 47 per cent among new admissions of cancer patients. The majority of these were cases of depression or anxiety judged to be treatable. Other studies (Hughes,

1981; Maguire *et al.*, 1978; Morris *et al.*, 1977) have shown the pre-valence to be between 20–35 per cent depending on the methods and timing of assessments. The vast majority of cases represent adjustment disorders and more recent surveys (Dean, 1987; Watson *et al.*, in press) suggest that serious disturbance is confined to between 5–15 per cent of recently diagnosed patients.

This observed morbidity is not confined to depression and anxiety. For example, a substantial number of patients with cancer of a sex organ go on to experience sexual and/or marital disruption (Dean, 1987; Morris *et al.*, 1977; Tross *et al.*, 1984). A significant number of patients being treated by chemotherapy will develop psychologically-based nausea and vomiting, often referred to as anticipatory nausea and vomiting. A survey of approximately 17 American studies (Burish and Carey, 1986) indicated an average combined prevalence rate of 32 per cent for patients receiving repeated cycles of chemotherapy. Pain too is a problem which is clearly capable of compromising the patient's quality of life and psychological treatments exist which can provide benefits when used alongside conventional methods of pain control.

In the area of terminal care important advances have been made. Much of this progress has sprung from the hospice movement and has brought a better understanding of the emotional and social, as well as the physical needs of the terminally ill. These issues and others relating to presenting problems are discussed in detail in the book.

Research in psychosocial oncology has made an important contribution by highlighting the range of problems. Perhaps as a result of this increasing evidence confirming the amount and extent of psychological morbidity, there is now a greater demand for psychological and psychiatric services for cancer patients and their families.

The need to address the patient's emotional well-being and adopt an holistic model of care goes beyond the domain of the specialist mental health professionals, however, to other professions involved in cancer patient care and the words of Peabody, some sixty years on, are still relevant:

> The good physician knows his patient through and through and his knowledge is bought dearly. Time, sympathy and understanding must be lavishly dispensed but the reward is to be found in that personal bond which forms the greatest satisfaction of the practice of medicine. One of the essential qualities of the clinician is interest in humanity, for the secret of the care of the patient is in caring for the patient. (Peabody, 1927)

AIMS

This book provides practical guidelines for improving the psychosocial services to cancer patients and their families.

Overall the book has three primary aims:

(1) To provide practical guidelines for psychosocial care based firmly on research.

(2) To encourage the implementation of psychological and psychiatric treatment methods and service recommendations, thereby providing patients with a more skilled and professional psychosocial service.

(3) To draw attention to the benefits for both patients and staff of allocating resources to this presently undersupported area of patient care.

Apart from the benefits received by patients in terms of improved quality of care it has been argued (Butcher, 1990; Schlesinger *et al.*, 1983) that psychosocial services can help reduce the utilization of hospital resources and financial benefits may accrue as a result. Any initial financial investment in providing psychosocial services will bring benefits in the longer term.

This book is not intended as a complete guide to implementing psychosocial services, indeed a number of the techniques described require supplementary training. The need for further training in this area is often undervalued. Here again, with few exceptions, the United States is ahead of Europe in providing 'highly developed programs for training health care professionals in the psychosocial aspects of cancer' (Ganz, *et al.*, in press). This book highlights the need for further training with the aim of providing a more skilled health care professional.

OVERVIEW OF THE CHAPTERS

The topics covered within this volume have been divided into two sections. The first part deals with specific problems and approaches which may be found throughout the many diagnostic groups. Particular techniques are outlined and although contributors may express a preference for one technique or another, they nevertheless describe excellent models for treating the specific problems. In some instances the contributors suggest a narrow range of treatment methods whilst others review a wide range of options. Some problem areas have received detailed and sustained research and others may have been only a limited focus for study. This is reflected to some degree in the descriptions of treatment techniques with some being narrow and highly specific and others more wide-ranging.

Basic communication skills are not covered in this volume, although a number of authors allude to these or describe some elements of these skills. In general this book is about specific techniques and models of care and assumes, to some extent, that the reader is already familiar with those skills which contribute to good doctor–patient or professional–client communication.

Because psychosocial oncology, in general, is not owned by any particular discipline, there is a tendency to avoid prescribing who should do what and instead, where roles *are* defined, these are usually recommendations about who might be best placed to provide a particular aspect of service. Some professional groups, such as clinical psychologists and psychiatrists will be able to draw upon a greater depth and range of skills and experience, thereby making some treatments more clearly their domain. However, the reviews of techniques described by the authors in this first section will be useful to all professions involved in cancer patient care by improving their knowledge of how these problems may be tackled either by themselves or others.

The second section of this volume concentrates on the problems which may arise within certain diagnostic groups. Some degree of overlap can be found between parts I and II because some of the difficulties described are common to all patients with a chronic life-threatening disease. However, the chapters in part II focus upon and highlight the problems specific to a particular type of cancer.

The chapter on children is exceptional in that it does not focus on a particular type of cancer. Children with cancer represent a separate group because although they share the experience of a life-threatening disease with adults, the problems they experience can be quite different and are worthy of separate attention.

Part of the reason for organizing chapters in part II according to diagnosis arises from the way in which psychosocial skills are developing. In the same way that oncologists tend to specialize in one diagnostic group or another, so too there is a tendency for mental health professionals to build up their knowledge of specific diagnostic groups. It seemed useful therefore, to devote a section of the book to service and treatment techniques relevant to these groups, and this also recognizes the special problems which arise because of the type of diagnosis.

This book has its gaps. The systemic cancers have been covered only in terms of the difficult, but increasingly utilized, bone marrow transplantation technique. The lack of anything on patients with brain, and head and neck tumours is an important omission. The whole range of diagnostic categories has not been covered and the problems which cancer patients present are not all dealt with in the same depth. There is still a great deal of research needed and some topics have received far more attention and provide a stronger data base than others. Where the evidence on psychological morbidity and evaluated intervention techniques is not clear or is lacking, then it is difficult to provide recommendations and therefore some diagnostic groups have not been covered. If the amount of research in this area continues at the present pace the next five to ten years should see an enrichment of our knowledge. If the *application* of this knowledge can follow the pace of the research we should see a continuing improvement in the psychosocial care of cancer patients.

The professionalization of this care should not necessarily mean increased limits and demarcations on who does what; rather it should serve to enhance skills (including the ability to recognize limitations in skills). Most important of all, clinical work in psychosocial oncology should be recognized as an area of skilled practice – the old adage that 'anyone who is sympathetic can do it' is simply not true. Once this has been accepted then it must follow that staff should be thoroughly trained in the techniques available so that they may practise these skills with success and confidence.

Cancer is a disease surrounded by myths and those caring for patients are not necessarily immune from irrational reactions or fears. W.H. Auden's poem 'Miss Gee' (Mandelson, 1977) reflects some of the mystery, misconceptions and emotional overtones surrounding cancer. Cancer is represented in the poem as a disease which befalls repressed spinster ladies or elderly gentleman and is some kind of perverse outcome of the victim's 'foiled creative fire'. The doctor who examined Miss Gee later sitting at dinner with his wife and ponderously rolling his bread declares 'Cancer's a funny thing': a hidden assassin waiting to strike. The frightened spinster, taken off to hospital, lies 'a total wreck', blankets pulled up to her neck; discussed by the doctors, not as a person, but as a sarcoma and ending her life finally on the anatomy table. Such are the myths of cancer and the attitudes to the 'victims'.

Professionals involved in the care of cancer patients have to deal with these myths and are not themselves unaffected by them. As pointed out by Ray *et al.* (1984) there is 'an inevitable conflict between detached professionalism and personal involvement'. This is not helped by the increasing pressure to provide a service which is both broader and deeper, encompassing elements of psychosocial, as well as the traditional physical care. But, like everything in life we will cope better if we are well prepared. It is hoped that this book will be a valuable resource for all who are interested in psychosocial oncology and wish to improve their skill in dealing with this other important side of cancer patient care.

References

AARONSON, N.K., BULLINGER, M. and AHMEDZAI, S. (1988) A modular approach to quality of life assessment in cancer clinical trials. *Recent Results in Cancer Research*, Vol III. Heidelberg: Springer-Verlag.

ALDERSON, P. (1988) Survey of cancer support and self help groups. *Cancerlink Newsletter*, 12, 10–13.

BARDELLI, D. and SARACCI, R. (1978) Measuring the quality of life in cancer clinical trials. Methods and impact of controlled therapeutic trials in cancer. *UICC Technical Report Series*, 36, 75–97.

BURISH, T.G. and CAREY, M.P. (1986) Conditioned aversive responses in cancer chemotherapy patients: Theoretical and developmental analysis. *Journal of Consulting and Clinical Psychology*, 5, 593–600.

BUTCHER, P. (1990) The clinical contribution and cost-effectiveness of a medical psychologist: Making a case for a sensible use of resources. *Clinical Psychology Forum*, 27, 25–27.

CANCER RESEARCH CAMPAIGN (1988) Breast Cancer Factsheet 6.1.

CANCER RESEARCH CAMPAIGN (1989) Mortality. Factsheet 3.1.

CASSILETH, B.R. (1987) Sociological implications of Mind-Body Cancer Research. In J.C. Holland and M.J. Massie (Eds) *Current Concepts in Psycho-Oncology and AIDS*. New York: Memorial Sloan-Kettering Cancer Center.

DEAN, C. (1987) Psychiatric morbidity following mastectomy: Preoperative predictors and types of illness. *Journal of Psychosomatic Research*, 31, 385–392.

DE HAES, J.C.J.M. (1988) Quality of Life: Conceptual and theoretical considerations. In M. Watson, S. Greer and C. Thomas (Eds) *Psychosocial Oncology*. Oxford: Pergamon.

DEROGATIS, L.R., MORROW, G.R., FETTING, J., PENMAN, D., PIASETSKY, S., SCHMALE, A.M., HENRICKS, M. and CARNICKE, C. (1983) The prevalence of psychiatric disorders among cancer patients. *Journal of the American Medical Association*, 249, 751–757.

GANZ, P.A., BERNHARD, J. and HÜRNY, C. (in press) Quality of life and psychosocial research in oncology in Europe: State of the art. *Journal of Psychosocial Oncology*.

HIRAYAMA, T., WATERHOUSE, J.A.H. and FRAUMENI JR., J.F. (1980) *Cancer Risks by Site*, UICC Technical Report Series, Vol. 41. Geneva: UICC.

HUGHES, J. (1981) Emotional reactions to the diagnosis and treatment of early breast cancer. *Journal of Psychosomatic Research*, 21, 277–285.

MENDELSON, E. (1977) *The English Auden: Poems, essays and dramatic writings 1927–1939*. London: Faber & Faber.

JEWSON, N.D. (1976) The disappearance of the sick-man from medical cosmology 1770–1870. *Sociology*, 10, 225–244.

MAGUIRE, G.P., LEE, E.G., BEVINGTON, D.J., KUCHEMANN, C.J., CRABTREE, R.J. and CORNELL, C.E. (1978) Psychiatric problems in the first year after mastectomy. *British Medical Journal*, 1, 963–965.

MORRIS, T., GREER, S. and WHITE, P. (1977) Psychological and social adjustment to mastectomy. *Cancer*, *40*, 2381–2387.

MOULD, R.F. (1983) *Cancer Statistics*. Bristol: Adam Hilger Ltd.

PEABODY, C. (1927) The care of the patient. *Journal of the American Medical Association*, *88*, 877–882.

RAY, C., FISHER, J. and LINDOP, J. (1984) The surgeon–patient relationship in the context of breast cancer. In C. Ray and J. Weinman (Eds) *Psychological Aspects of Serious Physical Illness*. London: Sage.

ROSSER, J.E. and MAGUIRE, P. (1982) Dilemmas in general practice: The care of the cancer patient. *Social Science and Medicine*, *16*, 323–331.

SCHLESINGER, H.J., MUMFORD, E., GLASS, G.V., PATRICK, C. and SHARFSTEIN, S. (1983) Mental health treatment and medical care utilization in a fee-for-service system: Outpatient mental health treatment following the onset of chronic disease. *American Journal of Public Health*, *73*, 422–429.

SLEVIN, M., STUBBS, L., PLANT, H., GREGORY, W. and MASSEY, L. (1989) 'Cost benefit' calculations in cytotoxic chemotherapy treatments – Decisions made in a hypothetical situation by cancer patients, controls, cancer nurses, cancer doctors and general practitioners. (Paper presented at European Society of Psychosocial Oncology and British Psychosocial Oncology Group Conference, London.)

TROSS, S., HOLLAND, J., BOSL, G. and GELLER, N. (1984) A controlled study of psychosocial sequelae in cured survivors of testicular neoplasms. *Association of the Society of Clinical Oncology*, *3*: 74 (abstract C-287).

WATSON, M., GREER, S., ROWDEN, L., GORMAN, C., ROBERTSON, B., BLISS, J. and TUNMORE, R. (in press). Relationships between emotional control, adjustment to cancer and depression and anxiety in breast cancer patients. *Psychological Medicine*.

WEISMAN, A.D. (1981) Understanding the cancer patient: The syndrome of caregiver's plight. *Psychiatry*, *44*, 161–168.

ACKNOWLEDGEMENTS

Thanks are due to all the contributors who have so willingly accepted the difficult task of providing guidelines on the different aspects of cancer patient care. Their knowledge and expertise have been gained by many years of working with cancer patients and I am honoured that they agreed to share this in the book.

Thanks must also go to the patients seen over the years, who have brought joy, pleasure, sadness and regrets but have allowed me to learn through their experience of having cancer. Working with cancer patients and their families does not have to be a depressing experience, as is often assumed; it can be filled with challenge and a sense of fulfillment, with always something new to learn just around the corner.

I would like to acknowledge the help of Gillian Chesney and Tereza Gladwell who helped organize and carry out the secretarial work and to Clare Moynihan for her helpful comments and Jan for his encouragement. Permission to reproduce Richard Lansdown and Ann Goldman's chapter was generously granted by the Editor of the *Journal of Child Psychology and Psychiatry* and Pergamon Press plc. Finally, I gratefully acknowledge the support of the Cancer Research Campaign.

Part I

Problem-specific treatment methods

PAIN: A COGNITIVE-BEHAVIOURAL PERSPECTIVE

Dennis C. Turk and Ephrem Fernandez

Every year, more than 15 million people receive a diagnosis of cancer (Bonica, 1979). Historically, being informed that one had cancer was tantamount to a death sentence. Advances in early detection and new and aggressive treatments (for example, chemotherapy, radiotherapy, immunotherapy and surgery) however, have increased life expectancy and even cure among patients who formerly would have been expected to die shortly after receiving the diagnosis. A paradox raised by the greater life expectancy, however, is that aggressive treatments can have severe iatrogenic consequences. Moreover, living longer can result in living with the consequences of disease progression such as increased tissue pathology and the concomitant nociceptive stimulation and resulting pain.

Pain is often inextricably intertwined with neoplastic disease. Bonica (1979) has reviewed existing data and concluded that moderate to severe pain is reported by 40–45 per cent of patients immediately after diagnosis, 35–45 per cent at intermediate stages of the disease, and 60–85 per cent in advanced stages of the disease. Pain can also be an unfortunate consequence of cancer treatment. The presence of unremitting and possibly intensifying pain is capable of compromising the patient's quality of life. In this latter instance, pain becomes an important issue in its own right.

In the two preceding paragraphs we have used the terms 'nociception' and 'pain'. It is important to differentiate between these two terms. Nociception refers to sensory information *capable* of being perceived as pain. Pain, however, can be experienced and reported even in the absence of nociceptive stimulation. Moreover, the association between report of pain and identifiable tissue pathology is less than perfect and less than might be expected.

Despite the magnitude of the problem, pain *per se* has received disproportionately little attention in oncology. Cancer is viewed primarily as a potentially lethal disease and thus eradication of the disease is the central concern. As such, the immediate concern is aetiologic, focusing on the isolation of a treatable cause. Pain is merely a sympton supposedly indicating disease progression. Once it is determined that the cause of pain is either untreatable, a consequence of treatment or unrelated to disease progression, it is viewed as a nuisance and subsequently relegated to a distant concern.

More recently, the quality of life of cancer patients has been recognized and palliation of pain symptoms, even when eradication of the cause is not possible, has been raised as an appropriate target for palliative treatment. Many papers (for example, Foley and Inturrisi, 1987; Portenoy, 1988; WHO, 1986) have focused on diverse interventions to control cancer pain – systemic analgesics, anti-inflammatory drugs, palliative radiotherapy and chemotherapy, neurosurgical procedures, regional anaesthesia. Accompanying these papers have been polemic debates about dependence, tolerance and addiction and the appropriate uses of narcotic medication. These issues have received much attention (see Portenoy, 1988 for a review) and hence will not be discussed in this chapter. Psychological factors as well as nonpharmacological interventions in cancer pain management, although acknowledged, have largely been ignored. Thus, we will direct our discussion to these topics. It should not be assumed from this that we see somatic therapies as dispensable or in any way inferior to psychological ones. On the contrary, we believe that they are essential but not the only modalities in the pain control armamentarium. A broader perspective is needed whereby psychological concepts, variables and treatment modalities receive greater consideration in keeping with their recognized contributions to pain, and the promise they hold for future advances in alleviating suffering (Turk and Fernandez, 1990).

DIVERGING PERSPECTIVES ON CANCER AND CHRONIC PAIN

It is interesting to observe how the pain literature has evolved over the past quarter century. Historically, pain was viewed as a sensory phenomenon directly linked to somatic perturbations. A common assumption that is pervasive in oncology is that pain associated with cancer is unique, directly linked to tissue pathology and less subject to the same psychological variables implicated in other classes of clinical pain (see, for example, McGuire, 1989). The assumption seems to be that if a cancer patient reports pain, this subjective report is a veridical reflection of an objective state of their anatomy and physiology. The cancer pain literature has tended to ignore research on chronic pain and continues to be guided by sensory models. The implicit sensory assumption influences how health care providers as well as patients think about pain and consequently how pain associated with cancer is reported as well as treated (Turk and Fernandez, 1990).

Although nonphysiological factors are acknowledged in cancer pain rarely do they receive serious attention; instead, they tend to be appended at the end of papers detailing pharmacological treatment for cancer pain. When nonpharmacological modalities of pain control are mentioned, they are explained in terms of physiological processes. Thus, biofeedback and relaxation are recommended to reduce muscle tension that might exacerbate pain associated with tumours impinging on physical structures. Hypnotic effects are occasionally attributed to endorphinergic mediation and cognitive coping strategies are characterized as distractors from nociceptive stimulation.

But various clinical findings are not handled well by a simple sensory-physiological model. For example, this model cannot explain why many individuals: (a) with the same extent of tissue pathology differ so widely in their report of pain intensity; (b) do not report any pain despite objective radiographic evidence of bony degenerative changes; (c) complain of severe pain in the absence of significant physical pathology; and (d) with the same physical diagnosis and identified tissue pathology respond in distinctly different ways when treated with the same intervention.

Psychological factors such as anxiety, expectancy, cognitive appraisal, self-efficacy, perceived control, along with principles of operant conditioning and observational learning have been shown to influence reports and experience of acute pain, acute recurrent pain, and chronic pain not associated with cancer, but these factors have been largely disregarded in the cancer pain literature. The influential gate control model of pain (Melzack and Casey, 1968; Melzack and Wall, 1965) postulating motivational-affective, cognitive-evaluative, as well as sensory-discriminative contributions to the perception of pain appears to have had relatively little impact in cancer pain. In short, the fund of knowledge about pain in general seems to be under-utilized in the cancer pain arena.

Inconsistencies in the pain literature outlined above have resulted in the development of a multidimensional perspective that incorporates both physical and psychological factors (Melzack and Wall, 1965), at least in chronic pain not associated with metastatic disease. The inadequacy of pure sensory models of pain has resulted in an explosion of research examining the role of psychological and social factors in pain perception and response. It is at this point where research on chronic pain and research on pain associated with malignancies appear to diverge.

PSYCHOLOGY OF CANCER AND CANCER PAIN

Cancer is a unique disease, more feared than any other malady. It conjures overwhelmingly negative images and beliefs (Turk and Rennert, 1981). The major sources of distress for cancer patients are their uncertain medical status, fear of physical and functional deterioration, the threat of aggressive anti-cancer treatments and the fear of intensifying pain, and ultimately death. Many of these beliefs are shared by health care professionals, cancer patients, as well as the general population (Turk et al., 1986).

Over time, health care providers have come to share the belief that cancer patients will experience severe pain (Levin et al., 1985). They are not surprised when patients report pain. Since complaints of pain fit the health care providers' expectancies, they are quite willing to accept the patient's report as an indication of nociception justifying an increase in the dosage of analgesic medication or other invasive medical interventions. The patient's beliefs about the severity of pain from cancer are confirmed by the prescription of larger doses of medication and aggressive treatment. This circularity reinforces the perceived link between pain and cancer, despite the fact that significant numbers of cancer patients do not report severe pain, or any pain for that matter (see, for example, Ahles et al., 1984; Turnbull, 1979).

The tendency for health care providers to accept cancer pain reports at face value can be contrasted with self-reports of pain in non-cancer, chronic pain patients. In this latter group, subjective reports are considered to be biased by many nonphysical factors, notably, desire for attention, fear, demoralization. Many of these same factors are operative in cancer pain to at least the same, if not greater extent. The nonphysical factors can influence behavioural communications of distress and suffering as well as 'pain behaviours' (for example requests for medication, grimacing, moaning). Overt communications of suffering elicit responses from health care providers as well as family and friends.

We anticipate that our comments about pain behaviour will provoke anger if not outright hostility. But we wish to have the reader stop, take a deep breath, and then examine his or her own assumptions. Our comments are not meant to imply that health care providers should trivialize cancer patients' reports of pain but rather to reiterate that factors other than nociception may *contribute to* and *modulate* patients' reports.

The nature of cancer pain presents a particular dilemma that has greatly contributed to the diverging views of cancer pain and pain not associated with malignancies. In chronic pain not associated with malignancies, complaints of pain can result from a range of possible reinforcers (for example attention, avoidance of undesirable activities). In these instances, where continuous reporting of pain contributes little information that is diagnostically or therapeutically useful, treatment efforts are often directed towards discouraging patients from reporting pain or engaging in behaviours (pain behaviours) that communicate distress and suffering (for example, grimacing, wincing, limping) and positive reinforcement for activity ('well behaviours') and stoicism. In cancer patients, however, report of pain may signal change in disease status and reporting of pain is necessary for proper titration of treatment for both the disease and pain. Thus, cancer patients are encouraged to focus on symptoms and to report exacerbations of pain to family members and medical staff. Attention may lead to increased reporting. This difference between cancer and non-cancer pain is an important one, and needs to be considered in assessing reports of pain, but it does not remove the probability of operant factors influencing the report of pain. The dilemma is how to differentiate appropriate reports of pain from maladaptive pain behaviours. We will return to this point later.

Does the evidence support a simple one-to-one relationship between physical pathology and report of pain? In the non-cancer pain literature, it has become clear that the direct link between pathology and pain is quite tenuous (for example, Beecher, 1946; Schmidt, 1985). In the oncology literature, there is also some evidence that challenges the isomorphic association. As early as 1920, Simmons and Daland noted that many patients indicated that the reasons they had delayed in seeking treatment for what were determined to be cancerous lesions was that they did *not* experience any pain. Only rarely is pain the primary symptom bringing cancer patients to physicians initially. However, the frequency of pain complaints appears to be significantly increased following the diagnosis of cancer (Black, 1975; Woodforde and Fielding, 1979). Cassell (1982) cited an example of a patient whose pain could easily be controlled with codeine when the patient attributed it to sciatica, but required significantly greater amounts of medication to achieve the same degree of relief when he was told that the pain was due to metastatic cancer. And, even after the diagnosis, contrary to what might be expected from the sensory view, Greenwald *et al.* (1987) found only a weak association between pain intensity and stage of disease (stage is associated with disease progression and concomitant pathology).

A range of psychological variables has been identified that influence patients' perceptions and reports of pain. This body of literature has tended to focus on pain unrelated to cancer and, as noted, the literature has tended to be ignored by oncologists. Space does not permit a detailed review of this literature (see Dolce, 1987; Skevington, 1983; Thompson, 1981; Turk and Rudy, 1986) thus we will only highlight some findings that carry implications for cancer pain management.

Expectancy

Anticipation of pain can lead to catastrophizing responses that augment perceived pain. Hall and Stride (1954), for instance, showed that when the word 'pain' was included in their instructions to laboratory subjects the latter demonstrated significantly lower thresholds for and greater sensitivity to a noxious thermal stimulus than when exposure was preceded by a neutral instructional set omitting the word pain. Byron and Yonemoto (1975) reported that 77 per cent of patients with advanced cancer obtained complete relief for four hours or more from pharmacological preparations that included *no* active analgesic medication. This well-known placebo effect has been observed across diverse pharmacological preparations and even surgery (Beecher, 1955, 1961).

These data provide support that patients' beliefs can influence both the perception of pain and response to pharmacological agents. And cancer patients expect to experience pain (Levin *et al.*, 1985) despite the fact that over half of breast cancer patients, 80 per cent of lymphoma patients, and 95 per cent of leukaemia patients do not report pain (Foley, 1984). Overall, nearly two thirds of all hospitalized cancer patients and one third of terminally ill patients do not require analgesic medication (Foley, 1979). Moreover, when pain is reported, the severity reported tends, even at its worst, to be moderate (Daut and Cleeland, 1982) and significantly lower than the pain reported by patients with chronic non-cancer pain. We do not mean to suggest that pain is not a problem for cancer patients but rather that the misconceptions of both patient and health care providers can affect how they think and respond to cancer and pain.

Fear and Anxiety

Anxiety has been demonstrated to be both a cause and correlate of pain reports. Anxiety can initiate a sequence of physiological changes instigating nociception through heightened sympathetic nervous system activity that provokes muscle spasm, vasoconstriction, visceral disturbances, and release of pain-producing substances (for example substance P, Bradykinen). Furthermore, in an anxious state, patients may not be able to differentiate signs of sympathetic arousal from nociceptive stimulation. Thus, anxiety may exacerbate pain by altering the discriminability of physical sensations, so that a lower threshold is used for *labelling* sensory events as pain (for example Mallow *et al.*, 1986; Yang *et al.*, 1983).

Over the past 30 years, a number of investigators (for example Bowers, 1968; Jones *et al.*, 1968) have demonstrated that level of anxiety can modulate subjective pain reports. Barber (1959) concluded:

> It appears that some procedures that are said to reduce pain actually reduce anxiety, fear, worry, and other emotions that are usually intermingled with pain. For instance, the pain relief that follows the administration of morphine and other opiates may be closely related to the reduction of anxiety or fear. Although the patient who has received the opiate may still experience pain sensations, the reduction in anxiety, fear or other emotions apparently leads him to report that pain is reduced.

Some of the pain and physical side-effects that accompany cancer treatments may be exacerbated by emotional distress. For example, Spiegel and Bloom (1983) found that mood disturbance and the meaning of pain to a patient predicted patients' reported pain intensity in a sample of 86 women with metastatic breast cancer. They reported that greater mood disturbance and the *belief* that pain signaled a worsening of their disease were significantly correlated with reported pain intensity. The authors concluded that since the patient sample was homogeneous with regard to medical status, the differential pain experiences reported were due in large part to the patients' emotional status.

The influence of the situation in which the pain occurs on the perceived level of pain is particularly important in cancer patients because of the fear and anxiety often evoked by the diagnosis. This is demonstrated by the observation in a study of 667 cancer patients in which pain was perceived as interfering with activity and enjoyment of life (as reported by patients) to a greater degree when pain was perceived to be caused by cancer than when it was thought to have another cause (Daut and Cleeland, 1982). Ahles *et al.* (1984) noted that 61 per cent of patients studied were afraid that pain signified a progression of their disease. These patients had significantly higher scores on several measures of anxiety and depression than the group that did not consider pain as indicative of worsening or progressive disease. Similarly, Easterling and Leventhal (1989) found that among patients who believed that cancer posed an imminent threat (i.e. who knew that the disease had metastasized), distress about cancer was found to be highly related to the number of chemotherapy side-effects. These same somatic sensations did not predict distress about cancer for women who had undergone 'successful' surgery and were receiving chemotherapy in the adjuvant situation, that is as a means of preventing recurrence.

Perceived Controllability

Attribution of control is another factor implicated in non-cancer pain research (Thompson, 1981). Several clinical studies indicate that perceived control, that is, the belief that one has control (whether veridical or not) is sufficient to produce significant pain relief (for example Holroyd et al., 1984). Hill et al. (1986) used patient-controlled analgesia (a patient-controlled drug infusion pump) for cancer patients undergoing painful bone marrow transplantation. The pain produced by this procedure is very severe and persists for up to four weeks. The authors found that those with the pump used approximately one third as much morphine to achieve equivalent levels of pain control compared to those who received narcotics administered by nurses. Thus, perception as well as actual ability to control pain appears to be capable of alleviating the intensity of the pain experienced.

Self-Efficacy

A central construct in the cognitive-behavioural model of chronic pain is self-efficacy (Bandura, 1977). A self-efficacy expectation is defined as a personal conviction that one can successfully perform certain required behaviours in a given situation. It has been suggested that given sufficient motivation to engage in a behaviour, it is an individual's self-efficacy beliefs that determine whether that behaviour will be initiated, how much effort will be expended, and for how long effort will be sustained in the face of obstacles and aversive experiences. From this perspective, the coping behaviours are conceptualized as mediated by individuals' beliefs that situational demands do not exceed their coping resources. Individuals with weak efficacy expectancies are viewed as less likely than those with strong expectancies to make coping responses or persist in the presence of obstacles and aversive consequences.

Mastery experiences gained through performance accomplishments are hypothesized to have the greatest impact on establishing and strengthening expectancies because they provide the most information about actual capabilities. Successful versus unsuccessful physical therapy may be distinguised by the presence versus the absence of changes in perceived self-efficacy in conjunction with physical improvements in tolerance, strength, and endurance. Patients need to learn to make a distinction between hurt and harm. One group of pain patients may stop an activity when it hurts often for fear of exacerbating the physical injury (they also stop because they wish to avoid the noxious sensations per se).

Thus, techniques that enhance mastery experiences (for example, graded task accomplishments with both physical and verbal feedback) will, according to Bandura (1977), be powerful tools for bringing about behaviour change. Moreover, the patient's self-attribution of task accomplishment should enhance maintenance of improvements (Kopel and Arkowitz, 1975). In this way, cognitive variables are the primary determinants of behaviour, but these variables are altered most effectively by performance-based accomplishments. If cancer patients feel there is little they can do to control pain, they will expend minimal effort in trying to use self-control techniques, may become more emotionally distressed, which in turn, may amplify the pain experienced.

Symptom Preoccupation

A physical symptom is the awareness of some aspect of internal state. Note that this definition does not mean that there necessarily is any physiological concomitant of the symptom. The symptom is a perception. A stomach ache may signal indigestion, food poisoning, intestinal flu, appendicitis, or anxiety.

Imagine a patient with breast cancer who notices pain in her leg several days after chemotherapy. The pain cues evoke emotional and perceptual memory images of her mother, who had similar pain from bone metastases of breast cancer. The knowledge of her mother's decline and death, particularly the perceptual memories of the change in her physical appearance, is extremely fear-provoking. The patient becomes agitated and concerned that the pain may represent a spread of the cancer, even though she knows that cancer only occasionally produces pain similar to what she is experiencing.

After a brief period, the patient takes two aspirins and hopes that the pain will diminish. She still remains upset about the possible meaning of her pain however, and calls two friends, describing her experience and soliciting advice. When these calls fail to calm her, she goes to see her local physician, who examines the site of pain and suggests the pain is muscular and not due to cancer. After some reassurance and instructions to use aspirin and try muscle relaxation, the visit is concluded.

The patient may become more relaxed and comforted by the physician's lack of concern. On returning home, she decides that the pain really is much less severe than it was before she took the aspirin. She chides herself for becoming so upset by a minor pain and decides that in the future she will take aspirin for such pain and continue her daily routine. In this example, the following sequence has occurred: symptom perception – interpretation – coping with the objective (sensation) and emotional (fear of cancer spread) factors – symptom monitoring – feedback – reinterpretation.

The very act of monitoring sensations for signs of change increases the probability that expected changes (*ipso facto* exacerbation of pain) will be perceived. The cancer patient may become increasingly isolated, self-centered, and preoccupied with his or her body. Constant monitoring of the body will likely lead to identification of bodily signs that in other situations might be ignored or never even be perceived. There may even be a tendency to report the presence of symptoms believed related to physical limitations and chronic conditions based on prior experience. Thus, there may be anticipation of noxious stimulation and reports of such sensation even in their absence.

Much of the diversity of people's responses to threatening events or ambiguous sensations is attributable to variations in the appraisal process. An individual's appraisals influence emotional arousal and the behavioural response to a situation. The more ambiguous the event the greater the reliance on subjective interpretations and appraisals and subsequent responding. Cancer is, by its very nature, an ambiguous disease. It is often of unknown origin, its course is unpredictable and erratic, the likelihood of arresting the disease progression is uncertain, and the physical sensations created by the disease, treatment, and physiological arousal in response to the diagnosis are often vague and diffuse. When an individual has cancer, he or she becomes sensitized to, continually monitors, and preoccupies himself or herself with bodily sensations. Physical sensations serve as a constant reminder of the disease, with all that it connotes, and are capable of being interpreted or misinterpreted as 'pain' (Ahles *et al.*, 1984; Pennebaker, 1982) as well as leading to over-reaction and outright panic (Rachman *et al.*, 1987). Continual vigilance and monitoring of noxious stimulation and the belief that it signifies disease progression may render even low intensity nociception less bearable.

As we have asserted, the difference between pain from cancer and pain related to non-malignant conditions may be more apparent than real. The differences are continuous rather than categorical. Both are subject to the same principles of pain management. We next turn our attention to the operant factors that have been studied in the non-cancer pain literature but viewed with some hostility in the cancer world (Chapman, 1979).

OPERANT CONDITIONING AND CHRONIC PAIN

Fordyce (1976) observed that all communication of pain takes place through some form of behaviour. Distinguished from the private experience of pain, pain behaviours are observable and quantifiable. They include moaning, grimacing, limping, seeking analgesic medication, and other overt communications of suffering.

The basic principles underlying the operant model have been summarized succinctly by Fowler *et al.* (1969):

1. Behavior is largely a function of its consequences.
2. Behavior which is followed by positive or rewarding consequences will tend to be maintained or to increase in rate.
3. Behavior which is followed by neutral [or negative] consequences will tend to diminish or drop out altogether.

These principles suggest that if behaviours signaling pain result in positive consequences, the frequency of these pain behaviours will increase. The patient may receive attention (often sympathy) and frequently is relieved of their usual responsibilities when such behaviours are displayed. Attention and legitimized abdication of responsibility are all presumably rewarding experiences. Thus, pain behaviours originally elicited reflexively or emitted randomly may come to occur, totally, or in part, in response to reinforcing environmental events. Elimination of positive reinforcement of pain behaviours in conjunction with positive reinforcement of well behaviours should, according to the 'law of effect', lead to extinction of maladaptive pain behaviours and increased activity.

Several studies provide evidence supporting the underlying assumptions of the operant conditioning model. Cairns and Pasino (1977) and Doleys *et al.* (1982) demonstrated that pain behaviours can be decreased by verbal reinforcement and the setting of exercise quotas. Block *et al.* (1980) demonstrated that pain patients reported differential levels of pain in an experimental situation depending on whether they were observed by their spouses or ward clerks. Pain patients with non-solicitous spouses reported more pain when neutral observers were present than spouses. When solicitous spouses were present, pain patients reported more pain than in the neutral observer condition. Flor *et al.* (1987) noted that chronic pain patients reported more intense pain and less activity if they indicated their spouses were solicitous. The latter two studies suggest that spouses, at least solicitous ones, can serve as discriminative stimuli for the display of pain behaviours by chronic pain patients, including reports of pain intensity.

Treatment Based on Operant Conditioning

Treatments based on the operant model include: (a) positive reinforcement for activity, and inattention to extinguish learned maladaptive behaviours; (b) use of medication on a time-contingent rather than on an as needed basis, with gradual reductions in the quantity of analgesic medications; (c) physical activity to increase strength, endurance, and flexibility that should also lead to corrective neuro-muscular feedback, and (d) assertiveness and social skills training to provide patients with more appropriate means of securing rewards or avoiding punishment in situations where they have become accustomed to displaying pain behaviours.

Partner participation is strongly encouraged because the partner is probably the most important reinforcing agent and he or she can facilitate transfer of new behavioural patterns to the home environment. The methods of achieving these goals include withdrawal of attention for pain behaviours, and attention and reinforcement of well behaviours. Increased activity levels are promoted by establishing exercise quotas and reinforcing activity using time-contingent or task completion-contingent rest, rather than pain-contingent rest, and praise and attention for effort and goal accomplishments. Rewards for requesting medications are eliminated by altering administration of medication from the usual *prn* (as needed, and thus pain-contingent) to a fixed interval (time-contingent) schedule.

Treatment based on the operant model has targeted patients with chronic pain unrelated to malignancies. Several reports of the efficacy of operant treatment have appeared in the literature (for example Anderson *et al.*, 1977; Fordyce *et al.*, 1973; for recent reviews see Linton, 1986; Turner and Romano, 1984). Until recently, however, little attention was given to operant factors as they might relate to cancer pain (see Keefe *et al.*, 1985).

There is no intrinsic reason why the same behavioural principles of managing pain unrelated to malignancies should not be pertinent to cancer pain. It is quite plausible that positive reinforcement (for example, attention, concern, support) might have the effect of maintaining and increasing the behavioural manifestations of distress. The maladaptive illness behaviour of cancer pain patients is often reinforced by well-meaning significant others and may be extinguished using the same operant principles described above. Reports of pain should not be ignored as they may be related to increased nociception or disease progression; however, once these possibilities are ruled out, then the role of operant factors needs to be entertained. Thus the clinician may wish to examine the consequents that follow complaints of pain. If significant others provide attention when the patient reports pain and no physical basis is identified, the clinician may consider discussing more appropriate ways to obtain attention with both the patient and those who might provide the attention desired by the patient.

Vicarious learning may also play an important role in cancer pain. Craig (1986; 1988) has demonstrated the role of modeling in the behavioural expression of experimental and acute pain. In one study, Fagerhaugh (1974) noted the potent effects of observational learning on pain behaviour and distress on a burn unit. In this study, patients who had been on the unit longer 'modeled' appropriate behaviours for newly-admitted patients. Appropriate behaviours included suppression of overt distress except at times of designated treatments (i.e. debridement of the burn sites). Similar modeling principles might be considered and utilized for cancer patients on palliative care units and hospices; conversely, the negative effects of modeling pain behaviours by patients needs to be examined in any clinical situation that brings patients into interaction with one another (for example while waiting for radiation therapy).

CLASSICAL CONDITIONING AND PAIN

Gentry and Bernal (1977) were the first to suggest that classical conditioning of pain and tension may occur in an acute pain state due to some form of physical damage leading to a pain–tension–pain cycle. This model views pain both as a response to and antecedent of specific autonomic activity. Lenthem *et al.* (1983) postulated that once an acute pain problem exists, conditioned fear of movement may develop and motivate avoidance of activity, and thereby lead to immobilization. Individuals who suffer from acute pain, regardless of the cause, may adopt specific protective and adaptive behaviours (for example limping, reclining) in order to avoid pain and, therefore, may never obtain 'corrective feedback' because they fail to perform more natural movements (Philips, 1987; Rachman and Lopatka, 1988). Reduction in physical activity may subsequently result in muscle atrophy, increased impairment and increased disability. In this manner, the physical abnormalities may actually be secondary to changes in behaviour initiated through a learning process.

As the pain symptoms persist, more and more situations may elicit anxiety and pain. Dependence on medication and depression may follow, further intensifying the pain–tension cycle. Thus, psychological expectations may lead to modified behaviour that, in turn, may produce physical changes leading to still further physical deconditioning. With chronic pain, the anticipation of suffering or prevention of pain may be sufficient for the long-term maintenance of the maladaptive avoidance behaviours.

Treatment Based on Respondent Conditioning

The respondent model described above gives priority for the maintenance of pain to the psychological principles of classical conditioning. In contrast to the operant view of physical causation, the respondent model emphasizes the learned contingency of movement and nociception and subsequent behavioural response. Treatment from this model focuses upon extinguishing the connection by exposure and disconfirmation. Specifically, the respondent model would explain part of the efficacy of physical therapy, for example, on the basis of exposure to the feared activities and the breaking of the association between hurt and harm (Fordyce, 1988).

The theoretical basis for biofeedback and relaxation training based on the respondent conditioning model assumes that the bracing and muscle spasm seen in many pain patients represents a conditioned response either to external stimuli or to internal nociceptive stimuli (interoceptive conditioning). From this perspective, biofeedback or relaxation have a clinical effect by reducing the presumed maladaptive physiological response and subsequent experiencing of pain through counterconditioning.

COGNITIVE-BEHAVIOURAL PERSPECTIVE ON CANCER

Specific cognitive variables such as expectancy and controllability have already been the subject of our discussion. The cognitive-behavioural approach, however, is a broader one that warrants mention here because of its focus on variables that may be particularly relevant for patients with cancer. It incorporates information-processing principles while recognizing the intimate association between cognition, affect, behaviour, and physiology.

The role of cognitive factors has been emphasized in perception and behavioural response to nociception (Turk *et al.*, 1983). From the cognitive-behavioural perspective, people who experience chronic or recurrent pain are viewed as having negative expectations about their own ability to execute certain motor skills without pain (Schmidt, 1985), adopt a negative set about pain and how pain will affect their lives, and appraise their situation as one in which there is little they can do to cope with the nociception experienced. Such negative, maladaptive appraisals about the situation and personal efficacy may reinforce the experience of demoralization and dysphoric mood, symptom preoccupation, inactivity, and overreaction to nociceptive stimulation, which in turn will influence behavioural response.

The cognitive-behavioural perspective has two basic assumptions. First, individuals are active processors of information rather than passive recipients of environmental stimuli. People attempt to make sense of, understand, predict and control their lives. When they are confronted with stimuli that interrupt ongoing behaviour, they attempt to appraise their resources for responding and behave accordingly. The amount of threat, arousal, or stress they experience is a joint function of the idiosyncratic appraisals of the novel stimuli and their adaptive resources. Second, cognitions, emotions, behaviours, and the social environment are to some extent causally related. Cognitions can elicit feelings, potentiate emotions, reduce arousal, and serve as an impetus for behaviour. Conversely, feelings and behaviours can facilitate or inhibit the production of cognition, and behaviours and emotions can influence the type of response from the environment. Thus, behaviour is reciprocally determined by both the individual and his or her environment.

The application of the cognitive-behavioural perspective to cancer patients and cancer pain has been described by several authors (for example, Cleeland and Tearnan, 1986; Fishman and Loscalzo, 1987; Turk and Rennert, 1981); however, empirical research on the efficacy of this approach is lacking. Turk and Rennert (1981) recognized the value of multicomponent treatment regimens tailored to specific stages in the course of pain. They proposed a treatment package in which rational self-statements, attention-diversion, relaxation, problem-solving, operant conditioning, and self-regulation techniques are carefully integrated with somatic treatments to deal with nociception, pain, and suffering. As Turk and Rudy (1989) suggest, the cognitive-behavioural perspective that focuses on individual appraisals, interpretations, and expectancies, as well as physiology and environmental influences may be more essential than any specific technique.

COGNITIVE-BEHAVIOURAL INTERVENTION

Cognitive-behavioural interventions are active, time-limited, structured forms of treatment that can be administered on either an individual or group basis. They are designed to help patients identify, reality test, and correct maladaptive, distorted conceptualizations and dysfunctional beliefs, by cognitive restructuring, problem-solving, and coping skills training. In addition, environmental variables are manipulated using behavioural methods such as reinforcement and exposure.

Drawing from earlier applications to anxiety disorders, depression, and chronic pain, cognitive-behavioural intervention for cancer pain has three foci: (1) alteration of maladaptive behaviours; (2) alteration of ongoing self-statements, images, and feelings that interfere with adaptive functioning, and (3) alteration of cognitive schema (tacit assumptions and beliefs) that give rise to habitual ways of construing the self (i.e. as helpless) and cancer (as uncontrollable, inevitably causing excruciating pain). The objective of intervention is not to abolish pain altogether but to promote well behaviours that facilitate physical reconditioning, as well as teach patients to cope with varying degree of discomfort, disfigurement, and potential lethality so that they can continue to lead effective lives.

The intervention begins from the moment of diagnosis, at which juncture much information is brought in to dispel myths about cancer and to instill a set of accurate facts antithetical to the development of dysfunctional cognitions. This information is accompanied by a skills-training programme that extends throughout the course of the disease. It is once again underscored that cognitive-behavioural therapy does not supplant other treatment modalities, but serves as a complement to regular physical therapy, occupational therapy, as well as appropriate medical care.

The specifics of treatment share much in common with most psychological treatments for chronic pain. As outlined by Turk and Holzman (1986) they are as follows:

(1) Reconceptualize the cause of patients' pain so that it is consistent with the rationale underlying the treatment.
(2) Foster a sense of optimism.
(3) Individualize the treatment to match the needs of each patient.
(4) Emphasize active patient participation and responsibility.
(5) Provide skills acquisition.
(6) Orchestrate perceptions of self-efficacy throughout treatment.
(7) Emphasize that the patient should attribute goal accomplishments to him or herself.

These are organized into a programmatic form of intervention. The programme consists of five overlapping stages (Turk and Meichenbaum, 1989):

(1) The initial assessment.
(2) Reconceptualization of the patient's view of pain.
(3) Skills acquisition and consolidation.
(4) Generalization and maintenance.
(5) Follow-through and follow-up.

Although listed separately, the stages overlap. There is a logical sequence to the programme but it must not be implemented with rigid invariance. Patients proceed at varying paces, and the therapist must remain sensitive to these differences. The separation of different stages is designed solely to highlight the different components of the multidimensional treatment. There is no one lock step cognitive-behavioural protocol. A wide range of strategies and techniques is available to the cognitive-behavioural therapist and treatment should be individualized for each patient. More important than any particular technique or tactic is the overall goal of enhancing self-control. It is critical for the therapist to keep in mind the patient's perspective and how he or she perceives each aspect of the treatment. In short, therapists must realize that flexibility and clinical skills have to be brought into play throughout the treatment programme.

Collaborative Therapeutic Relationship

The collaborative therapeutic relationship is a critical ingredient of successful intervention and failure of this relationship will doom any psychological intervention, no matter how potent. In the collaborative therapeutic relationship, the therapist is an ally who is primarily the disseminator of options and a confidant and facilitator of the treatment process. Treatment is designed to assist patients to relinquish the passive, helpless victim role, and to accept an active, self-management role. Therapists can assist but they do not dictate or control. The therapist attempts to enhance patients' commitment by involving them in all phases of the treatment.

The listening and observational skills of the therapist become quite important because they will influence subsequent strategies, revisions of goals and methods. These clinical skills and the relationship that is established between the therapist and the patient become the lubricant that keeps the gears of treatment (i.e. techniques) moving and without which treatment will come to a grinding halt.

Stage 1:   Assessment

The assessment and reconceptualization phases listed above are interdependent. The assessment phase serves several distinct functions:

(1) To establish the extent of physical impairment.
(2) To provide baseline material against which the progress and success of treatment can be compared.
(3) To provide the therapist with detailed information about the nature of the patient's medical condition, previous treatments, perception of their medical condition, expectations about treatment, resources, competencies, as well as deficiencies for handling pain, and their view of various aspects of their lives (for example marital, social, vocational).
(4) To assist in the establishment of appropriate treatment goals.
(5) To begin the reconceptualization process by assisting patients and significant others to become aware of the situational variability and psychological and social factors that influence the nature and degree of pain.
(6) To examine the important role of significant others in the maintenance of maladaptive behaviours and as resources in the change process.

To accomplish these functions, cognitive-behavioural therapists rely on structured interviews, standardized assessment instruments (for example the West Haven-Yale Multidimensional Pain Inventory, Kerns *et al.*, 1985; the Mental Adjustment to Cancer Scale, Greer and Watson, 1987; and the Pain Related Self Statement and Coping Scales, Flor and Turk, 1988), and self-monitoring using self-report diaries (Turk *et al.*, 1983). It is worth noting that these instruments and procedures are not designed to identify psychopathology but rather to focus on impact on various domains of the patient's life, such as alterations in social activities, change in marital interactions.

One question that is particularly suited to providing examples of how cognitive and affective factors, such as appraisal of the situation and coping resources, contribute to the pain experience simply involves asking the patient to imagine the last time they experienced pain of 6 or more on a 10 point scale (10 being the worst pain imaginable) and to recall the thoughts and feelings they can remember experiencing at that time. One colon cancer patient provided the following response:

> How much longer do I have to live this way? I have outlived my capabilities. . .the hours feel aimless and I feel alone. I wish someone could just cut out the pain like they cut out the tumour. . .I am incapable of everything I used to do. How am I going to fill the rest of my life: unemployed, disfigured, dependent but increasingly alone.

The patient obviously feels helpless, views her situation as hopeless, and appraises her situation as one of deterioration and over which she has limited control. In such situations, patients can be asked to consider the impact of such thoughts and feelings on the experience of pain and what they can do in such circumstances. They can be asked how such thinking might exacerbate pain and to consider alternative coping strategies.

Negative thoughts and pain-engendering appraisals are reviewed in treatment so that the patient is not surprised when they do arise. They are not the only ones to have these thoughts. The patient is encouraged to use the negatively valenced cognitions and feelings as cues to instigate more adaptive strategies. For example, patients who report thoughts that they are incompetent and helpless in controlling their pain are encouraged to become aware of when they engage in such thinking and to appreciate how such thoughts may exacerbate their pain and become a self-fulfilling prophecy. Alternative thoughts such as realistic appraisal of the situation will be taught.

Stage 2:   Reconceptualization

A central emphasis of the cognitive-behavioural treatment is to facilitate the emergence of a new conceptualization of pain over the course of treatment, thereby permitting the patient's symptoms to be translated into difficulties that can be pinpointed and viewed as circumscribed and addressable problems, rather than as vague, undifferentiated and overwhelming experiences. The reconceptualization process is designed to prepare the patient for future therapeutic interventions in a way designed to anticipate and minimize patient resistance.

The therapist attempts to alter the patient's conceptualization of his or her pain from the usual sensory view to a more multifaceted one that acknowledges the contributions of cognitive, affective, and socioenvironmental factors to the experience of pain and suffering. The therapist must deal with the patient's conviction that (a) pain inevitably signifies that the disease is progressing; (b) activity that increases pain should *always* be avoided; (c) avoidance of activity will prevent pain, and (d) the patient is helpless when it comes to controlling pain. These beliefs may contribute to inactivity, physical deconditioning, disability, suffering, and prohibit corrective feedback. 'Imaginary patients' may be invoked to bring up fears that may be difficult for the patient to vocalize. For example, the therapist might say, 'Some patients are concerned that if they learn some ways to control their pain, others will think that the pain was all in their head. Let me assure you that learning to control pain by psychological means in no way implies that psychological factors caused the pain'. Through an educational process, the patients are encouraged to think in terms of a treatment that will be effective in enhancing and providing them with greater control over their lives.

Cognitive restructuring refers to identifying and modifying anxiety-engendering cognitive events, processes, and structures. Common cognitive restructuring procedures include: (a) evaluating the validity and viability of thoughts and beliefs; (b) eliciting and evaluating predictions; (c) exploring alternative explanations; (d) attribution retraining, and (e) altering an absolutist, catastrophic thinking style. The therapist encourages the patients to test the adaptiveness (not the so-called rationality) of individual thoughts.

Cognitive restructuring is designed to make patients aware of the role cognitions and emotions play in potentiating and maintaining stress. The therapist elicits the patient's thoughts, feelings, and interpretations of events, gathers evidence for or against such interpretations, identifies habitual self-statements, images and appraisals that occur, tests the validity of these interpretations, identifies automatic thoughts that set up an escalating stream of negative, catastrophizing ideation, and helps examine how such habitual thoughts exacerbate stress and interfere with performance of adaptive coping responses. What are the circumstances when these thoughts and feelings occur and what alternatives are available?

Beecher's (1946) discussion of pain experienced by wounded

soldiers can be used as an example of how appraisal and meaning systems affect the perception of pain. He noted that many soldiers did not report experiencing intense pain despite having incurred life-threatening wounds. Beecher attributed these responses to individuals' appraisals which in turn influenced how much they perceived pain.

The therapist can make use of imagery recall to assist in this process. For example, the patient may be asked to relive in their mind's eye one or more recent experiences of stress as if they were running a movie in slow motion, eliciting thoughts and feelings around specific events and responses. The therapist can then perform a situational analysis with the patient to identify common themes.

Through self-monitoring, the therapist helps patients identify when they are becoming stressed, assists them to become aware of low-intensity cues, then examines the contribution of their thoughts, and deautomatizes the connection between events and arousal or distress. The therapist may ask patients to monitor symptoms but not to over-react by assuming that all unusual or noxious sensations are attributable to worsening of disease – catastrophizing, symptom preoccupation.

A conceptualization of pain loosely based on the gate control model of pain (Melzack and Wall, 1965) can be outlined and then contrasted with the conventional sensory-physiological model that most patients have accepted. The interaction of cognitions, affect, and sensory aspects of a situation are presented in a clear, understandable fashion – for example, the impact of anxiety is described as it relates to exacerbations of pain. In addition, patients review recent stressful events and examine the course of their pain at the time. One breast cancer patient, who had been aware of a connection between periods of tension and intensity of her pain, attributed the pain to spread of the cancer. As the details of her situation were examined, an alternative explanation emerged, namely that the exacerbation of pain was stress-related. The patient's misattribution prevented appropriate action being taken to reduce the muscle contraction that aggravated the chest-wall pain. Biofeedback was used to make her aware of the relationship between stress and muscle tension. Moreover, the reappraisal of the pain stimulus improved her ability to control the pain through timely and target-appropriate interventions, which in turn reinforced her sense of self-efficacy.

Stage 3:   Skills Acquisition and Consolidation

The skills acquisition and consolidation phase begins once the basic goals of the programme have been agreed upon. During this phase, the therapist provides education, guidance and practice in the use of a range of specific cognitive and behavioural coping skills geared toward both the alteration of maladaptive responses to environmental contributors to pain and to coping with specific symptoms.

Coping can occur prior to a stressful event (anticipatory coping) or in response to a confrontation with harm. In cancer, teaching about coping has to be reactive rather than anticipatory, as it is only after the diagnosis that the patient must cope with having a life-threatening disease. Anticipatory coping concerns the way individuals engage in the active regulation of emotional reactions, selecting their environment, planning, choosing, tolerating, and avoiding. Some cognitive-behavioural approaches also focus on trying to prevent the occurrence of stressful transactions, rather than just improving the ways individuals deal with those transactions once they have occurred.

The order in which the various cognitive and behavioural strategies are covered can be varied. In addition to helping the patients develop specific coping skills, this phase is designed to help the patients use skills that they already possess and to enhance their belief in their ability to exercise control, increasing their sense of self-efficacy. The point to be emphasized is that the cognitive-behavioural approach does not deal exclusively with the pain symptoms *per se*, but with those self-statements and environmental factors that may instigate or maintain less than optimal functioning and pain exacerbations.

Problem solving. Cancer patients do not simply have to cope with cancer but with a range of separate problems (for example emotional, social, financial, marital problems and their symptoms). Thus, it is helpful to assist patients to identify some of the problems, help them to label them as such, and to keep them manageable and in perspective. We have found the following algorithm to be useful. It can be anchored to specific problems identified by patients.

(1) Define the source of distress or stress reactions as a problem to be solved.
(2) Set realistic goals as concretely as possible by stating the problem in behavioural terms and delineating steps necessary to reach each goal.
(3) Generate a wide range of possible alternative courses of action.
(4) Imagine and consider how others might respond if asked to deal with a similar problem.
(5) Evaluate the pros and cons of each proposed solution and rank order the solutions from least to most practical and desirable.
(6) Rehearse strategies and behaviours by means of imagery, behavioural rehearsal, and graduated practice.
(7) Try out most acceptable and feasible solution.

(8)   Expect some failures, but reward yourself for having tried.
(9)   Reconsider the original problem in light of the attempt at problem solving.
(10) Repeat as needed.

The goal of this process is to make patients better problem-solvers, able to deal with future stressful events as they arise.

Relaxation and controlled breathing.   Relaxation and controlled breathing exercises are especially useful in the skills acquisition stage because they can be readily learned by almost all patients and are credible since they focus on physiological activity. There is a range of relaxation strategies that can be used and there is little evidence to recommend one method over another. More important is the message to the patient that relaxation is a skill that can be learned and that there are a wide range of relaxation techniques available. The therapist will help patients find one or more that are most helpful for them.

The therapist can discuss with patients how to identify bodily signs of physical tenseness, the stress–tension cycle, how occupying one's attention can short-circuit stress, how relaxation can reduce anxiety because it enables patients to exert control, how relaxation and tension are incompatible states, and finally, how unwinding after stressful experiences can be therapeutic.

Instruction in the use of relaxation is designed not only to teach an incompatible response, but also as a way of helping patients to develop a set of behavioural coping skills that can be employed in any situation in which adaptive coping is required. The practice of relaxation and controlled breathing strengthens patients' beliefs that they can exert control during periods of stress and pain and that they are not helpless or impotent. Patients are asked to practise relaxation at home on a regular basis and in situations where they perceive themselves becoming tense, anxious, or experiencing pain, such as prior to chemotherapy, following radiation treatments, during bone marrow aspirations and other unpleasant diagnostic procedures.

The therapist teaches patients that one can relax not only by tensing and releasing muscle groups or by means of some passive activity such as meditation, but also by means of absorbing activities such as walking, swimming, knitting, gardening, expressing their feelings to others, and so forth. All too often therapists fail to underscore the fact that relaxation is as much a state of mind as it is a physical state.

The therapist works with the patients to anticipate potential problems before they arise and to communicate to patients that they are capable of generating alternative solutions to the problems.

Attentional training. The role of attention is a major factor in perceptual activity and therefore of primary concern in examining and changing behaviour. The act of attending has both a selective and amplifying function. Attention-diverting strategies (such as visualizing a pleasant scene) have probably been employed since humans first experienced pain. It is important to emphasize that the patient is viewed as a collaborator in the selection of specific coping strategies that he or she will use. A number of types of cognitive coping strategies are available and patients are encouraged to choose among these and to develop specific ones that are personally relevant.

Prior to the description of any specific cognitive coping strategies, the therapist prepares the patient for intervention. In this case the therapist describes how attention influences perception. The therapist notes that people can focus their attention on only one thing at a time and that although people control, to some extent, what they attend to, this may be more difficult at some times than at others. This should be illustrated with examples, for example, the analogy of the simultaneous availability of all channels on a TV when only one channel can be fully attended to at any one time, or a searchlight that can only illuminate a small section of available area. The therapist might state: 'Attention is like the TV or searchlight; we can control what we attend to and what we avoid. With instruction and practice, you can learn how to gain greater control over your attention.'

Guided imagery training is used in order to enhance patients' ability to employ *all* sensory modalities (i.e. sight, sound, smell, taste and feel) and thereby increased absorption. The therapist may ask the patient to imagine such scenes as a pleasant day at the beach or an engaging tennis match. Such practice can be of assistance to patients by providing them with opportunities to try out a range of different scenes so that they can learn to use all senses and to generate a set of images that is of particular use for them. It is important that the therapist assists the patient discover personally relevant attention-diverting scenes rather than imposes a specific and predetermined set.

Attempts should be made to involve patients actively in their own treatment. As is the case with relaxation, the data do not unequivocally support the effectiveness of any one strategy compared to any other (Fernandez and Turk, 1989). What appears to be more important is the extent to which patients can become actively absorbed in any imaginary scene. Six categories of attention-diverting strategies have been identified (Wack and Turk, 1984) and these can be reviewed and discussed, with the patients proposing additional examples for each category. Some patients may have difficulty generating sufficiently engaging scenes and the therapist may use pictures, videotapes, or audiotapes to assist in the focusing of attention.

It is important at the outset for the therapist to explain to the patient that because they can distract themselves from pain in no way negates the reality of their pain. We have found that failure to discuss this directly can lead to patient resistance.

Stage 4:   Generalization and Maintenance

Generalization and maintenance are fostered throughout treatment by means of guided exercises, rehearsals, and other homework assignments to increase the patient's sense of self-efficacy. Following the skills acquisition and consolidation phase, patients are encouraged to try out the various skills that have been covered during the treatment in a broad range of situations and to identify and report any difficulties that arise. During these sessions, the patient is encouraged to consider potentially problematic situations and is helped to generate plans for how he or she might handle these difficulties, should they arise. Plans are also formulated with the patient for how he or she might handle lapses or relapses. The therapist attempts to anticipate problems and helps the patient to generate solutions – in a sense to inoculate the patient against difficulties that may occur (see Marlatt and Gordon, 1985 for a discussion of relapse prevention). Finally, the patient is encouraged to evaluate progress, review homework assignments, to reinforce him or herself for the efforts expended and success, and most importantly, to attribute progress and success to his or her own efforts.

Stage 5:   Follow-through and Follow-up

Follow-through and follow-up are not phases that are tied to a time interval. Rather, patients are scheduled for check-in and booster sessions and are encouraged to stay in contact with the therapist, on a *prn* basis. Patients should be provided with non-technical written materials highlighting specific components that have been covered during treatment. They should be encouraged to review these as needed.

Maximizing Treatment Effectiveness

Perhaps the more important and appropriate questions for treatment studies are not whether the treatment is successful but how successful the treatment is for which patients with what characteristics (Turk and Rudy, 1988). The most appropriate strategy might be to maximize the commonalities (non-specifics) for all patients but simultaneously individualize treatments to specific physiological, psychosocial, and behavioural characteristics. The exclusive reliance on group effects may mask important subject-by-treatment interactions.

Psychological interventions based on the operant, respondent, and cognitive-behavioural conceptualizations each have useful implications for treatment and recommend helpful strategies that are effective with samples of patients with recalcitrant chronic pain. Matching patients to treatments, focusing on alterations of self-efficacy, and involvement of significant others should augment these outcomes and foster maintenance of post-treatment gains.

SUMMARY AND CONCLUSIONS

In summary, psychological principles and variables have been found to be important in the perception of and behavioural responses to diverse pain syndromes, acute and chronic. Moreover, cognitive and behavioural modalities have been effectively used in the management of pain not associated with malignancies. However, these approaches and principles have seldom been systematically and consistently incorporated into treatments of patients with cancer pain. We have argued (Turk and Fernandez, 1990) that this is primarily a result of some misconceptions regarding cancer pain as unique by virtue of its organicity and association with impending death. Pain, however, as discussed throughout this chapter, is a perception that is subject to modulation by numerous psychological variables, prominent among which are controllability, expectancy, anxiety, appraisal processes, perceived self-efficacy, and contingencies of reinforcement. The manipulation of such variables can help patients to reinterpret noxious sensations as less intense, to relabel physical perturbations in terms other than pain, and to engage in coping and other well behaviours. The successful use of such techniques also adds to a sense of control over what many treat as an uncontrollable disease and thus can further alleviate suffering.

It must be added that cognitive and behavioural approaches to cancer pain management are likely to be time-consuming and involved for both patient and practitioners. Some patients may be resistant to such intervention for fear that it connotes that their pain is 'all in their head.' On the contrary, it must be emphasized that pain is a multidimensional experience with sensory as well as cognitive and affective components affected by environmental contingencies, and that each of these needs to be addressed by a multifaceted approach giving broader consideration to both biomedical and psychosocial contributors. It is important to acknowledge that the association between pain and psychological distress in cancer patients may be one of reciprocal causality (Davis *et al.*, 1987). The occurrence of pain may contribute to the patient's psychological distress; conversely, the occurrence of psychological distress may amplify the patient's perception of pain. When patients report exacerbation of pain, this often has several indistinguishable causes, including progression of the disease and an increase in the level of psychological distress. Both of these contributors need to be addressed. The techniques described above should help the clinician who treats cancer patients. In the cancer literature, the former has been addressed repeatedly but the latter is rarely given sufficient emphasis.

We believe that the most appropriate treatment of cancer pain is by an interdisciplinary team that includes psychologists along with a range of other health care professionals (for example, physicians, nurses, physical therapists, social workers, pharmacologists (see also Cleeland et al., 1986). Psychologists should be encouraged to address not only traditional psychological issues of depression and should not be brought in to intervene as a last resort when all physical modalities have been exhausted. Instead they can play an important role simultaneous with the use of somatic modalities as well as to assist patients in understanding the role of appraisal processes, body preoccupation, environmental contingencies, along with how such factors can contribute to pain perception and suffering. Psychologists can also teach patients a range of cognitive and behavioural techniques to increase their sense of control over the disease and thereby reduce the demoralization frequently encountered in cancer patients. Furthermore, psychologists may serve as consultants to other members of the pain treatment team by alerting them to the role of cognitive and behavioural factors in the report, maintenance, and exacerbation of suffering.

Acknowledgement. Preparation of this article was supported in part by Grants ARNS38698 from the National Institute of Arthritis and Musculoskeletal and Skin Diseases and DE07514 from the National Institute of Dental Research.

References

AHLES, T.A., RUCKDESCHEL, J.C. and BLANCHARD, E.B. (1984) Cancer-related pain – I. Prevalence in an outpatient setting as a function of stage of disease and type of cancer. *Journal of Psychosomatic Research, 28,* 115–119.

ANDERSON, T.P., COLE, T.M., GULICKSON, G., HUDGENS, A. and ROBERTS, A.H. (1977) Behavior modification of chronic pain: A treatment program by a multidisciplinary team. *Clinical Orthopaedics, 129,* 96–100.

BANDURA, A. (1977) Self-efficacy: Toward a unifying theory of behavioral change. *Psychological Review, 84,* 191–215.

BARBER, T.X. (1959) Toward a theory of pain: Relief of chronic pain by prefrontal leucotomy, opiates, placebos, and hypnosis. *Psychological Bulletin,* 56, 430–460.

BEECHER, H.K. (1946) Pain in men wounded in battle. *Annals of Surgery, 123,* 96–105.

BEECHER, H.K. (1955) The powerful placebo. *Journal of the American Medical Association, 159,* 1602–1606.

BEECHER, H.K. (1961) Surgery as placebo: Quantitative study of bias. *Journal of the American Medical Association, 176,* 1102–1107.

BLACK, R.G. (1975) The chronic pain syndrome. *Surgical Clinics of North America, 55,* 999–1011.

BLOCK, A.R., KREMER, E.F. and GAYLOR, M. (1980) Behavioral treatment of chronic pain: Variables affecting treatment efficacy. *Pain, 8,* 367–375.

BONICA, J.J. (1979) Cancer pain: Importance of the problem. In J.J. Bonica and V. Ventafridda (Eds) *Advances in Pain Research and Therapy Vol. 2.* New York: Raven Press.

BOWERS, K.S. (1968) Pain, anxiety and perceived control. *Journal of Consulting and Clinical Psychology, 32,* 596–602.

BYRON, R. and YONEMOTO, R. (1975) Pain and malignancy. In B. Crue, Jr. (Ed) *Pain Research and Treatment.* New York: Academic Press.

CAIRNS, D. and PASINO, J. (1977) Comparison of verbal reinforcement and feedback in the operant treatment of disability of chronic low back pain. *Behavior Therapy, 8,* 621–630.

CASSELL, E.J. (1982) The nature of suffering and the goals of medicine. *New England Journal of Medicine, 306,* 639–645.

CHAPMAN, C.R. (1979) Personal communication.

CLEELAND, C.S. and TEARNAN, B.H. (1986) Behavioral control of cancer pain. In A.D. Holzman and D.C. Turk (Eds) *Pain management: A handbook of psychological treatment approaches.* New York: Pergamon Press.

CLEELAND, C.S., ROTONDI, A., BRECHNER, T., LEVIN, A., MACDONALD, N., PORTENOY, R., SCHUTTA, H. and MCENIRY, M. (1986) A model for the treatment of cancer pain. *Journal of Pain and Symptom Management, 1,* 209–215.

CRAIG, K.D. (1986) Social modeling influences: Pain in context. In R.A. Sternbach (Ed) *The Psychology of Pain.* New York: Raven Press.

DAUT, R.L. and CLEELAND, C.S. (1982) The prevalence and severity of pain in cancer. *Cancer, 50,* 1903–1908.

DAUT, R.L., CLEELAND, C.S. and FLANERY, R.C. (1983) Development of the Wisconsin Brief Pain Questionnaire to assess pain in cancer and other diseases. *Pain, 17,* 197–210.

DAVIS, M., VASTERLING, J., BRANSFIELD, D. and BURISH, T.G. (1987) Behavioural interventions in coping with cancer related pain. *British Journal of Guidance and Counselling, 15,* 17–28.

DOLCE, J.J. (1987) Self-efficacy and disability beliefs in behavioral treatment of pain. *Behaviour Research and Therapy, 25,* 289–299.

DOLEYS, D.M., CROCKER, M. and PATTON, D. (1982) Response of patients with chronic pain to exercise quotas. *Physical Therapy, 62,* 1111–1115.

EASTERLING, D.V. and LEVENTHAL, H. (1989) Contribution of concrete cognition to emotion: Neutral symptoms as elicitors of worry about cancer. *Journal of Applied Psychology, 74,* 787–796.

FAGERHAUGH, S. (1974) Pain expression on a burn care unit. *Nursing Outlook, 22,* 645–650.

FERNANDEZ, E. and TURK, D.C. (1989) The utility of cognitive coping strategies for altering pain perception: A meta-analysis. *Pain, 38*, 123–136.

FISHMAN, B. and LOSCALZO, M. (1987) Cognitive-behavioral interventions in management of cancer pain: Principles and applications. *Medical Clinics of North America, 71*, 271–287.

FLOR, H. and TURK, D.C. (1988) Chronic back pain and rheumatoid arthritis: Predicting pain and disability from cognitive variables. *Journal of Behavioral Medicine, 11*, 251–265.

FLOR, H., KERNS, R.D. and TURK, D.C. (1987) The role of the spouse in the maintenance of chronic pain. *Journal of Psychosomatic Research, 31*, 251–260.

FOLEY, K.M. (1979) Pain syndromes in patients with cancer pain. In J.J. Bonica and V. Ventafridda (Eds) *Advances in Pain Research and Therapy, Vol. 2.* New York: Raven Press.

FOLEY, K.M. (1984) Assessment of pain. *Clinical Oncology, 3*, 17–31.

FOLEY, K.M. and INTURRISI, C.E. (1987) Analgesic drug therapy in cancer pain: Principles and practice. *Medical Clinics of North America, 71*, 207–232.

FORDYCE, W.E. (1976) *Behavioral Methods for Chronic Pain and Illness.* St Louis, MO: Mosby.

FORDYCE, W.E. (1988) Pain and suffering: A reappraisal. *American Psychologist, 43*, 276–282.

FORDYCE, W.W., FOWLER, R.S., LEHMANN, J.F., DELATEUR, B.J., SAND, P.L. and TRIESCHMAN, R.B. (1973) Operant conditioning in the treatment of chronic pain. *Archives of Physical Medicine and Rehabilitation, 54*, 399–408.

FOWLER, R.S., FORDYCE, W.E. and BERNI, R. (1969) Operant conditioning in chronic illness. *American Journal of Nursing, 69*, 1226–1228.

GENTRY, W.D. and BERNAL, G. (1977) Chronic pain. In R. Williams and W.D. Gentry (Eds), *Behavioral Approaches to Medical Treatment.* Cambridge, MA: Ballinger.

GREENWALD, H.P., BONICA, J.J. and BERGNER, M. (1987) The prevalence of pain in four cancers. *Cancer, 60*, 2563–2569.

GREER, S. and WATSON, M. (1987) Mental adjustment to cancer: Its measurement and prognostic importance. *Cancer Surveys, 6*, 439–453.

HALL, K. and STRIDE, E. (1954) The varying response to pain in psychiatric disorders: A study in abnormal psychology. *British Journal of Medical Psychology, 27*, 48–60.

HILL, H.F., SAEGER, L.C. and CHAPMAN, C.R. (1986) Patient controlled analgesia after bone marrow transplantation for cancer. *Postgraduate Medicine,* August, 33–40.

HOLROYD, K.A., PENZIEN, D.B., HURSEY, K.G., TOBIN, D.L., ROGERS, L., HOLM, J.E., MARCILLE, P.J., HALL, J.R. and CHILA, A.G. (1984) Change mechanisms in EMG biofeedback training: Cognitive changes underlying improvement in tension headache. *Journal of Consulting and Clinical Psychology, 52*, 1039–1053.

JONES, A., BENTLER, P. and PETRY, G. (1968) The reduction of uncertainty concerning future pain. *Journal of Abnormal Psychology, 71*, 87–94.

KEEFE, F.J., BRANTLEY, A., MANUEL, G. and CRISSON, J.E. (1985) Behavioral assessment of head and neck cancer patients. *Pain, 23*, 327–336.

KERNS, D.C., TURK, D.C. and RUDY, T.E. (1985) The West Haven-Yale Multidimensional Pain Inventory (WHYMPI) *Pain, 23*, 345–356.

KOPEL, S. and ARKOWITZ, H. (1975) The role of attribution and self-perception in behavior change: Implications for behavior therapy. *Genetic Psychology Monographs, 92*, 175–212.

LENTHEM, J., SLADE, P.D., TROUP, J.D.G. and BENTLEY, G. (1983) Outline of a fear-avoidance model of exaggerated pain perception. *Behaviour Research and Therapy, 21,* 401–408.

LEVIN, D.N., CLEELAND, C.S. and DAR, R. (1985) Public attitudes toward cancer pain. *Cancer, 56,* 2337–2339.

LINTON, S.J. (1986) Behavioral remediation of chronic pain: A status report. *Pain, 24,* 125–141.

MALOW, R.M., WEST, J.A. and SUTKER, P.B. (1986) A signal detection analysis of anxiety and pain responses in chronic drug abusers. Paper presented at the annual meeting of the American Psychological Association, Washington, D.C.

MARLATT, G.A. and GORDON, J.R. (1985) *Relapse prevention: Maintenance strategies in the treatment of addictive behaviors.* New York: Guilford.

MCGUIRE, D.B. (1989) Cancer pain: Pathophysiology of pain in cancer. *Cancer Nursing, 12,* 310–315.

MELZACK, R. and WALL, P.D. (1965) Pain mechanisms: A new theory. *Science, 50,* 971–979.

MELZACK, R. and CASEY, K.L. (1968) Sensory, motivational and central control determinants of pain: A new conceptual model. In D. Kenshalo (Ed) *The Skin Senses.* Springfield, IL: Thomas.

PENNEBAKER, J.W. (1982) *The Psychology of Physical Symptoms.* New York: Springer.

PHILIPS, H.C. (1987) Avoidance and its role in sustaining chronic pain. *Behaviour Research and Therapy, 25,* 273–279.

PORTENOY, R.K. (1988) Practical aspects of pain control in the patient with cancer. *CA, 36,* 327–352.

RACHMAN, S. and LOPATKA, C. (1988) Accurate and inaccurate predictions of pain. *Behaviour Research and Therapy, 26,* 291–296.

RACHMAN, S., LEVITT, K. and LOPATKA, C. (1987) Panic: The links between cognitions and bodily symptoms. *Behaviour Research and Therapy, 25,* 411–423.

SCHMIDT, A.J.M. (1985) Cognitive factors in the performance of chronic low back pain patients. *Journal of Psychosomatic Research, 29,* 183–189.

SIMMONS, C.C. and DALAND, E.M. (1920) Cancer: Factors entering into the delay in its surgical treatment. *Boston Medical and Surgical Journal, 183,* 298–303.

SKEVINGTON, S.M. (1983) Social cognitions, personality, and chronic pain. *Journal of Psychosomatic Research, 27,* 421–428.

SPIEGEL, D. and BLOOM, J.R. (1983) Pain in metastatic breast cancer. *Cancer, 52,* 341–345.

TEARNAN, B.H., WARD, C.H. and CLEELAND, C.S. (1989) Psychological management of malignant pain. In C.D. Tollison (Ed) *Handbook of Chronic Pain Management.* Baltimore: Williams & Wilkins.

THOMPSON, S.C. (1981) Will it hurt less if I can control it? A complex answer to a simple question. *Psychological Bulletin, 90,* 89–101.

TURK, D.C. and RENNERT, K.S. (1981) Pain and the terminally-ill cancer patient: A cognitive social learning perspective. In H. Sobel (Ed) *Behavior Therapy in Terminal Care: A humanistic approach.* Cambridge, MA: Ballinger.

TURK, D.C. and HOLZMAN, A.D. (1986) Commonalities among psychological approaches in the treatment of chronic pain: Specifying the meta-constructs. In A.D. Holzman and D.C. Turk (Eds) *Pain Management: A handbook of psychological treatment approaches.* Elmsford, NY: Pergamon Press.

TURK, D.C. and RUDY, T.E. (1986) Assessment of cognitive factors in chronic pain: A worthwhile enterprise? *Journal of Consulting and Clinical Psychology*, 54, 760–768.

TURK, D.C. and MEICHENBAUM, D. (1989) Cognitive-behavioral approach to the management of chronic pain. In P.D. Wall and R. Melzack (Eds) *Textbook of Pain*, 2nd edn. New York: Churchill Livingstone.

TURK, D.C. and RUDY, T.E. (1989) An integrated approach to pain treatment: Beyond the scalpel and syringe. In C.D. Tollison (Ed) *Handbook of Chronic Pain Management*. Baltimore, MD: Williams & Wilkins.

TURK, D.C. and FERNANDEZ, E. (1990) On the putative uniqueness of cancer pain: Do psychological principles apply? *Behaviour Research and Therapy*, 28, 1–13.

TURK, D.C., MEICHENBAUM, D. and GENEST, M. (1983) *Pain and Behavioral Medicine: A cognitive-behavioral perspective*. New York: Guilford Press.

TURK, D.C., RUDY, T.E. and SALOVEY, P. (1986) Implicit models of illness: Description and validation. *Journal of Behavioral Medicine*, 9, 453–574.

TURNBULL, F. (1979) The nature of pain that may accompany cancer of the lung. *Pain*, 7, 371–375.

TURNER, J.A. and ROMANO, J.M. (1984) Evaluating psychologic interventions for chronic pain: Issues and recent developments. In C. Benedetti, C.R. Chapman and G. Moricca (Eds) *Advances in Pain Research and Therapy*, Vol. 7. New York: Raven Press.

WACK, J.T. and TURK, D.C. (1984) Latent structure in strategies for coping with pain. *Health Psychology*, 3, 27–43.

WOODFORDE, J.M. and FIELDING, J.R. (1970) Pain and cancer. *Journal of Psychosomatic Research*, 14, 365–370.

WORLD HEALTH ORGANIZATION (1986) CANCER PAIN RELIEF. Geneva: World Health Organization.

YANG, J.C., WAGNER, J.M. and CLARK, W.C. (1983) Psychological distress and mood in chronic pain and surgical patients: A sensory decision analysis. In J.J. Bonica, U. Lindblom and A. Iggo (Eds) *Advances in Pain Research and Therapy*. New York: Raven Press.

ANTICIPATORY NAUSEA AND EMESIS: BEHAVIOURAL INTERVENTIONS

Peter M. Black and Gary R. Morrow

Although medical science has made great strides in the treatment of morbidity and prevention of mortality through the use of various techniques, virtually all medical treatments have some type of side-effect. This is especially true of the treatment of cancer by chemotherapeutic agents. For a potentially curative course of chemotherapy to have its maximum effect for cure or control of disease, the patient must be able to tolerate the various side-effects that result from the treatment. The success of the treatment depends both on the health care provider's success in managing those side-effects and the patient's ability to tolerate side-effects that cannot be successfully managed.

Nausea and vomiting are among the most prevalent, persistent, and undesirable side-effects of cancer chemotherapy treatment. In addition to being a wholly unpleasant experience in themselves, they can affect the chemotherapy treatment. For example, nausea and/or vomiting can promote such treatment complications as anorexia, dehydration, metabolic imbalance, and psychological depression (Harris, 1978; Morrow, 1987). Additionally, the aversive side-effects of standard chemotherapy treatment may encourage patients to seek unorthodox and less efficacious treatments in a search for side-effect reduction.

Two types of chemotherapy nausea and vomiting have been identified: Post-treatment nausea and vomiting (PNV) and anticipatory nausea and vomiting (ANV). PNV is primarily thought to be a function of the chemotherapeutic drugs damaging healthy tissue, while ANV has been characterized as a learned or classically conditioned response to the chemotherapy procedure (Burish and Carey, 1986). Here we present an overview of the available behavioural treatments for ANV and other psychological side-effects, an evaluation of their efficacy, and both methodological and theoretical considerations for future studies and applications.

BEHAVIOURAL TREATMENT OF SIDE-EFFECTS

Neither anticipatory nor post-treatment nausea and vomiting are completely controlled by antiemetic medications (Laszlo, 1983; Morrow, 1982; 1984b; Morrow *et al.*, 1984). Additionally, a number of the agents have side-effects of their own (for example, sedation) and have been known to worsen already existing symptoms such as anxiety (Zeltzer *et al.*, 1984). Various interventions (for example EMG biofeedback, progressive muscle relaxation training and systematic desensitization) have been examined as either primary or adjunctive methods in the control of anticipatory nausea and vomiting. Appendix 1 summarizes selected aspects of case studies and controlled investigations of these interventions. This comprehensive list is provided so that the reader can make his or her own judgements regarding the weight of the evidence for each intervention. Within this chapter itself we have chosen to discuss specific studies which we feel represent both the strengths, and in some cases, the weaknesses of each particular type of intervention.

This chapter does not represent a 'how to' approach. Rather, we wish to present the sum of the evidence for each intervention and let the would-be practitioner decide. There are two specific reasons for this: (1) the state of the art is not that well developed for some of these interventions and new information is constantly being added to the literature; in view of this, we feel a static prescription is not wise and; (2) possibly more important, many of the techniques (for example, hypnosis, EMG biofeedback) do not lend themselves to a simple 'how to' approach. Indeed, specialized therapeutic or technique training is needed to utilize successfully many of these interventions (the one exception being progressive muscle relaxation training). As a consequence, we have included some general guidelines on the consideration of individual differences and their possible interactions with a given technique and have provided an example of the progressive muscle relaxation training used in our work in Appendix 2.

Progressive Muscle Relaxation Training

One of the most widely used and efficacious behavioural interventions is progressive muscle relaxation training (PMRT). PMRT is a behavioural technique which involves the patient actively learning to relax by tensing and relaxing selective muscle groups. An individual is usually taught deep muscle relaxation by a therapist, a training audiotape is made, and the individual is requested to practise PMRT at home in order to acquire the skill. At least four case studies and six controlled investigations of PMRT have been reported thus far. Results from case studies (Burish and Lyles, 1979; Cotanch, 1983; Weddington *et al.*, 1983) have suggested that PMRT can benefit cancer patients by reducing side-effects such as postchemotherapy nausea and vomiting, and negative states such as depression and anxiety.

Lyles *et al.* (1982) conducted a study of cancer patients experiencing anxiety, depression, nausea, and vomiting. Fifty patients were randomly assigned to one of three treatment conditions: (a) PMRT with guided imagery; (b) a therapist control, in which a therapist spent an equal amount of time with the patients as in condition (a), and, (c) a no-treatment control. Patients who received PMRT were found to be less anxious and nauseated both during and following their chemotherapy treatment sessions compared to the patients in the therapist control and no-treatment control groups. Furthermore, the authors report that patients receiving PMRT manifested less physiological arousal (lower pulse rates) and were less depressed following chemotherapy. The differential effects found between the treatment conditions (PMRT vs. therapist control), suggest that the improvements were not simply the result of 'nonspecific' treatment factors.

The findings of Lyles *et al.* (1982) were supported by Cotanch (1983) in a controlled study in which 43 cancer patients were randomly assigned to one of three conditions: (1) PMRT, provided by audiotape; (2) tape control, in which patients listened to soothing music and were requested to focus on positive thoughts, and (3) no-treatment control. Patients took part in one baseline session and 'varying numbers' of training sessions. Results showed that 67 per cent of the patients in the PMRT conditions showed increases in postchemotherapy nausea and vomiting (PCNV), whereas 85 per cent of the patients in the two control groups showed increase in PCNV. This 18 per cent difference between the groups suggests that PMRT can be helpful even with a minimal amount of therapist contact.

Burish, Carey, Krozely, and Greco (1987) investigated whether PMRT could be used to prevent or ameliorate chemotherapy side-effects through early intervention. Thirty-two cancer patients about to start their first course of emetogenic chemotherapy were randomized to either a PMRT group or a no-treatment control group. PMRT sessions were held prior to the beginning of chemotherapy and progressed through the first five chemotherapy treatments. Patients in the PMRT group reported feeling less nauseated during and following chemotherapy. Additionally, these patients reported fewer occurrences of vomiting and lower physiological arousal (for example, heart rate and blood pressure) compared to the patients in the control group. PMRT also resulted in less dysphoria and a progressive reduction in PCNV symptoms as treatment with chemotherapy continued over time. Reportedly, by the fifth session only 10 per cent of the PMRT patients experienced PCN whereas 54 per cent of the control patients experienced PCN. Preliminary data from a study by Blumberg and colleagues (1989) found similar results. One hundred and eighteen patients were randomly assigned to an experimental condition consisting of written materials, live instruction and an audiotape of the session or a standard treatment control group. Preliminary results showed that the experimental group had greater pre-to-post decline in both systolic and diastolic blood pressure and significant reductions in nervousness and nausea.

In conclusion, the evidence regarding the use of PMRT with cancer chemotherapy patients indicates that this type of intervention can be effective in reducing side-effects which are present during and after cancer chemotherapy sessions. Since nausea symptoms occurring before a treatment session were not assessed in the early work carried out by Burish and his associates (Morrow, 1986a; Morrow and Morrell, 1982), any potential impact PMRT has on ANV symptoms defined strictly as pre-treatment remains a potentially fruitful area of investigation. For example, in view of the relationship between post-chemotherapy side-effects and the subsequent development of ANV, using this technique before the initial chemotherapy treatment could potentially block the conditioning process and thereby prevent its occurrence.

Systematic Desensitization

Systematic Desensitization (SD) is a well-developed, standardized behavioural technique shown to be useful in altering a number of maladaptive learned responses such as phobias (Wolpe, 1983). In SD, patients are first taught a response incompatible with the maladaptive response they presently have to particular stimuli. This alternative response is then paired cognitively with the original stimuli so as to countercondition the maladaptive response.

At the University of Rochester Cancer Center, patients with anticipatory nausea/vomiting have been taught a modified version of progressive muscle relaxation training as a competing response to the maladaptive response of anticipatory nausea/vomiting. The PMRT technique is outlined in Appendix 2. During the systematic desensitization treatment, patients imagine scenes from a hierarchy of events related to chemotherapy treatment (for example, driving to the cancer centre) while in a deeply relaxed state. In this way, treatment stimuli become associated with relaxation so that when the patient encounters stimuli (for example, the clinic nurse or clinic odours), they respond with a counter-conditioned relaxation response rather than nausea and vomiting.

Two case studies and four controlled investigations of SD have been reported (Dobkin, 1987; Haily and White, 1983; Hoffman, 1983;

Meyer, 1982; Morrow, 1986a; Morrow and Morrell, 1982). In a study designed to examine the antiemetic efficacy of SD for the control of ANV, Morrow and Morrell (1982) randomly assigned 60 patients with ANV to one of three groups: (a) SD; (b) counselling, based on a Rogerian, client-centered approach, and (c) no-treatment control. Results revealed that only patients in the SD group showed a significant reduction in the frequency, severity, and duration of ANV. The efficacy of SD was unrelated to type or dose of antiemetic medications used by the patients. Furthermore, patients in the SD group reported no greater expectation for improvement than did the patients in the counselling group, thus reducing the possibility that nonspecific therapy effects (for example, attention) were responsible for the reported positive effects.

In a follow-up study, Morrow (1986b) compared the effectiveness of SD to three conditions: (a) relaxation only; (b) counselling, and (c) no-treatment control in order to examine the essential treatment components in the SD procedure. Relative to the other three groups, patients treated with SD reported a significant decrease in the severity and duration of anticipatory nausea from baseline to follow-up sessions. SD and relaxation patients had a significantly greater decrease in the duration and severity of post-treatment nausea compared to patients who were in the other two groups. These findings were independent of patients' ratings of their expectations for success or the credibility of the experimenter. These results support a view that *both* the cognitive stimulus hierarchy and relaxation response are necessary components for the successful treatment of ANV.

In a prevention study, Dobkin and Morrow (1985) examined the possibility of reducing, retarding, or preventing the development of both post- and anticipatory side-effects in cancer patients who were new to chemotherapy. Forty consecutive patients were randomly assigned to either SD or a waiting-list control group. SD was taught in two separate one-hour sessions prior to the second chemotherapy cycle. A repeated measures design was employed with one baseline and three follow-up periods; dependent measures included: postchemotherapy nausea and vomiting, anticipatory nausea and vomiting, anxiety (trait at baseline, state at all periods), and tension level postchemotherapy.

A reduction in the SD patients' PNV side-effects was found. Nausea and vomiting were less frequent, severe, and of shorter duration as chemotherapy progressed. Conversely, there was an upward trend for the control group patients' PNV side-effects in that nausea and vomiting were more frequent, severe, and of longer duration as chemotherapy progressed. In addition, the control patients reported higher levels of tension following chemotherapy compared to SD patients. These preliminary findings suggest that the introduction of

SD early in treatment can reduce and/or retard the development of conditioned side-effects resulting from chemotherapy in cancer patients; however, replications and extensions of this work are needed before firmer conclusions can be reached.

In summary, consistent findings regarding the effectiveness of SD have been reported in both case and controlled studies. Although the majority of the SD investigations have been carried out in one research centre, two case studies and one controlled investigation (Meyer, 1982) in other geographical locations have replicated the basic results.

Hypnosis

Hypnosis has been defined as a state of intensified attention and receptiveness and an increased responsiveness to an idea or set of ideas (Erickson, 1959). Seven case histories of hypnotherapy with cancer patients have reported generally positive results (for example, Dempster et al., 1976; Ellenberg et al., 1980; LaBaw et al., 1975; Margolis, 1983; Olness, 1981; Zeltzer et al., 1983; Walker et al., 1988). However, caution is warranted in the interpretation of these studies because the majority have been carried out with a paediatric population, probably since children are more readily hypnotized than adults (Olness, 1981). In addition, children often experience a greater number of undesirable side-effects from antiemetic drugs then do adults, and thus some antiemetics are not used with this population (Cotanch et al., 1985).

LaBaw et al. (1975) studied 27 children and adolescents, aged 4–20 years, who were treated with self-hypnosis over a two-year period (the exact number of treatment sessions per patient was not specified). 'Progressive body relaxation' was employed as an inductive technique which was followed by 'psychic imagery' of fantasized idyllic scenes common in the patient's experience. Dependent measures included patients' self-report and therapist observations. Results indicated that 'varying degrees of success' were obtained where 'success' was defined as improved sleep, increased caloric intake and retention, increased fluid intake, and greater tolerance for therapeutic procedures. In general, few objective data were collected from this series of case studies. The 'hypnotic' intervention was not standardized and sometimes not described.

Three controlled studies have examined hypnotherapy. Redd et al. (1982) treated six patients experiencing ANV with hypnosis in a multiple baseline design. During treatment, each patient was individually instructed in focusing attention, achieving deep muscle relaxation, and imagining pleasant scenes. The training sessions were audiotaped and patients were instructed to practise the treatment daily. Due to study problems, the hypnotic intervention was temporarily interrupted for several of the patients. At this time, the symptoms which had been apparently controlled by hypnosis reappeared, suggesting that the intervention was involved in the initial positive effects. Given the small sample size, these findings require replication before conclusions can be drawn.

Cotanch *et al.* (1985) also combined relaxation training with hypnosis in a study of 12 paediatric inpatients (aged 10–18 years) who were referred by oncologists for treatment since they were experiencing troublesome chemotherapy-related nausea and vomiting. The children were randomly assigned to an experimental group (*n*=6), or a control group (*n*=6) who received standard care. On the day of chemotherapy, the children in the experimental group were trained by a therapist in self-hypnosis. Both groups were followed through two consecutive chemotherapy cycles. Child self-report and nurse observations were obtained on the parameters of nausea and vomiting (intensity, severity, frequency) and on the amount of oral intake 24 hours postchemotherapy. Data were collected by staff nurses and research assistants who did not know which group the child was assigned to. In the intervention group, there was a significant reduction in nausea and vomiting both in terms of intensity and severity, as well as a significant increase in oral intake. These changes were not evident in the control group.

Although this study is suggestive regarding the effectiveness of hypnotherapy, the results could be explained in terms of an attention effect. The children in the experimental group received 'extra' attention from a therapist whereas the children in the control group did not. While these initial findings are encouraging, they require replication with an attention-placebo group to rule out the alternative hypothesis or attention effect.

Zeltzer, LeBaron, and Zeltzer (1984) compared hypnotherapy to supportive counselling and suggested that nonspecific therapy effects such as demand characteristics and/or attention may contribute to treatment changes found. In their study, 19 children, aged 6–17 years, were randomly assigned to a hypnotherapy or a supportive counselling group. Children in both groups reported reductions in nausea and vomiting and rated chemotherapy as 'less noxious' following intervention. There were, however, no statistically or clinically significant differences in outcome found between the two approaches.

In conclusion, it appears that studies using hypnosis for ANV control have shown that this intervention may be beneficial for children. Less evidence is available demonstrating its usefulness for adults. In order to establish the effectiveness of hypnotherapy for cancer chemotherapy patients, studies with larger sample sizes in which patients are randomly assigned to treatment or appropriate control groups and the use of standardized outcomes are needed.

Miscellaneous Behavioural Interventions

Five studies have used behavioural interventions other than those previously discussed. Moore and Altmaier (1981) reported in a pilot study of nine cancer patients (6 females and 3 males, with a mean age of 47 years) treated with *stress inoculation training* (the six-session treatment 'package' consisted of cognitive behaviour modification combined with PMRT and education). Prior to the intervention, patients were interviewed and completed the Multiple Affect Adjective Checklist (MAACL; Zuckerman *et al.*, 1964) which is designed to measure anxiety, depression, and hostility. Five of the nine patients exhibited ANV prior to treatment. Since the authors discontinued monitoring the patients at the last training session lack of follow-up data means that it is not possible to determine the effectiveness of this approach. Three patients did report, however, that they felt less anxious prior to treatment having learned effective coping skills.

Burish *et al.* (1981) treated a 44-year-old female cancer patient with *EMG biofeedback combined with relaxation* in order to help control anticipatory and post-treatment symptoms. Baseline measures of affect (anxiety, depression, and hostility, MAACL; Zuckerman *et al.*, 1964), muscle tension, pulse rate, and blood pressure were taken. After ten training sessions, the patient was able to reduce her physiological arousal levels (as measured by EMG, pulse rate, and blood pressure) and reported feeling less nauseated. These changes were maintained during three follow-up periods. There were no reported improvements in affect. These results, which are similar to those found for PMRT, suggest that EMG biofeedback may be another means of teaching relaxation to cancer patients although it is somewhat time and labour intensive.

Three studies by LeBaron and Zeltzer (1984), Kolko and Rickard-Figueroa (1985) and Redd *et al.* (1987) have investigated interventions based on *cognitive diversion* or distraction techniques. The former study involved directing adolescents' attention away from the treatment by having them play games and be actively engaged with a therapist (modified relaxation training was also included in some cases). The latter two studies involved the use of video games to distract paediatric and adolescent patients.

LeBaron and Zeltzer (1984) reported a decrease in postchemotherapy nausea, vomiting, and 'bother' (as measured by reports of fewer disruptions in daily activities post-treatment) during the intervention. These improvements were maintained at follow-up (time period not reported). They concluded that 'since a repeated measures design found no symptom reductions prior to intervention, it can be assumed that some aspects of the intervention itself were responsible for the reductions found, rather than attention or expectations related to assessment alone'. This conclusion seems premature given a sample size of eight, no control groups, and no theoretical rationale of how distraction alone could reduce chemotherapy-related side effects.

Kolko and Rickard-Figueroa (1985) used a multiple-baseline (ABAB) design (Kazdin, 1982) with three paediatric oncology patients (all male, aged 11, 16, and 17 years). Anticipatory 'distress', PNV and state anxiety (State–Trait Anxiety Inventory; Spielberger *et al.*, 1968) measures were taken. A Modified-Procedure Behavioral Rating Scale (Katz *et al.*, 1980) was used to gather observational data just prior to chemotherapy. The introduction of video games concurrent with the administration of chemotherapy was associated with the reduction of self-reported and observer-reported anticipatory symptoms (not ANV) as well as postchemotherapy distress. These improvements were reversed when the return-to-baseline phase was initiated. Symptoms decreased again when the video game procedure was reintroduced in two of the three cases (the third case could not be evaluated due to admission of the patient just before the final condition).

Kolko and Rickard-Figueroa's study (1985) addressed the relaxation versus distraction issue regarding the therapeutic mechanisms underlying behaviour therapy. Although the results imply that distraction may effectively reduce symptomatology, ANV and PCNV side-effects *per se* were not reduced, only 'distress' levels were altered.

Redd *et al.* (1987) conducted two experiments, one of which employed an ABAB design, to evaluate the effect of video-game playing in paediatric oncology patients with anticipatory nausea and anxiety. In the first experiment, patients were alternately assigned to either the experimental group or to the control condition. In the second experiment, patients from the first experiment were carried over and exposed to an ABAB design presentation of the video games. Unlike Kolko and Rickard-Figueroa's (1985) study, the ABAB presentation took place within the same chemotherapy session, that is, after a no-video-game baseline assessment (A), patients played video games for 10 minutes (B), followed immediately by a 10-minute no-video-game period (A), and then a second 10-minute video game period (B). Nausea and anxiety were assessed using a 10 cm Visual Analogue Scale; pulse rate and blood pressure measures were taken to assess physiological indices. Results indicated that anticipatory nausea but not anxiety decreased significantly following video games playing in both studies. Reportedly pulse rates and systolic/diastolic blood pressure rates were variable, with one measure (systolic blood pressure) showing a significant increase from the previous no-game level following the second exposure to video games within the session. The authors interpreted these findings as support for the hypothesis that cognitive distraction, and not relaxation, is the critical component of the intervention. These findings by Redd *et al.* (1987) complement Kolko and Rickard-Figueroa's investigation quite well. However, this conclusion may be somewhat premature in view of the methodological constraints of these studies.

Hypothetical Mechanisms of Action

Behavioural interventions can reduce chemotherapy side-effects. What are the 'active ingredients' in the behavioural interventions? Carey and Burish (1988) propose five specific factors: (1) non-specific factors; (2) counter-conditioning; (3) attentional diversion/redirection; (4) perceived sense of control; and (5) physiological relaxation.

Non-specific factors. This refers to the basic phenomenon that many investigations in the behavioural science area need to consider – factors extraneous to the treatment or intervention itself, yet related to the delivery of that intervention, may account for part of the observed variance in the outcome. Examples of this would be the novelty effect of video games with a paediatric population (Redd *et al.*, 1987) or expectancies of the patient in regard to treatment outcome. The existence of this phenomenon has been studied by several researchers in studies involving both the placebo effect (Morrow and Morrell, 1982; Lyles *et al.*, 1982) and possible expectancy effects (Morrow, 1986a, 1986b; Carey and Burish, 1987). In these studies the researchers controlled for placebo/attention effect by including appropriate control groups. Overall, results indicated that the experimental interventions had a greater effect on symptom reduction than either placebo controlled or the non-treatment controlled conditions. Thus, although not ruling out completely the effect of non-specific factors, the studies do reduce the plausibility of this alternative hypothesis.

Counterconditioning. Another possible explanation for the 'success' of behavioural treatments is tied to the theory that many of the chemotherapy side-effects manifest themselves through an associative learning process similar to Pavlovian conditioning (Burish and Carey, 1986). This counterconditioning hypothesis states that by pairing previous negative stimuli with feelings of relaxation and comfort, the noxious side-effects of chemotherapeutic treatment will be reduced or counterconditioned, and future experiences with the conditioned stimuli will be less likely to produce the noxious side-effects. From a learning perspective this is indeed an attractive explanation. However, there have been a number of objections to this hypothesis (see Carey and Burish, 1988) and to our knowledge, none of the studies conducted to date provide specific empirical support for this hypothesis.

Attentional distraction. This hypothesis states that behavioural techniques distract the patients' awareness from the conditioning process by engaging their attention on either external events (for example, video games or music) or internal stimuli (for example, imagery) instead of the stimuli that serve as the cues for conditioning the side-effects. Support for this contention comes from two studies cited earlier in this paper (Kolko and Rickard-Figueroa, 1985; Redd et al., 1987). However, as Morrow (1986a) notes, behavioural techniques (such as PMRT and hypnosis) that are successful, not only divert the patients' attention away from possible conditioning stimuli, but some (for example, SD) actually focus the patients' attention on these stimuli as part of the intervention itself. If the counterconditioning phenomenon were operating one would expect that techniques such as SD would not be successful in reducing side-effects such as ANV and dysphoria in view of the use of a cognitive hierarchy which would include the actual conditioned stimuli from the clinic.

Perceived sense of control. The concept of self-efficacy (Bandura, 1977) has received much attention of late in regard to its applicability to the field of health care. As Carey and Burish (1988) note, all of the behavioural intervention techniques mentioned thus far can be conceptualized as allowing the patient more perceived control over their situation in that they take an active part in the behavioural intervention. This participation reportedly reduces the sense of helplessness and improves the patients' 'psychological state'. Although an appealing idea, this concept lacks empirical support when applied to the control of side-effects stemming from chemotherapy. In fact, two studies actually supply evidence to refute this hypothesis. Morrow and Morrell (1982) measured the perceived sense of control of a group of patients undergoing chemotherapy using the Health Locus of Control Scale (Wallston et al. 1978). They found that reductions in the frequency of ANV were not associated with change in locus of control. Similarly, Burish et al. (1984) found that patients with a high external health locus of control were more likely to benefit from a behavioural intervention than those high on the internal dimension. Thus, although the perceived sense of control construct has yielded positive results in other health care domains, this phenomenon has not yet been replicated in the chemotherapy side-effect control area. However it should be borne in mind that the studies cited were in fact secondary analyses of the data and were not therefore specifically designed to measure the perceived sense of control construct. Further and more refined studies will be needed in order to make definitive statements regarding the role that a perceived sense of control plays in the efficacy of behavioural interventions in controlling chemotherapy side-effects.

Physiological relaxation response.   The final, and possibly unifying, hypothesis is that behavioural interventions induce an overall relaxation response. This relaxation response could serve to reduce physiological arousal which may set the stage for the conditioning of side-effects. Some researchers (Redd and Andrykowski, 1982) propose that this physiological relaxation response may inhibit gastric contractions that precede vomiting and thereby reduce or prevent the incidence. However, work by Morrow (1986a) suggests that although relaxation is indeed a necessary component in reducing nausea and vomiting, it is not by itself sufficient, and that the use of cognitive elements (for example, the cognitive hierarchy constructed in SD) in conjunction with the induction of a relaxation response are more efficacious in treating chemotherapy side-effects such as ANV.

In conclusion there are a number of hypotheses which suggest various mechanisms by which behavioural interventions reduce ANV and other 'psychological' side-effects of cancer chemotherapy regimens. Although initial studies support various aspects of these hypotheses, no one hypothesis seems to be able to adequately explain the 'active ingredients' in the behavioural interventions. However, various studies have shown that these hypotheses are not necessarily in competition with each other and indeed they may form an interactive mechanism that differentially operates depending upon the individual differences of the patient, the chemotherapeutic setting, and/or past experiences with chemotherapy regimens.

FUTURE DIRECTIONS

Individual differences.   Once it has been demonstrated that a particular technique is effective, the next logical question is whether it is differentially more effective for people with specific characteristics than for others. Although behavioural interventions in chemotherapy have not yet been shown to be more effective than pharmacological or other techniques, it might be helpful to look at the possible interactions between individual differences and specific techniques. For example, while hypnosis has been found to have some effectiveness in controlling adversive side-effects of chemotherapy for adults and children, it is much more useful for children than for adults because adults do not accept being hypnotized at a high enough rate to make it clinically relevant. On the other hand, systematic desensitization is much more appropriate for adults than for children due to the greater ease with which adults can cognitively construct the needed hierarchy of events (Morrow, 1986a).

A variety of individual characteristics seems to influence chemotherapy induced side-effects (Morrow, 1984a; Morrow, 1985). For example, elderly patients seem to have fewer chemotherapy related side-effects than younger patients. Similarly, patients who are susceptible to motion sickness report more side-effects and more nausea and vomiting than other patients. They are also more prone to developing anticipatory side-effects.

The degree to which individual differences may prove critical in tailoring specific interventions to specific patients or patient populations is an area rich with opportunities for controlled specific investigation. For example, it is a common clinical observation that patients want different amounts of control over their treatment situation (Rodin *et al.*, 1980). In addition, there seems to be marked differences in the amount of information patients wish to receive about the treatment and its options (Morrow *et al.*, 1983). The degree to which any of these potential individual differences may affect a particular behavioural intervention and the subsequent impact on compliance is a question of practical as well as theoretical importance.

SERVICE PROVISION

As is apparent from the above brief literature review, behavioural techniques of various types have been found to be effective with differing populations. However, one question that arises is who can deliver these techniques, under what conditions, and using what methods? The majority of studies reported have used trained psychologists or therapists to administer the intervention. Can paraprofessionals, oncology nurses and/or lay people use these techniques without a reduction in effectiveness and within a feasible cost/benefit ratio? Furthermore, can techniques such as audiotapes be as successful as procedures taught by 'live' instructors?

Carey and Burish (1987) conducted a study examining the use of three different delivery techniques for relaxation training to a population of cancer chemotherapy patients. Forty-five patients were randomly assigned to one of four treatment conditions: 1) PMRT training and guided relaxation imagery (GI) with a professional therapist; 2) PMRT and GI using a paraprofessional; 3) PMRT and GI using audiotapes; or 4) standard antiemetic treatment. Patients were assessed by self-report of psychological symptoms, physiological measures (systolic/diastolic BP) and nurse observation during the first five chemotherapy sessions. Results indicated that the professionally administered relaxation group were better able to reduce both physiological arousal and anxiety (patient self-reports) both pre- and post-chemotherapy when compared to patients receiving the paraprofessional or the audiotape condition. Both the audiotape condition and the paraprofessional condition did no better than the standard antiemetic control condition. One explanation for these findings could be that professional therapists have greater technical skill in inducing a relaxation state in the patient. Alternatively, it may be that the volunteer paraprofessionals had greater difficulty in coping with the medical context of the treatments (Burish and Carey, 1987). A third alternative is that subjects were aware that the paraprofessionals were in fact paraprofessionals or community volunteers and therefore 'discounted' them as being less effective at administering relaxation therapy. This third alternative is supported somewhat by some preliminary data from Morrow (1990).

Morrow (1990) randomly assigned 72 consecutive cancer patients with ANV to a no-treatment control or to a SD treatment group. The SD condition was administered by one of three groups: a) a behavioural trained clinical psychologist; b) a clinical oncologist, or c) oncology nurses. Overall, the SD treatment condition was found effective in reducing both ANV and PNV symptoms compared to controls. Additionally, there were no significant differences found in effectiveness between any of the three groups administering the SD treatment. This study, as well as supporting the contention that various health professionals can successfully administer behavioural interventions, also sheds light on the work of Carey and Burish (1987) in regards to the use of paraprofessionals in administering behavioural interventions. It shows that after minimal training the oncology staff, both nurses and doctors, were just as able to administer successfully behavioural interventions as compared to trained clinical psychologists, thus supporting the hypothesis that the use of paraprofessionals in a medical setting may not be successful because of the medical context, and that, for the same reason, clinical oncology personnel can work successfully in this context.

In a study designed to examine the possibility of reducing professional time to administer SD Morrow (1984a) randomized patients to a live instructor condition where lessons were given in PMRT, the session was audiotaped and the tape was given to the patient for subsequent practice. In the second condition the patient was provided with a prerecorded audiotape with instructions for PMRT. Patients in both conditions were instructed to practice the PMRT daily. Morrow reported that 80 per cent of the patients in the audiotape only condition reported that listening to the audiotape produced a nauseous response. This phenomenon was found in none of the five patients who were in the *in vivo* and tape condition. Morrow explains this phenomenon within a conditioning paradigm – that is, the prerecorded voice on the tape acted as a novel stimulus which may have been incorporated into a stimulus configuration facilitating a conditioned nausea response. Similar findings that the therapist's voice on audiotapes can become a conditioned stimulus eliciting nausea and/or distress has been supported by work from Redd *et al.* (1983).

In conclusion, preliminary results suggest that various health care professionals can indeed administer behavioural interventions as successfully as trained psychologists and that paraprofessionals because of their status or their unfamiliarity with the chemotherapeutic/medical setting may not be successful in this endeavour. Furthermore, various studies suggest that using audiotape alone may not be a successful mode for the application of behavioural interventions and may in fact be counterproductive.

Summary and Conclusions

The data reviewed indicate that the use of behavioural interventions in reducing psychological side-effects including ANV and in some cases PNV can indeed be successful. Research with both children and adults across a variety of settings, techniques, and research designs support this contention. Although we have made great strides in the use of behavioural interventions in the reduction of cancer chemotherapy side-effects in the last few years, there is still much to learn. Further research in the use of behavioural interventions to ameliorate cancer chemotherapy side-effects can be potentially useful as a paradigm or model for addressing a number of theoretical issues as well as the practical and important concerns of patient care. To maximize the full potential of behavioural interventions in this area there are a number of issues that need to be considered, such as individual differences, delivery techniques and the possibility of relapse. One caveat is called for however, and that is that we should not concentrate on behavioural interventions to the exclusion of examining their theoretical underpinnings. We need to remember that science is indeed a building block approach and that putting the cart before the horse can be detrimental to a relatively young and promising area.

Acknowledgement. Preparation of this article was supported in part by Research Career Development Award K04-CA01038 from NCID-HHS, Grant R01–NR01905 from the National Center for Nursing Research DHH and Grant PBR 42D, PBR 43 from the American Cancer Society.

APPENDIX 1   Biobehavioural intervention with cancer chemotherapy: case and controlled studies

(See page 68 for key to abbreviations.)

	N.	Design	Demographic/Clinical data	Protocol	Measures	Results
CASE STUDIES						
			RELAXATION TRAINING			
Burish & Lyles (1979)	1	Pt referred Single case	Gender: F Age: 30 Status: Outpt Dx: Lymphoma	1 BL 11 Tx (PMRT)	Anxiety, depression PR BP N/V	N reduced during Tx. Negative affect reduced during Tx. V eliminated. Physiological arousal reduced.
Cotanch (1983)	12	Pts referred Serial case studies	Gender: 5F; 7M Age: 17–49 (X = 34) Status: Outpt 4 Inpt 8 Dx: Melanoma 3 Soft cell 5 Adenocystic 1 Breast 1 Testicular 2	I BL I Tx (audiotaped) 6 FU	Anxiety N/V Caloric intake PR, BP	All patients – reduced PCNV. All patients – increased caloric intake – decrease in pulse rate. (Anxiety – reductions suggested.)
Scott et al. (1983)	10	'Convenience' sample Serial case studies	Gender: All F Age: 42–67 Status: Stage III or IV/Inpts Dx: Ovarian	No BL 1 Tx	Observations of emesis Diarrhoea Pt 'perception of the experience'	Reduction in duration, frequency, and intensity of emesis; in diarrhoea. Improved pt perception of experience.

Study	N	Sample	Subjects	Design	Measures	Results
Weddington et al. (1983)	2	Pts referred	Gender: M Age: Pt 1 = 58, Pt 2 = 46 Status: Outpt Dx: Lung	No BL Pt 1: 10 Tx Pt 2: 4 Tx	Pt 1: Pt self-report of ANV and PCNV Anxiety – self-report Pt 2: Pt self-report of ANV and PCNV	Pt 1: ANV reduced by 50% (intensity) Anxiety reduced. Pt 2: ANV reduced by 60% (severity).
Johanssen et al. (1989)	80	'Convenience' sample Hospital pts	Gender: Not reported Age: 25–80 Status: Inpts Dx: Not reported	4 Tx 1. Antiemetic and relaxation 2. Relaxation alone	Pt self-report of N and V	N and V were significantly reduced in the experimental group.
CONTROLLED STUDIES						
Burish et al. (1981)	16	Pt referred Stratified according to Dx and Rx Random assignment to: (1) PMRT (2) Control	Gender: 14 F; 2M Age: Not reported Status: Outpt Dx: Mixed	1 BL 2 Tx (written instructions only) 2 FU	Anxiety, depression PR, BP, N/V Nurse observations	*PMRT group:* During and post-Rx – less distress and nausea. Post-Rx – reduction of PR and BP. (Nurse and pt reports agreed.) (No changes in V.)
Lyles et al. (1982)	50	Pt referred Stratified according to Dx and Rx Random assignment to: (1) PMRT (2) Attention-control (3) NTC	Gender: 31 F; 19 M Age: Not reported Status: Outpt Dx: Breast 14, Lung 10, Ovarian 10, Testicular 5, Lymphoma 5, Hodgkin's disease 3, Other 3	3 Tx 1 FU	Anxiety, depression PR, BP, N/V Nurse observations	*PMRT group:* During Rx – reduction in anxiety and N. Post-Rx – reduction of PR and BP. N – less severe, shorter duration.

continued on page 62

Relaxation Training cont.

	N.	Design	Demographic/Clinical data	Protocol	Measures	Results

Burish et al. (1987)	24	'Select' sample* Stratified according to Dx and Rx
		
		Random assignment to:
		(1) PMRT
		(2) NTC
		
		(*based on chemotherapy emetogenic values)
			Gender: 19 F; 5 M
			Age: 23–69
			Status: Outpt
			Dx: Breast 9
			     Lung 4
			     Ovarian 10
			     Hodgkin's disease 1
				No BL*
				6 Tx
				
				(*pts seen at Rx1)
					Anxiety, depression, PR, BP, N/V
					Nurse observations
						PMRT group:
						During Rx – reduction in anxiety and N
						Post-Rx – reduction in anxiety, N, PR, BP (ANV did not develop in PMRT pts).
						NTC group:
						ANV developed in 'majority'.

Carey & Burish (1985)	45	Stratified according to Dx and Rx
		
		Random assignment to:
		(1) Professional
		(2) Volunteer
		(3) Audiotape
		(4) NTC
			Gender: 25 F; 20 M
			Age: 25–73
			Status: Not reported
			Dx: Breast 9
			     GYN 10
			     Haematological 10
			     Lung 9
			     Other 7
				1 BL
				3 Tx
				1 FU
					Anxiety, depression PR, BP
					Nurse observations
						Pts treated by professional experienced less distress than did pts treated by volunteers or with audiotape.

Cotanch & Strom (1985)	60	Random assignment:
		(1) PMRT (audiotape)
		(2) placebo (music)
		(3) NTC
			Gender: 28 F; 32 M
			Age: 17–68
			Status: Not reported
			Dx: Breast 11
			     Haematological 17
			     Melanoma 10
			     Testicular 11
			     Other 11
				1 BL
				3–4 FU
					Anxiety
					Respiration rate
					N, V
					Calorie count
					Skin fold
					Body weight
						PMRT group:
						Lower BP, PR, RR, V and anxiety (trait).
						Increased caloric intake.
						(Data for NTC not reported.)

Carey & Burish (1987)	45	Randomized clinical trial	Gender: Mixed
			Age: 25–73
			Status: Outpt
			Dx: GYN
			     Haematological
			     Lung
			     Other
				1 BL
				3 Tx
				
				(1) PMRT – GI/professional
				(2) PMRT – GI/volunteer
				(3) PMRT –
					Self-report of dysphoria, N, V, anxiety
					BP, breathing ratio
					Nurse observations
						Professionally administered PMRT and GI reduced emotional distress, and physio. arousal.
						Professionally administered relaxation

Study	N	Design	Sample	Conditions	Measures	Results
Blumberg et al. (1989)	14	Serial case studies	Gender: Not reported Age: Not reported Status: Not reported Dx: Breast, Lung, Lymphoma	GI/audiotape (4) Control (antiem) 4 Tx 1 Relaxation and audiotape 2 Control	Pt self-report BP	was superior to both audiotape and volunteer condition. No significant differences between conditions or post-chemo, N and V. Reduction in pre-treatment nausea and nervousness. Reduction in pre- to post-treatment blood pressure.

SYSTEMATIC DESENSITIZATION

Study	N	Design	Sample	Conditions	Measures	Results
CASE STUDIES						
Hailey & White (1983)	1	Pt referred	Gender: M Age: 28 Status: Outpt Dx: Lymphoma	No BL 10 SD sessions (No FU due to Rx change)	Pt self-report of distress, N/V, ANV, self-control	Elimination of ANV. Reduction in severity of PCN. Increased sense of self-control. Results generalized to hospital environment.
Hoffman (1983)	1	Pt referred	Gender: M Age: 'mid 40s' Status: Inpt Dx: Hodgkin's disease	No BL 4 Tx (hypnosis and SD) 1 FU (3 month)	Self-report of emesis Spouse-report of eating behaviour	Elimination of ANV. Increase caloric intake. Results generalized to hospital enviroment.
CONTROLLED STUDIES						
Meyer (1982)	37	Pt referred Random assignment to: (1) SD (2) PMRT (3) NTC	Gender: 25 F; 12 M Age: 18–67 (X = 43) Status: Not reported Dx: Breast 8 Lung 8 GYN/Genital 8 Haematological 4 Other 9	1 BL 2 Tx 2 FU	Pt self-report N, V, and anxiety Locus of control Nurses ratings N, V	Less severe PCN for 2 Tx groups (SD sooner than PMRT). Decrease in duration of PCN for SD. Decrease in frequency of PCV for SD. Decrease in anxiety for both Tx groups.

continued on page 64

Systematic Desensitization cont.

	N.	Design	Demographic/Clinical data	Protocol	Measures	Results
Morrow & Morrell (1982)	60	Consecutive pts (with ANV) Random assignment to: (1) SD (2) Counselling (3) NTC	Gender: 42 F; 18 M Age: 19–76 Status: Outpt Dx: Breast 29 Haematological 13 Lung 8 Other 10	2 BL 2 Tx 2 FU	Pt self-report N, V, ANV Anxiety Health locus of control	Pts in the SD group reported less severe ANV of shorter duration than the pts in the other 2 groups. No group differences in anxiety or locus of control.
Dobkin & Morrow (1985)	40	Consecutive pts Random assignment to: (1) SD (2) NTC	Gender: 26 F; 8 M Age: X = 52.2 Status: Out- and Inpt Dx: Breast 15 Lung 4 Lymphoma 5 Ovarian 7 Other 4	1 BL 2 Tx 3 FU	Pt self-report N/V Physical symptoms checklist Self-monitoring N/V, tension Anxiety	*Preliminary data:* Downward trend for SD pts' PCNV. Upward trend for NTC pts' PCNV. Anxiety higher in NTC than SD at FU3.
Morrow (1986a) * Some overlap with patients from Morrow & Morrel (1982).	92*	Consecutive pts (with ANV) Group assignment to: (1) SD (2) PMRT (3) Counselling (4) NTC	Gender: 66% F; 33% M Age: Mn > 50 yrs. Status: Inpt Dx: Mixed: maj. = breast	2 BL 2 Tx 2 FU	Pt self-report N, V Anxiety	*SD group:* ANV reduced in terms of severity and duration. *SD & PMRT group* PCN reduced in severity and duration.

HYPNOSIS

	N.	Design	Demographic/Clinical data	Protocol	Measures	Results
CASE STUDIES						
LaBaw et al. (1975)	27	Serial case studies	Gender: Mixed (about 50–50) Age: 4–20 Status: Not reported Dx: Not reported	Unspecified number of Tx	Pt self-report Therapist observations	Varying degrees of 'success' reported ('success' defined as: improved sleep, increase caloric intake and retention, increase fluid intake, and greater tolerance for therapeutic procedures).

Study	N	Design	Patient characteristics	Number of Tx	Measures	Outcomes
Dempster *et al.* (1976)	1	Case study	Gender: F Age: 21 Status: Stage IV Dx: Hodgkin's disease	Unspecified number of Tx	Pt self-report	ANV extinguished. Reduction in duration of PCN. Increases in 'quality of life'.
Dash (1980)	4	Pts referred	Gender: 2 F; 2 M Age: 7–13 (X = 11) Status: Not reported Dx: Leukaemia Lymphoma Hodgkin's disease Ewing's sarcoma	1–4 Tx	No objective data	Anecdotal reports of improvement.
Ellenberg *et al.* (1980)	1	Pt referred Case study	Gender: F Age: 12 Status: Inpt Dx: Leukaemia	1 BL 1 Tx	Self-report of anxiety, pain, anorexia, N, V Nurse observations	Reduction of PCNV frequency (but Rx also reduced). Reduction of pain and anxiety associated with medical procedures.
Olness (1981)	25	Consecutive referrals Serial case studies	Gender: Not reported Age: 3–18 Status: Inpt Dx: Leukaemia 15 Lymphoma 4 Other 6	No BL 4–7 Tx (+ optimal group work)	Self-report of pain, N, V	Reduction in pain, N, V for 10 pts.
Redd *et al.* (1982)	6	Single subject Multiple baseline (ABAB design) Pts referred for ANV	Gender: All F Age: 24–54 Status: Not reported Dx: Lung 1 Haematological 1 Breast 4	7–14 BL 5–7 Tx	Pt self-report of N Nurse observations of V	Decreased N/V during all Rx sessions for all pts. Elimination of ANV.
Margolis (1983)	6	Pt referred Serial case studies	Gender: 3 F; 3 M Age: 27–54 (X = 39) Status: In- and Outpt Dx: Lymphoma 1 Lung 1 GYN 3 Pancreas 1	No BL Tx varied across pts	Self-report of N, V, insomnia, pain	Reduction in suffering (no objective data).

continued on page 66

Hypnosis cont.

	N.	Design	Demographic/Clinical data	Protocol	Measures	Results
Zeltzer et al. (1983)	12	Pt referred Serial case studies	Gender: 5 F; 7 M Age: X = 14.2 Status: Not reported Dx: Hodgkin's disease 4 Haematological 2 GYN 1 Brain 3 Other 2	1 BL 1–3 Tx 1 FU (6M)	Pt self-report of V Anxiety Health locus of control Illness impact Self-esteem	(25% of pts received Tx.) 73% reduced – PCV frequency – PCV intensity. Reduction in trait anxiety. (No changes in health locus of control, impact of illness, self-esteem.)
Walker et al. (1988)	14	Serial case studies	Gender: Mixed (Approx. 50–50) Age: 9–64 Status: Not reported Dx: Breast Lymphoma Ewing's sarcoma Leukaemia	2–6 (hypnosis + cue control)	Pt self-report Therapist observations	Improvement in pharmacological PNV and conditioned ANV. Improvement in insomnia, irritability, concern over medical procedures.
CONTROLLED STUDIES						
Zeltzer et al. (1984)	19	Time series design Stratified (age & severity) Random assignment: (1) Hypnosis (n = 9) (2) Supportive counselling (n = 10)	Gender: Not reported Age: 6–7 (X = 11.3) Status: Not reported Dx: Haematological 11 Lymphoma 3 Bone 5	2 BL 2 Tx FU (n = 9)	Pt self-report 'bother' Parent report	*Both groups:* reductions in N, V, and 'bother'.
			OTHER INTERVENTIONS			
CASE STUDIES						
Burish et al. (1981)	1	Single subject Multiple baseline	Gender: F Age: 44 Status: Not reported Dx: Adenocarcinoma	3 BL 4 Tx (EMG biofeedback) 3 FU	Anxiety N, V, BP, PR, EMG	Reduced BP, PR, EMG levels. Reduced anxiety and N.

	N	Design	Characteristics	Conditions	Measures	Results
Moore & Altmaier (1981)	9	Serial case studies	Gender: 6 F; 3 M Age: 19–66 (X = 47) Status: Outpt Dx: Breast 4 Sarcomas 3 Other 2	6 Tx (Stress inoculation including PMRT)	Structured interview Anxiety	Reduction in anxiety.
LeBaron & Zeltzer (1984)	8	Single subject Multiple baseline	Gender: Not reported Age: 10–17 (X = 12) Status: Not reported Dx: Haematological 6 Bone 2	2–3 BL 2–3 Tx (distraction)	Pt self-report of N, V, 'bother', 'disruption' Parent report, N, V, 'bother', 'disruption'	Reduced N/V, bother and disruption of activities.
Kolko & Richard-Figueroa (1985)	3	Serial single case Multiple baseline (ABAB)	Gender: M Age: 11–17 Status: Outpt Dx: Haematological	3–5 BL 3 Tx (video game – distraction) 3 Withdrawal 3 Tx	Pt self-report of anxiety, distress, and chemo-related symptoms Observer rating of distress	Reduction in ANV and severity of PCNV.
Redd *et al.* (1982)	15	Serial single case Multiple baseline (ABAB)	Gender: Mixed Age: 9–18 Status: Outpt Dx: Leukaemia Lymphoma Brain tumour Sarcoma	2 BL 2 Tx	Visual analogue scales of nausea and anxiety	No significant reduction in anxiety. Significant reductions in conditioned N.
Redd *et al.* (1987)	26	Randomized trial	Gender: Mixed Age: 9–20 Status: Not related Dx: Leukaemia Lymphoma Sarcoma Taratoma Brain tumour	1 Tx 1 Video game 2 Control	Visual analogue scales of nausea Observational checklist of nausea behaviour	Significant decrease in N for experimental group.

Key to abbreviations in Appendix 1

ANV	anticipatory nausea and vomiting
BL	baseline
BP	blood pressure
D(x)	disease(s)
F	female
FU	follow-up (e.g. FU3)
GYN	gynaecological
Inpt	inpatient
M	male
maj.	majority
N	nausea
n	number
NTC	no treatment control
Outpt	outpatient
PCN	postchemotherapy nausea
PCNV	postchemotherapy nausea and vomiting
PCV	postchemotherapy vomiting
PMRT	progressive muscle relaxation training
PR	progressive relaxation
Pt	patient
R(x)	prescription(s)
SD	systematic desensitization
T(x)	treatment(s)
V	vomiting
X	mean

APPENDIX 2   *Progressive muscle relaxation training*

This is a synopsis of the PMRT technique that we have utilized successfully in our previous and ongoing research. It is provided because the technique is relatively simple to use and we have had few, if any problems, with its implementation. The session should take place in a semi-dark, quiet room, preferably with the patient in a comfortable chair. The patient is told that this technique is not hypnosis and that they will have complete control. Tight-fitting clothing, such as a tie, should be loosened and glasses and contact lenses removed. The patient is asked to close their eyes and breath slowly, in through their nose and out through their mouth. The patient is allowed to get used to this procedure for about 1–1½ minutes and then the therapist begins:

I am going to teach you a way to relax.
    This will be done by first tensing, then relaxing, each group of muscles progressively. Have you any questions?
    You will tense each of the following muscle groups for about ten seconds, then say the word 'RELAX' to yourself and focus on the difference between the relaxed state and tensed state.

(Each of the actions listed below should be completed successively, with 10–15 seconds of the tension phase followed by 10–15 seconds of the relaxation phase.)

- *make a tight fist with your right hand;*
- *make a tight fist with your left hand;*
- *make a tight fist with your right hand (you shouldn't feel as much tension);*
- *make a tight fist with your left hand (again, not as much tension);*
- *hold your right arm straight out, palm towards the floor and point your fingers toward the ceiling;*
- *hold your left arm straight out, palm towards the floor and point your fingers toward the ceiling;*
- *raise your eyebrows to touch your hair;*
- *press your eyes tightly together;*
- *press your lips tightly together;*
- *push your tongue against the roof of your mouth;*
- *push your tongue against the roof of your mouth again;*
- *raise your shoulders and try to touch your ears (relax-move your head side to side);*
- *take a deep breath and hold it (feel the muscles in your chest, pulling on your ribs);*
- *pull in your stomach and try to touch the back of your chair with your belly button;*
- *spend some time listening to your own easy breathing.*

Words and phrases to use as the patient is being treated
(during tensing state)   (during relaxing state)

- feel the tension   - listen to your breathing
- tight   - getting deeper and deeper relaxed
- tense   - feel tension leaving your body
- unpleasant   - calm and peaceful

- warm and gentle
- very pleasant

Now that you are completely relaxed, I am going to count backwards from three to one. With each number you will feel more and more relaxed. When I reach one, you will open your eyes when you choose. You will feel refreshed and remember everything in exact detail.

3 — *very calm, very relaxed with each gentle breath you take;*
2 — *totally in control, peaceful, gentle, relaxed;*
1 — *with each gentle breath, very peaceful, very pleasant.*

References

BANDURA, A. (1977) Self-efficacy: Toward a unifying theory of behavioral change. *Psychological Review*, 85, 191–215.

BLUMBERG, B., LERMAN, C., RIMER, B., KUNTZ, M., SERY, J., CRISTIZIO, S., ENGSTROM, P., and LEVY, B. (1989) Chemotherapy management through relaxation education. *Proceedings of the American Society of Clinical Oncology, Abstract 322.* American Society of Clinical Oncology.

BURISH, T.G., LYLES, J.N. (1979) Effectiveness of relaxation training in reducing the aversiveness of chemotherapy in the treatment of cancer. *Journal of Behavior Therapy and Experimental Psychiatry*, 10, 357–361.

BURISH, T.G. and CAREY, M.P. (1986) Conditioned aversive responses in cancer chemotherapy patients: Theoretical and developmental analysis. *Journal of Consulting and Clinical Psychology*, 5, 593–600.

BURISH, T.G., SHATNER, C.D. and LYLES, L.N. (1981) Effectiveness of multiple-site EMB biofeedback and relaxation in reducing the aversiveness of cancer chemotherapy. *Biofeedback and Self-Regulation*, 6, 523–535.

BURISH, T.G., CAREY, M.P., KROZELY, M.G. and GRECO, F.A. (1987) Conditioned side effects induced by cancer chemotherapy: Prevention through behavioral treatment. *Journal of Consulting and Clinical Psychology*, 55, 42–48.

BURISH, T.G., CAREY, M.P., WALLSTON, W.A., STEIN, M.J., JAMISON, R.N. and LYLES, J.W. (1984) Health locus of control and chronic disease: An external orientation may be advantageous. *Journal of Social and Clinical Psychology*, 21, 326–332.

CAREY, M.P. and BURISH, T.G. (1985) Etiology and treatment of psychological side effects associated with cancer chemotherapy: A critical review and discussion. *Journal of Consulting and Clinical Psychology*, 104, 307–325.

CAREY, M.P. and BURISH, T.G. (1987) Providing relaxation training to cancer chemotherapy patients: A comparison of three delivery techniques. *Journal of Consulting and Clinical Psychology*, 55(5): 732–737.

CAREY, M.P. and BURISH, T.G. (1988) Etiology and treatment of the psychological side effects associated with cancer chemotherapy: A critical review and discussion. *Psychological Bulletin*, 106(3), 307–325.

COTANCH, P.H. (1983) *Muscle relaxation versus 'attention – placebo' in decreasing the aversiveness of chemotherapy.* Unpublished manuscript, Duke University, Durham.

COTANCH, P.H. and STROM, S. (1987) Progressive muscle relaxation as antiemetic therapy for cancer patients. *Oncology Nursing Forum*, 14(1), 33–37.

COTANCH, P.H., HOCKENBERRY, M. and HERMAN, S. (1985) Self-hypnosis as anti-emetic therapy in children receiving chemotherapy. *Oncology Nursing Forum*, 12, 41–46.

DASH, J. (1980) Hypnosis for symptom amelioration. In J. Kellerman (Ed.), *Psychological Aspects of Childhood Cancer*. Springfield, IL: Charles C. Thomas.

DEMPSTER, C.R., BALSON, P. and WHALEN, B.T. (1976) Supportive hypnotherapy during the radical treatment of malignancies. *The International Journal of Clinical and Experimental Hypnosis*, 24, 1–9.

DOBKIN, P. (1987) *The use of systematic desensitization, a behavioral intervention, in the reduction of aversive chemotherapy side effects in cancer patients*. Unpublished doctoral dissertation, University of Georgia, Athens.

DOBKIN, P.L. and MORROW, G.R. (1985) *Prevention of chemotherapy induced nausea and vomiting*. Paper presented at the meeting of Biobehavioral Oncology, 6th Eupsyca Symposium, Zaragoza, Spain.

ELLENBERG, L., KELLERMAN, J., DASH, J., HIGGINS, G. and ZELTZER L. (1980) Use of hypnosis for multiple symptoms in an adolescent girl with leukemia. *Journal of Adolescent Health Care*, 1, 132–136.

ERICKSON, M.H. (1959) Hypnosis in painful terminal illness. *American Journal of Clinical Hypnosis*, 1, 117.

HAILEY, B.J. and WHITE, J.G. (1983) Systematic desensitization for anticipatory nausea associated with chemotherapy. *Psychosomatics*, 24, 287–291.

HARRIS, J.G. (1978). Vomiting and cancer treatment. *Cancer*, 28, 196–201.

HOFFMAN, J.L. (1983) Hypnotic desensitization for the management of anticipatory emesis in chemotherapy. *American Journal of Clinical Hypnosis*, 25, 173–176.

JOHANNSON, S., FREDERIKSON, M., FURST, C.J., HURSTI, T., PETERSON, C. and STEINECK, G. (1989) Poster presented at the Joint ESPO-BPOG Conference, Royal College of Physicians, London.

KATZ, E.R., KELLERMAN, J. and SIEGEL, S.E. (1980) Behavioral distress in children with cancer undergoing medical procedures: Developmental considerations. *Journal of Consulting and Clinical Psychology*, 48, 356.

KAZDIN, A.E. (1982) *Single-case Research Designs*. New York: Oxford University Press.

KOLKO, D.J. and RICKARD-FIGUEROA, J.L. (1985) Effects of video games in the adverse corollaries of chemotherapy in pediatric oncology patients: A single-case analysis. *Journal of Consulting and Clinical Psychology*, 53, 223–225.

LABAW, W., HOLTON, C., TEWELL, K. and ECCLES, D. (1975) The use of self-hypnosis by children with cancer. *American Journal of Clinical Hypnosis*, 17, 233–238.

LASZLO, J. (1983) *Antiemetics and cancer chemotherapy*. Baltimore: Williams and Wilkins.

LEBARON, S. and ZELTZER, L.K. (1984) Behavioral intervention for reducing chemotherapy-related nausea and vomiting in adolescents with cancer. *Journal of Adolescent Health Care*, 5, 178–182.

LYLES, J.N., BURISH, T.G., KROZELY, M.G. and OLDHAM, R.K. (1982) Efficacy of relaxation training and guided imagery in reducing the aversiveness of cancer chemotherapy. *Journal of Consulting and Clinical Psychology*, 50, 509–524.

MARGOLIS, C.G. (1983) Hypnotic imagery with cancer patients. *American Journal of Clinical Hypnosis*, 25, 128–134.

MEYER, J. (1982) Systematic desensitization versus relaxation training and no treatment (controls) for the reduction of nausea, vomiting, and anxiety resulting from chemotherapy. Unpublished doctoral dissertation, Virginia Commonwealth University, Richmond.

MOORE, K. and ALTMAIER, E.M. (1981) Stress inoculation training with cancer patients. *Cancer Nursing, October*, 389–393.

MORROW, G.R. (1982) Prevalence and correlates of anticipatory nausea and vomiting in chemotherapy patients. *Journal of the National Cancer Institute, 68*, 585–588.

MORROW, G.R. (1984a) Clinical characteristics associated with the development of anticipatory nausea and vomiting in cancer patients undergoing chemotherapy treatment. *Journal of Clinical Oncology, 10*, 1170–1176.

MORROW, G.R. (1984b) Prevalence, etiology and treatment of chemotherapy induced anticipatory nausea and vomiting. *Proceedings of the American Cancer Society 4th National Conference on Human Values and Cancer*.

MORROW, G.R. (1985) The effect of susceptibility to motion sickness on the side-effects of cancer chemotherapy. *Cancer, 55*, 2766–2770.

MORROW, G.R. (1986a) Effect of the cognitive hierarchy in the systematic desensitization treatment of anticipatory nausea in cancer patients: A component comparison with relaxation only, counseling, and no treatment. *Cognitive Therapy and Research, 10*, 421–446.

MORROW, G.R. (1986b) Behavioral management of chemotherapy-induced nausea and vomiting in the cancer patient. *The Clinical Oncologist, 113*, 11–14.

MORROW, G.R. (1987) Predicting the development of anticipatory nausea and vomiting in cancer patients: A prospective validation. (Manuscript submitted for publication.)

MORROW, G.R. (1989) Anticipatory nausea. *Cancer Investigation, 6*(3), 327–328.

MORROW, G.R. A comparison of the effectiveness of behavioral treatment to reduce chemotherapy-induced nausea/vomiting in cancer patients when administered by oncology nurses, medical oncologists or clinical psychologists. (Manuscript submitted for publication.)

MORROW, G.R. and MORRELL, C. (1982) Behavioral treatment for the anticipatory nausea and vomiting induced by cancer chemotherapy. *New England Journal of Medicine, 307*, 1476–1480.

MORROW, G.R., CARPENTER, P.J. and HOAGLAND, A.C. (1983) Improving physician-related communication in cancer treatment. *Journal of Psychosocial Oncology, 1*, 93–101.

MORROW, G.R., LOUGHNER, J. and BENNETT, J.M. (1984) Prevalence of nausea and vomiting (N&V) and other side effects in patients receiving Cytoxan, Methotrexate, Fluorouracil (CMF) therapy with and without Prednisone. *Proceedings of the American Society for Clinical Oncology, 3*, 105.

MORROW, G.R., ASBURY, R., CARPENTER, P.J., CARUSO, L., CORY, S., DOBKIN, P., HAMMON, S., PANDYA, K. and ROSENTHAL, S. (1990) A comparison of the effectiveness of behavioral treatment to reduce chemotherapy-induced nausea/vomiting in cancer patients when administered by oncology nurses, medical oncologists or clinical psychologists. (Paper submitted to the Lancet.)

OLNESS, K. (1981) Imagery (self-hypnosis) as adjunct therapy in childhood cancer: Clinical experience with 25 patients. *American Journal of Pediatric Hematology/Oncology, 3*, 313–321.

REDD, W.H. and ANDRYKOWSKI, M.A. (1982) Behavioral intervention in cancer treatment: Controlling aversion reactions to chemotherapy. *Journal of Consulting and Clinical Psychology, 50*, 14–19.

REDD, W.H., ANDERSON, G.U. and MINAGAWA, R.Y. (1982) Hypnotic control of anticipatory emesis in cancer patients receiving chemotherapy. *Journal of Consulting and Clinical Psychology*, 50, 14–19.

REDD, W.H., ROSENBERGER, P.H. and HENDLER, C.S. (1983) Controlling chemotherapy side effects. *American Journal of Clinical Hypnosis*, 25, 161–172.

REDD, W.H., JACOBSEN, P.B., DIE-TRILL, M., DERMATIS, H., McEVOY, M. and HOLLAND, J. (1987) Cognitive/attentional distraction in the control of conditioned nausea in pediatric cancer patients receiving chemotherapy. *Journal of Consulting and Clinical Psychology*, 55, 391–395.

RODIN, J., RENNERT, W. and SOLOMON, S.K. (1980) Intrinsic motivation for control: Fact or fiction? In A. Baum and J.E. Singer (Eds), *Advances in Environmental Psychology*, 2. Hillsdale, NJ: Erlbaum.

SCOTT, D.W., DONAHUE, D.C., MASTROVITO, R.C. and HAKES, T.B. (1983) The antiemetic effect of clinical relaxation: Report of an exploratory pilot study. *Journal of Psychosocial Oncology*, 1, 71–84.

SPIELBERGER, C.D., GORSUCH, R.L. and LUSHENE, R. (1968) *The state–trait anxiety inventory (STAI)*. Palo Alto: Consulting Psychologists Press.

WALKER, L.G., DAWSON, A.A., POLLET, S.M., RATCLIFFE, M.A. and HAMILTON, L. (1988) Hypnotherapy for chemotherapy side effects. *British Journal of Experimental and Clinical Hypnosis*, 5(2), 78–82.

WALLSTON, H.A., WALLSTON, B.S. and DeVILLIS, R. (1978) Development of the multidimensional health locus of control scales (MHLC). *Health Psychology*, 4, 189–202.

WEDDINGTON, W.W., BLINDT, K.A. and MCCRAKEN, S.G. (1983) Relaxation training for anticipatory nausea associated with chemotherapy. *Psychosomatics*, 24, 281–283.

WOLPE, J. (1983) *The Practice of Behavior Therapy*, (3rd edn.). New York: Pergamon Press.

ZELTZER, L., LEBARON, S. and ZELTZER, P.M. (1984) The effectiveness of behavioral intervention for reduction of nausea and vomiting in children and adolescents receiving chemotherapy. *Journal of Clinical Oncology*, 2, 683–690.

ZELTZER, L., KELLERMAN, J., ELLENBERG, L. and DASH, J. (1983) Hypnosis for reduction of vomiting associated with chemotherapy and disease in adolescents with cancer. *Journal of Adolescent Health Care*, 4, 77–84.

ZUCKERMAN, M., LUBIN, V., VOGEL, L. and VALERIUS, E. (1964) Measurement of experimentally induced affects. *Journal of Consulting and Clinical Psychology*, 28, 418–425.

COUNSELLING IN ROUTINE CARE: A CLIENT-CENTRED APPROACH

Mary V. Burton

The number of psychotherapeutic and counselling approaches to the cancer patient has grown enormously in recent years. There is now an extensive literature on individual counselling and psychotherapy with the cancer patient (for example: Bahnson, 1975; Burton and Parker, 1988; Fallowfield, 1988; Goldberg, 1981; Gordon et al., 1980; Greer, 1987, 1989; Greer and Moorey, 1987; Linn et al., 1982; Maguire et al., 1980; Maguire and Faulkner, 1988a&b; Moorey and Greer, 1989; Watson, 1983, 1987; Worden and Weisman, 1980; Vachon, 1985, 1987). When group, family, marital, psychosexual and behavioural approaches are considered, the range of techniques widens further. Some of the interventions described in the literature have been provided by staff with specialist training in psychotherapy, but elements of these counselling techniques can be taught to medical and nursing staff in hospital and community settings. General practitioners, social workers and medical staff in oncology and surgery can also profit from an understanding of counselling techniques in their work with cancer patients.

Communication between the cancer patient and health care providers is receiving an increasing amount of attention in the psychosocial oncology literature (Brewin, 1977; Buckman, 1986; Holland et al., 1987; Krant, 1976; Lichter, 1987; McIntosh, 1974, 1976, 1977; Reynolds et al., 1981; Slevin, 1987; Souhami, 1978). The problem of breaking bad news has received special attention (Buckman, 1984; Clark and LaBeff, 1982; Goldschmidt and Hess, 1987; Hogbin and Fallowfield, 1989; Hoy, 1985; Lind et al., 1989; Maguire and Faulkner, 1988a&b; Radovsky, 1985).

This chapter addresses the question of what health care professionals without specialized training in psychotherapy can reasonably undertake in a routine way in counselling the cancer patient.

Brewin (1977) describes five different patient attitudes to information about malignancy:

It is important to accept that you cannot soften the impact of bad news since it is still bad news however it is broken. The key to breaking it is to try to slow down the speed of the transition from a patient's perception of himself as being well to a realization that he or she has a life threatening disease. For example:

Doctor: *I'm afraid it's more than just an ulcer . . .*
Mr K: *What do you mean more than just an ulcer?*
Doctor: *Some of the cells looked abnormal under the microscope . . .*
Mr K: *Abnormal?*
Doctor: *They looked cancerous.*
Mr K: *You mean I've got cancer?*
Doctor: *I'm afraid so, yes.*

You should next explore how he feels about this information and why. This will usually reveal that there are good reasons for his responses.

Doctor: *How does this news leave you feeling?*
Mr K: *Terrified! I've always had this thing about cancer. I've always been frightened of getting it. Two of my uncles died of it. They both had a bad time. Suffered terrible pain and wasted away...to nothing.*
Doctor: *So you're frightened you're going to go the same way.*
Mr K: *I'm bound to be scared, aren't I?*
Doctor: *Yes, you are in view of those experiences. It must be hard for you. Any other reasons you are terrified?*
Mr K: *I hate being a burden. My wife has enough to contend with.*

Sometimes a patient's responses are better signalled by nonverbal behaviour [crying, going silent, shouting]. It then helps if you acknowledge this and invite him to discuss his feelings.

Doctor: *I'm sorry I've had to give you this news. I can see you're distressed. Would you like to talk about it?*
Mr C: *It is so incredibly unfair. I have always been careful with what I eat. I've not been a drinker. I have exercised regularly. To get cancer now, just when we're getting on our feet as a family, seems so unfair. It makes me feel very bitter.*

Having established his immediate responses you should establish any other concerns before attempting to give further information.

These other concerns can take many forms, for example moving house, taking on a new job, the effect of the illness on partner and children, fear of pain, fear of mutilating surgery, fear of secondaries, fear of radiotherapy or chemotherapy and the side-effects of treatments, fear of being a burden, fear of the outcome, fear of dying from the disease or fear of dying in the same terrible way the patient may have watched a close relative die. Sometimes the cancer is the latest in a disastrous string of stressful life events, a kind of 'last straw': 'First I lost my husband, then my son was killed in a car accident, my mother is dying of leukaemia, my daughter's husband has just walked out on her, my best friend moved away three months ago, and now this'. It is very supportive to discuss with the patient the meaning of the disease to his or her life. To some, for example, the knowledge one has cancer is the most devastating news; to others, the prospect of surgical mutilation is more terrifying.

PSYCHOLOGICAL REACTIONS TO SUDDEN LOSS

The news that one has or may have cancer is psychologically not dissimilar to being told suddenly and unexpectedly of the loss of a loved one. The trajectory of one's future years, which once stretched indefinitely into the future, is suddenly altered. The emotions experienced at this time can be extreme and very distressing, especially for people who have had little previous experience of loss. Although this news is not a loss of a loved one, there are other losses to be negotiated:

- the loss of the notion that one enjoys perfect health: '*my body has let me down*';
- the loss of an indefinite future stretching out ahead of one: '*how long do I have?*';
- the loss of a sense of invulnerability and omnipotence: '*my lifespan is now limited*';
- the loss of living to see one's children or grandchildren settled: '*I might not be here*';
- the loss of hard-earned retirement years: '*why now, of all times?*';
- in the case of mutilating surgery, the loss of a body part or body function affecting one's body image and self-esteem: '*how am I going to feel without a breast?*' or '*how am I going to cope with this colostomy?*';
- fears of losing one's partner's affection or sexual attentions because of mutilating surgery;
- fears of ill health from the side-effects of treatment (nausea, vomiting, hair loss, depression).

There may be unique and idiosyncratic losses an individual patient faces. For example: 'When I lost my first breast, my marriage was going through a bad patch. Now we have a wonderful sexual relationship, and I am going to have to lose the other breast. I feel absolutely devastated this time.' Some patients have an ill or handicapped family member to look after, and their first worry is for others. Other special circumstances in the life of the patient may create specific fears and concerns for an individual.

The emotions a patient experiences at the time of diagnosis and initiation of treatment may be powerful, upsetting and unfamiliar to them (Worden, 1983):

numbness	sadness	guilt	loneliness
anger	anxiety	panic	shock
helplessness	rage	fatigue	confusion
disbelief	preoccupation		

A patient may burst into unconsolable crying, become panic-stricken in the clinic, shout at staff in an uncontrollable rage, or scream out distress. Other patients become silent and withdrawn or evidence disbelief. Still others take the news apparently calmly and matter-of-factly and experience their emotional reaction when they get home, sometimes much later. Unpleasant physical sensations or altered behaviours associated with acute anxiety and panic may also occur and these may be distressing in themselves (Worden, 1983):

hollowness in the stomach	breathlessness
tightness in the chest	weakness in the muscles
tightness in the throat	lack of energy
dry mouth	sense of depersonalization
oversensitivity to noise	loss of appetite
sleep disturbance	restless overactivity
absent-minded behaviour	social withdrawal
crying for long periods	phobic behaviours

When these symptoms appear in the short term, they are features of normal grief and are not in themselves abnormal. They are none the less very painful feelings for us to respond to, and may cause staff as well as patients considerable distress.

Maguire (1975) describes typical patient reactions to learning the news:

> *I don't know whether it is me or not, but the feeling is just indescribable. Unless you've experienced it you just don't know...I was just so frightened. All I could think of was the children. If anything is going to happen to me, they are still so young. That's what I latched onto...My feelings were indescribable. I think I touched absolute hell. I didn't want to die, and I didn't know if I'd got cancer. It's the thing everyone dreads. At first you think it can't be happening to you. Then, my God – it is.*

> *I was so terrified of the result, I couldn't sleep, I just felt stunned. I just felt numb, I couldn't take it in.*

> *I felt so bitter and resentful, why me? Why should it happen to me? Why not someone else?*

Bard (1955) describes some of the reactions of women with breast cancer:

I'm scared out of my wits. I'm afraid of dying. Why should I be afraid of dying? I have to die sometime. Hospitals always worried me anyway. I guess I always thought hospitals were for dying.

I'm scared. I know it has to be done, but I'm afraid of the ordeal, the operation. My hands are shaking just talking about it. I'm scared but I can't say why.

I wouldn't care if it is just a cyst, but if it will be taken off, I'd mind. If they have to take my breast off, I would feel as though I'm losing part of myself, that I'd be disfigured. I'm not afraid of the operation, I'm more afraid of losing that part of myself. I know this has to be taken care of, but I'd rather die than to have them take it off.

I feel it's disgusting in a sense. It seems like you are sexless. That's why I worry about my husband's reaction. I feel it would be one of disgust, that he has to sleep with a sexless woman.

Would it make a difference to John? If it's a mastectomy, I'd feel funny about it. It's so important in our relationship. Ever since I discovered this, I keep staring at breasts everywhere I go. On the street, in the shop windows I look at brassières. All I can do is keep looking at breasts ever since I heard about this.

IDENTIFYING RISK FACTORS

The detection of psychiatric morbidity and an awareness of coping style, stressful life events and level of available social support will enhance the health care professional's ability to communicate effectively with the cancer patient.

In some patients, the news of having cancer leads to the development of *psychiatric morbidity* such as major depression or anxiety states. Several studies have shown that the detection of these disorders by health professionals is generally poor (Burton and Parker, in preparation; Hardman *et al.*, 1989; Maguire, 1985; Maguire *et al.*, 1978). The Hospital Anxiety and Depression Scale (Zigmond and Snaith, 1983), a 14-item paper and pencil measure, is well accepted by patients and provides a quick measure of caseness. Psychotropic medication may be indicated for some patients (Goldberg and Cullen, 1986; Massie and Holland, 1988).

We have also found it helpful to assess coping style, stressful life events and levels of social support in cancer patients in order to intervene psychologically (Burton and Parker, 1988; in preparation). Five *coping styles* have been studied recently in cancer patients: denial, fighting spirit, stoic acceptance, helpless/hopeless and anxious preoccupation (Watson *et al.*, 1988).

DENIAL: *I don't believe this really is cancer. I think it's just a cyst.*

FIGHTING SPIRIT: *I'm not going to let this thing beat me. I'm going to fight this.*

STOIC ACCEPTANCE: *This is something I am just going to have to learn to accept.*

HELPLESS/HOPELESS: *This is going to be the end of my life. There is nothing I can do.*

ANXIOUS PREOCCUPATION: *Every morning before breakfast I ask my husband to have a look: 'John, what do you think this is? Could it be another lump?'.*

If one adopts a client-centred approach to counselling the cancer patient, one does not attempt to alter the patient's coping style, but simply to reflect back to the patient what has been heard:

DENIAL: *So you're not sure you actually have cancer.*

FIGHTING SPIRIT: *It sounds like you're going to fight this.*

STOIC ACCEPTANCE: *You seem to be saying this is something you have decided to accept.*

HELPLESS/HOPELESS: *So the whole idea of this illness makes you feel hopeless and depressed.*

ANXIOUS PREOCCUPATION: *You seem to be spending a lot of time looking for lumps and worrying about recurrence.*

Such a technique allows the patient to say more about the coping style they have adopted, and to explore their feelings further. Recently cognitive-behavioural techniques have been used to teach cancer patients a fighting spirit attitude to their illness (Moorey, this volume; Moorey and Greer, 1989). A more prescriptive psychotherapeutic approach than that described here, it may be of considerable value to depressed cancer patients.

Severity of *stressful life events* may affect patients' needs for psychological support. Our work with breast cancer patients suggests that patients with high levels of perceived stress may profit more from psychological intervention than patients with mild or moderate stress (Burton and Parker, in preparation). An example of a patient with severe stressful life events was cited earlier: loss of husband, sudden death of son, break-up of daughter's marriage, mother's terminal illness, loss of best friend who has moved away, and now cancer.

Patients with few sources of *social support* may also be at risk for high levels of distress during and after treatment. The patient who was widowed recently, has no family and few or no friends, who belongs to no club, church or other social organization is especially vulnerable. 'No one would know if anything happened to me here. Sometimes no one comes here for days at a time', one patient told me anxiously at follow-up.

Clinicians caring for the cancer patient will be helped by learning to identify those patients with:

- high levels of perceived life stress;
- few social supports;
- significant psychological morbidity, and
- an attitude to the illness of helplessness, hopelessness or anxious preoccupation.

Such patients may particularly welcome an opportunity to discuss their feelings, and may profit more from psychological support and counselling than patients whose histories, at assessment, are without these risk factors.

THE PSYCHODYNAMIC LIFE NARRATIVE

In listening to the patient's story, it is possible to begin to place the illness in the context of the patient's life situation (Viederman and Perry, 1980). An example of such a psychodynamic life narrative follows:

'So you were happily married at 18 but then your mother developed motor neuron disease and died. You had twins, one of whom died and the second of whom was partially sighted. Then your husband developed uremia and died. You were by now only 24, a widow. At 26 you were in a road traffic accident, with no ill effects at first. The first marriage had been a good one but when your husband died your world fell apart. You married your second husband out of loneliness and to replace what you had lost. He treated you badly and was violent to both you and your daughter, who couldn't see the blows coming. Later you discovered that he raped your partially-sighted daughter, and you still feel very guilty about having brought him into your home. You blamed yourself for your daughter's divorce. After 10 years of suffering the violence of your ex-husband, even after your divorce from him, a new judge on the bench put him in prison. Then you became paraplegic as a result of the road traffic accident years before, and spent three years on your back until the neurosurgeons discovered that an operation would help you walk again. You were no sooner beginning to resume a normal life than you developed breast cancer. Facing mastectomy, it has been particularly difficult because your gentleman friend has stopped speaking to you since you learned the news. His lack of support at this time you feel very keenly. Given all these tragic losses in your life, it is not surprising that you are feeling very depressed about the disease, and about the operation. The cancer feels like a "last straw".'

It is not uncommon for patients to respond to such a reflection with the words, 'I never thought about it that way before, but that makes sense, doesn't it?' Note that no attempt is made here by the clinician to alter the patient's coping style. The current illness is placed in the context of the patient's life story and situation. Psychological morbidity, where it occurs, becomes more understandable in the light of events. This simple intervention can be of considerable comfort and support to the patient. We have found that the techniques required of listening to feelings and reflecting them back to the patient are readily taught to well-motivated medical and nursing staff through seminars and role-play training sessions.

COUNSELLING TECHNIQUES WITH CANCER PATIENTS

Klein (1971) suggests six principles for supporting the cancer patient:

- *help her to express her feelings*: nonjudgmentally allow her to talk about it;
- *help her to sort out the real from the unreal*: that cancer always recurs or kills, that she will be perceived by others as 'untouchable', or that she is somehow responsible for her cancer;
- *don't give false reassurances*: 'Don't worry, everything will be all right' is not a helpful intervention. It may not be all right at all for this patient in future;
- *help her to anticipate the future*: the depression she will feel for the next few months is part of the normal grieving process;
- *help the family to understand the patient's feelings and to express theirs;*
- *help the patient to consider how and what to tell those significant persons in her life.*

We shall focus in more detail on the first of these suggestions: 'help the patient to express her feelings'. Reflection of feelings techniques lie at the centre of client-centred counselling. They are also an essential component in both behavioural and psychodynamic approaches. Standing alone, reflection-of-feelings (Rogerian) methods are reasonably safe for relatively untrained staff to attempt in a routine way with patients.

TALKING WITH PATIENTS ABOUT THEIR FEELINGS

Talking with patients about their feelings need not take an hour's time. These are skills which can be used in very brief exchanges, even in a sentence or two. The aim is to help the other person feel understood and heard at the feeling level. These are skills which can be learnt, but to be effective they require a desire on our part to hear whatever the other person wants to tell us. People can tell if we are using a technique but don't really want to listen to them.

Talking with people about their feelings requires three basic attitudes in the listener (Rogers, 1951):

Empathy, the ability to sense the other person's world of felt meanings as if they were your own, but without ever losing the 'as if' quality; the ability to step into the other person's shoes for long enough to sense what life is like for him or her. Empathy is very different from sympathy, as sympathy more closely resembles pity or compassion. Empathy involves a greater risk that we might be changed by our experience.

Unconditional positive regard, a positive, warm, accepting response to the other person, regardless of how difficult his or her behaviour may be at the moment; the assumption that behind the difficult behaviour is a feeling and almost certainly suffering person; a respect and liking for the other person. With very difficult people, it may be essential to work hard at finding something one can like in the other person, and ally oneself with that.

Openness to feelings, communicating to the other person that whatever the feeling is, we can reply to that and deal with that. Any feeling can be talked about. Some feelings are very painful and we may be motivated to avoid discussing them. However we will make an effort not to avoid them with the other person if possible.

There is a substantial nonverbal component to the communication of empathy, unconditional positive regard, and openness to feelings. This is difficult to describe in words, and is probably best learnt through observation of others and if possible, videotape feedback on our own performance. People can tell whether we seem to be empathic, whether we like them or not, and whether certain feelings can be discussed with us. They probably could not say exactly how they know these things about us, but when patients are ill and feeling vulnerable, they often very rapidly assess those around them in just these terms.

Twelve Things We Often Do Instead Of Listening For Feelings

Here are twelve types of communication which are best avoided in client-centred counselling (Gordon, 1970).

(1) ORDERING, DIRECTING, COMMANDING: telling someone what to do:
    Don't speak to me that way!
    Stop complaining!

(2) WARNING, ADMONISHING, THREATENING: telling someone what consequences will occur:

If you carry on pulling those tubes out, you'll be sorry.
You'd better not do that if you know what's good for you.

(3) EXHORTING, MORALIZING, PREACHING: telling someone what he/she ought to do:

You shouldn't act like that.
If you want to get better, you'll do as I suggest.

(4) ADVISING, GIVING SOLUTIONS OR SUGGESTIONS: telling someone how to solve a problem, giving advice, providing answers:

I suggest you speak to your husband about that.
Why don't you try...

(5) LECTURING, TEACHING, GIVING LOGICAL ARGUMENTS: trying to influence a person with facts, logic, counterarguments or your own opinions:

If you'll just cooperate with what we're suggesting, things will go much better for you.

(6) JUDGING, CRITICIZING, DISAGREEING, BLAMING: making a negative judgment:

You're not thinking clearly at the moment.
You're very wrong about that. That's a ridiculous idea.

(7) PRAISING, AGREEING: offering a positive evaluation or judgment:

I don't think it looks bad at all [when the other person feels it looks terrible].

(8) NAME-CALLING, RIDICULING, SHAMING: making someone feel put down or foolish:

Look here, Mister Smarty.

(9) INTERPRETING, ANALYSING, DIAGNOSING: analysing why a person is doing what they are doing, telling them you have them all figured out:

You're doing this because you are a very aggressive sort of person.
You really don't believe that at all. What you really think is...

(10) REASSURING, SYMPATHIZING, CONSOLING, SUPPORTING: trying to make the person feel better:

It will soon feel better. You'll look at it differently tomorrow.
Don't worry, everything is going to turn out all right.

(11) PROBING, QUESTIONING, INTERROGATING: searching for more information to help you solve the problem for the other person:

When did you start feeling this way?
Is this the way you have responded to illness in the past?

(12) WITHDRAWING, DISTRACTING, HUMOURING, DIVERTING: pushing the problem aside:
Let's talk about something a bit more pleasant.

There is an alternative to the 'typical twelve': listening for the feeling in what the other person is saying and reflecting that feeling back to the person in a simple, accepting manner. You want to communicate to the other person that whatever the feeling is, you would like to hear about it. Listening in this way carries with it the risk that you might be changed or affected emotionally by what you hear. Because of this risk, you may close off this kind of conversation with a diversionary tactic such as one of the typical twelve. Many of these twelve approaches have a useful place in certain circumstances. However any one of them can be used by the counsellor defensively, to keep away from strong feelings.

Being Receptive to Feelings

Invitations for the other person to share their feelings ('door openers') include:

- silence;
- a nonverbal attending attitude: good eye contact, open body posture, communicating that you are there for the other person and want to hear what he has to say to you;
- encouraging noises: 'um hm', 'uh huh', 'ah', 'oh', 'right', 'yes', 'I see';
- 'It sounds like you have very strong feelings about that';
- 'It sounds like this must be very hard for you';
- 'Would you like to say a bit more about that?'.

When you use encouragements like this, it is important to keep the door open and accept whatever the feeling is that the other person would like to talk about.

Reflecting Feelings

When you are first learning how to reflect the feelings that the other person is communicating the following formulae may help:

It sounds like you're feeling _____ [naming the feeling in one word].
So you're feeling sort of _____.
You're feeling very _____ *because* _____.
So there's a feeling of _____.

Make your response tentative, so that the other person can either accept your comment or go on to say that it's really something else. It is alright to pick up the wrong feeling (and you *will* pick up the wrong feeling sometimes), as long as it is also alright for the other person to say, 'No, it's not that at all, it's more this other thing'. Then he or she will tell you what it is, and you can go on from there. Don't worry excessively about initially reflecting the wrong feeling back to the other person. If your reflection is made tentatively, you are letting the other person know that whatever the feeling is, you would like to hear about it. Sometimes you may have picked up the correct feeling but the person doesn't want to face that with you yet. You may be able to come back to it later on. He or she is more likely to come back to it if you make your first response a tentative one.

Some common feelings. Feelings are best reflected back to the other person as a single word or a very brief phrase. For example:

sad	miserable	disgusted
depressed	drained	repulsed
low	lonely	weak
down in the dumps	isolated	exhausted
disappointed	strange	numb
disillusioned	ugly	alone
unhappy	rotten	hopeless
worthless	guilty	helpless
unworthy	ashamed	bleak
down		
angry	resentful	end of rope
irritated	cheated	frustrated
furious	betrayed	going to put up a good fight
fearful	like jelly	edgy
apprehensive	anxious	butterflies in the stomach
terrified	worried	threatened
horrified	concerned	scared stiff
overwhelmed	nervous	uneasy
afraid	jittery	upset
spineless		
peaceful	over the moon	comforted
calm	pleased	confident
lucky	keen	hopeful
new lease of life	excited	
cautious	doubtful	stuck
uncertain	self-conscious	trapped
confused	shy	locked in

mixed up	respectful	surprised
puzzled	distant	relieved
bewildered	indifferent	determined
misunderstood	not bothered	foolish
not attended to		

The first section lists some depressive feelings; the second section angry and frightened feelings; the third column positive feelings, and the final section an assortment of other feelings. Those feelings we find most difficult to speak about in ourselves may well be the feelings we find hardest to explore with other people. When such feelings come up in conversation, we may use one of the 'typical twelve' to defend ourselves against getting in touch with our own discomfort.

Common Problems in Client-Centred Counselling

- If an issue has been identified and it is clear that the person doesn't want to talk about it:
  So you don't want to talk about that right now.
  If the answer is no, this should be respected. Your saying 'right now' leaves the door open to talk about it later, if the person wishes.

- If the person does seem to want to talk, but is having difficulty expressing him or herself:
  It seems as if this is very difficult to talk about, or
  All of this seems very painful, and very hard to talk about

- Sometimes people break down and cry, in which case it can help to offer a hanky and, after an appropriate interval, say something like:
  It seems like you've been needing to let go of some of these feelings.
  If the person apologizes for crying, you might say:
  It's alright for you to cry, you don't have to apologize.

- Sometimes people are very angry at us, but may feel they do not have permission to express it:
  It seems that you were very angry at me when I gave you the bad news, or
  So there's a lot of anger in you about this news that the cancer has spread.

- Sometimes feelings are being expressed quite freely up to some point, and then there seems to be a block. You can still reflect the feeling. It is a feeling of being blocked. For example:
  It seemed like it was easy for you to talk about this until you got on to the topic of telling your mother. Then it became very difficult for you to go on. OR:

So there's something difficult about talking about that, but you don't know what it is.
Sometimes just focusing on the block, or naming the 'something' that is blocking, can release it.

• Sometimes it can be helpful, especially if you are not sure what the feeling is, to repeat the last word or two, or some puzzling phrase from what the other person has said:
So you 'just don't know what's going on'.
So you're 'wondering what's going to happen now'.

Caution should be used with this last technique, however, because it can be overused.

How the Reflection of Feelings Response Works Therapeutically

When the counsellor has accurately reflected a feeling, there is an indication that the intervention has been successful when the patient says, 'That's right, and another thing is...'. Experiencing is always a felt complexity of feeling: there is always more than one feeling about a situation, and the therapeutic task is to explore as many of these as possible (Gendlin, 1962). One is on the right track therapeutically when the discussion moves from one feeling to another: 'So you feel very sad, but another part of you is very very angry'.

When a person expresses accurately in words for the first time how they are feeling, just then they are no longer that way. In the very act of sharing the feeling with another, the feeling has already changed. Also, only certain words will exactly fit the way a person feels at one time. When the right word is found, it is accompanied by the feeling, 'That's exactly right'. And when the feeling has become capable of being named, it has already changed and may lead to the discovery of other feelings: 'That's exactly right, and another thing is...'. This increased access to the range of one's feelings facilitates decision making and the resolution of crisis situations.

Even when the feeling is not exactly clear and no adequate words can be found, one can point to it as a 'that', or 'that feeling, whatever it is'. The expression, '...or something like that' can be very useful in such situations. It is as if one is pointing to a part of the patient's inner life as a part of the landscape: it may as yet have no name, but it can be identified as a 'that', or an 'over there', a 'that part' or 'that block I can't get past'. And the process moves on from there (Gendlin, 1967).

Client-Centred Counselling with Cancer Patients

The reflection of feelings technique can be taught to staff in medicine, surgery, general practice, nursing, social work, psychology, liaison psychiatry or allied professions who have not had a training in psychotherapy. Study days and workshops can be organized using a combination of written material, demonstrations, videotape exercises and role plays. Our work suggests that these are skills that can be learned by surgical staff, and that even very brief interventions of 30 minutes' duration can have lasting benefits three months and one year post-surgery in breast cancer patients (Burton and Parker, 1988).

From the initial outpatient appointment through the process of diagnosis and treatment, staff caring for the cancer patient need to be aware of the patient's emotional needs and reactions. This chapter has described the importance of:

- accurately assessing the patient's needs for information;
- adequate skills during the 'bad news' consultation;
- sensitivity to the common psychological reactions to sudden loss;
- skill in identifying psychiatric morbidity, coping style, stressful life events and levels of social support;
- the ability to formulate a psychodynamic life narrative, placing this illness in the context of the meaning of the patient's overall life trajectory; and
- the ability to help the patient express feelings about the illness.

Nondirective, Rogerian skills in reflecting feelings have been discussed in some detail. Specialist psychotherapeutic help may not be available in a hospital surgical or oncology unit, even on a liaison basis, in some centres. Nevertheless it is possible to train many existing staff to provide more sensitive psychological care to these vulnerable patients.

This chapter has focused largely on patients who have recently been diagnosed. The question of relapse or recurrence has not been addressed separately because (a) patients may experience fresh grief on learning of this further loss, not dissimilar to the grief they experienced at diagnosis; and (b) the reflection of feelings techniques required of the counsellor are exactly the same as those described here. The intensity of an individual patient's reaction to recurrence will be a function of variables specific to that person. Social support, stressful life events, coping style, previous psychiatric history, age, marital status, and a history of prior significant loss all play a role. The counsellor will take note of these factors and reflect back to the patient those feelings heard accordingly, at the time of relapse.

Inexperienced staff are always concerned about when to refer the patient for specialist psychotherapeutic help. When the reflection of feelings technique fails to contain adequately the patient's intense emotions; when listening uncovers a lifelong story of loss and inadequate means of coping with that loss; when helplessness and anxious preoccupation are extreme, leading to a clinical depression and/or anxiety state; when the patient is facing a series of devastating stressful life events in addition to the cancer, in the presence of few or no sources of social support; when the use of a psychodynamic life narrative approach is insufficient to contain the level of distress present; and (perhaps most important) when the patient indicates a desire to explore these issues in greater depth with a psychotherapist, referral to a specialist in psychotherapy should be arranged as a matter of urgency. Nevertheless, a great deal may be accomplished for a large percentage of patients in a routine way by utilizing supportively the client-centred techniques described here. With practice, health care professionals readily develop an intuitive ability to identify those patients in need of more in-depth assistance.

References

BAHNSON, C.B. (1975) Psychologic and emotional issues in cancer: The psychotherapeutic care of the cancer patient. *Seminars in Oncology, 2*, 293–309.

BARD, M. (1955) Psychological impact of cancer and its treatment. IV. Adaptation to radical mastectomy. *Cancer, 8*, 656–672.

BREWIN, T.B. (1977) The cancer patient: Communication and morale. *British Medical Journal, 2*, 1623–1627.

BUCKMAN, R. (1984) Breaking bad news: Why is it still so difficult? *British Medical Journal, 288*, 1597–1599.

BUCKMAN, R. (1986) Communicating with the patient. In B.A. Stoll and A.D. Weisman (Eds) *Coping with Cancer Stress*. Dordrecht: Martinus Nijhoff.

BURTON, M.V. and PARKER, R.W. (1988) A randomized controlled trial of preoperative psychological preparation for mastectomy: A preliminary report. In M. Watson, S. Greer and C. Thomas (Eds) *Psychosocial Oncology*. Oxford: Pergamon.

BURTON, M.V. and PARKER, R.W. (in preparation). A randomized controlled trial of preoperative psychological preparation for mastectomy.

CLARK, R.E. and LaBEFF, E.E. (1982) Death telling: Managing the delivery of bad news. *Journal of Health and Social Behavior, 23*, 366–380.

FALLOWFIELD, L.J. (1988) Counselling for patients with cancer. *British Medical Journal, 297*, 727–728.

GENDLIN, E.T. (1962) *Experiencing and the Creation of Meaning*. New York: The Free Press of Glencoe.

GENDLIN, E.T. (1967) Therapeutic procedures with schizophrenics. In C.R. Rogers (Ed) *The Therapeutic Relationship and its Impact: A Study of Psychotherapy with Schizophrenics*. Madison, Wisconsin: University of Wisconsin Press.

GOLDBERG, J.G. (Ed) (1981) *Psychotherapeutic Treatment of Cancer Patients*. New York: Free Press.

GOLDBERG, R.J. and CULLEN, L.O. (1986) Use of psychotropics in cancer patients. *Psychosomatics, 27*, 687–700.

GOLDSCHMIDT, R.H. and HESS, P.A. (1987) Telling patients the diagnosis is cancer: A teaching module. *Family Medicine, 19,* 302–304.

GORDON, T. (1970) *Parent Effectiveness Training.* New York: Wyden.

GORDON, W.A., FREIDENBERGS, I., DILLER, L., HIBBARD, M., WOLF, C., LEVINE, L., LIPKINS, R., EZRACHI, O. and LUCIDO, D. (1980) Efficacy of psychosocial intervention with cancer patients. *Journal of Consulting and Clinical Psychology, 48,* 743–759.

GREER, S. (1987) Psychotherapy for the cancer patient. *Psychiatric Medicine, 5,* 267–279.

GREER, S. (1989) Can psychological therapy improve the quality of life of patients with cancer? *British Journal of Cancer, 59,* 149–151.

GREER, S. and MOOREY, S. (1987) Adjuvant psychological therapy for patients with cancer. *European Journal of Surgical Oncology, 13,* 511–516.

HARDMAN, A., MAGUIRE, P. and CROWTHER, D. (1989) The recognition of psychiatric morbidity on a medical oncology ward. *Journal of Psychosomatic Research, 33,* 235–239.

HOGBIN, B. and FALLOWFIELD, L. (1989) Getting it taped: The 'bad news' consultation with cancer patients. *British Journal of Hospital Medicine, 41,* 330–333.

HOLLAND, J.C., GEAHY, N., MARCHINI, A. and TROSS, S. (1987) An international survey of physician attitudes and practice in regard to revealing the diagnosis of cancer. *Cancer Investigation, 5,* 151–154.

HOY, A.M. (1985) Breaking bad news to patients. *British Journal of Hospital Medicine, 34,* 96–99.

KLEIN, R. (1971) A crisis to grow on. *Cancer, 28,* 1660–1665.

KRANT, M.J. (1976) Problems of the physician in presenting the patient with the diagnosis. In J.W. Cullen, B.H. Fox and R.N. Isom (Eds) *Cancer: The Behavioral Dimensions.* New York: Raven Press.

LICHTER, I. (1987) *Communication in Cancer Care.* Edinburgh: Churchill Livingstone.

LIND, S.E., DELVECCHIO GOOD, M., SEIDEL, S., CSORDAS, T. and GOOD, B.J. (1989) Telling the diagnosis of cancer. *Journal of Clinical Oncology, 7,* 583–589.

LINN, M.W., LINN, B.S. and HARRIS, R. (1982) Effects of counseling for late stage cancer patients. *Cancer, 49,* 1048–1055.

MAGUIRE, P. (1975) The psychological and social consequences of breast cancer. *Nursing Mirror, 3 April,* 54–57.

MAGUIRE, P. (1985) Improving the detection of psychiatric problems in cancer patients. *Social Science and Medicine, 20,* 819–823.

MAGUIRE, P. and FAULKNER, A. (1988a) Communicate with cancer patients: 1. Handling bad news and difficult questions. *British Medical Journal, 297,* 907–909.

MAGUIRE, P. and FAULKNER, A. (1988b) Improve the counselling skills of doctors and nurses in cancer care. *British Medical Journal, 297,* 847–849.

MAGUIRE, P., TAIT, A., BROOKE, M., THOMAS, C. and SELLWOOD, R. (1980) The effects of counselling on the psychiatric morbidity associated with mastectomy. *British Medical Journal, 281,* 1454–1456.

MAGUIRE, P., LEE, E.G., BEVINGTON, D.J., KUCHEMANN, C.J., CRABTREE, R.J. and CORNELL, C.E. (1978) Psychiatric problems in the first year after mastectomy. *British Medical Journal, 1,* 963–965.

McINTOSH, J. (1974) Processes of communication, information seeking and control associated with cancer: A selective review of the literature. *Social Science and Medicine, 8,* 167–187.

McINTOSH, J. (1976) Patients' awareness and desire for information about diagnosed but undisclosed malignant disease. *Lancet, 7980*, 300–303.

McINTOSH, J. (1977) *Communication and Awareness in a Cancer Ward*. London: Croom Helm.

MASSIE, M.H. and HOLLAND, J.C. (1988) Assessment and management of the cancer patient with depression. *Advances in Psychosomatic Medicine, 18*, 1–12.

MOOREY, S. and GREER, S. (1989) *Psychological Therapy for Patients with Cancer: A New Approach*. Oxford: Heinemann Medical Books.

RADOVSKY, S.S. (1985) Bearing the news. *New England Journal of Medicine, 313*, 586–588.

REYNOLDS, P.M., SANSON-FISHER, R.W., POOLE, A.D., HARKER, J. and BYRNE, M.J. (1981) Cancer and communication: Information-giving in an oncology clinic. *British Medical Journal, 282*, 1449–1451.

ROGERS, C.R. (1951) *Client-Centered Therapy*. Boston: Houghton Mifflin.

SLEVIN, M.L. (1987) Talking about cancer: How much is too much? *British Journal of Hospital Medicine, 38*, 56–59.

SOUHAMI, R.L. (1978) Teaching what to say about cancer. *Lancet, 2*, 935–936.

VACHON, M. (1985) Psychotherapy and the person with cancer: An analysis of one nurse's experience. *Oncology Nursing Forum, 12*, 33–40.

VACHON, M. (1987) Unresolved grief in persons with cancer referred for psychotherapy. *Psychiatric Clinics of North America, 10*, 467–486.

VIEDERMAN, M. and PERRY, S.W. (1980) Use of psychodynamic life narrative in the treatment of depression in the physically ill. *General Hospital Psychiatry, 3*, 177–185.

WATSON, M. (1983) Psychosocial intervention with cancer patients: A review. *Psychological Medicine, 13*, 839–846.

WATSON, M. (1987) Supportive and psychotherapeutic services for cancer patients. *The Cancer Journal, 1*, 424–425.

WATSON, M., GREER, S., YOUNG, J., INAYAT, Q., BURGESS, C. and ROBERTSON, B. (1988) Development of a questionnaire measure of adjustment to cancer: The MAC Scale. *Psychological Medicine, 18*, 203–209.

WORDEN, J.W. (1983) *Grief Counselling and Grief Therapy*. London: Tavistock.

WORDEN, J.W. and WEISMAN, A.D. (1980) Do cancer patients really want counseling? *General Hospital Psychiatry, 2*, 100–103.

ZIGMOND, A.S. and SNAITH, R.P. (1983) The Hospital Anxiety and Depression Scale. *Acta Psychiatrica Scandinavica, 67*, 361–370.

ADJUVANT PSYCHOLOGICAL THERAPY FOR ANXIETY AND DEPRESSION

Stirling Moorey

The cognitive approach to emotional disorders is one of the most exciting psychological developments of the last decade. In several clinical trials cognitive therapy has established itself as an effective treatment for depression (Rush *et al.*, 1977; Blackburn *et al.*, 1981; Murphy *et al.*, 1984; Teasdale *et al.*, 1984). In all of these studies of depressed psychiatric outpatients cognitive therapy was consistently found to be as effective as standard treatment with tricyclic anti-depressants. Although not so well established as depression, the cognitive therapy of generalized anxiety disorders is attracting increasing attention, with some evidence that cognitive behaviour therapy is more effective than behaviour therapy alone (Butler *et al.*, 1987; Durham and Turvey, 1987).

A focused, short-term psychotherapy for anxiety and depression is of interest to mental health professionals who work with oncology patients for two reasons. First, research into the prevalence of psychiatric disorders in oncology outpatients (Farber *et al.*, 1984) and inpatients (Derogatis *et al.*, 1983) has shown that symptoms of anxiety and depression are common. These are often part of an 'adjustment disorder' – most patients go through a period of distress while coming to terms with the impact of cancer, but for some the degree of disturbance is so severe that work and personal relationships are affected. Symptoms may persist for some time: in 22–25 per cent of women with breast cancer they can persist for one to two years after mastectomy (Morris *et al.*, 1977; Maguire *et al.*, 1978). Second, the use of psychotropic medication is often problematic in cancer patients. As Scott (1989) has observed, antidepressants may be associated with more side-effects in this group of patients, they may interact with other drug treatments, and the mixture of anxiety and depression encountered in adjustment disorders may not be readily amenable to pharmacological treatment (Hughes describes the indications and contraindications for psychopharmacological treatment in cancer patients in this volume.)

This chapter will describe a form of psychological treatment for patients with cancer, based largely on Beck's cognitive therapy for depression and anxiety (Beck *et al.*, 1979; Beck and Emery, 1985), which has been developed by Greer and Moorey at the Royal Marsden Hospital (Moorey and Greer, 1989). It is intended as a treatment which can be delivered alongside and as a complement to medical treatments, and for this reason has been called adjuvant psychological therapy (APT).

THE COGNITIVE MODEL OF ADJUSTMENT TO CANCER

The cognitive approach views the individual's perceptions, interpretations and evaluations as the central mediating factor in adjustment to threat. It is not the situation *per se*, but the meaning it has for the person concerned which determines how that person feels and behaves. A diagnosis of cancer presents a different type of threat to each patient. Two women with breast cancer may undergo similar treatments and have a similar prognosis. One sees cancer as a death sentence and feels hopeless and depressed, while the other believes that the treatment will be successful and expresses cheerful optimism. In order to understand the patient's experience and reactions it is necessary to know the personal meaning that cancer holds for them.

Lazarus (1984) has suggested that in response to a possibly threatening situation the individual first makes a primary appraisal of the nature and degree of threat. A situation can be seen as harmless, threatening, a challenge or a loss. For example, following an amputation, fear of the effect of this on one's social relationships would result from a primary appraisal of threat to one's social role; depression and a conviction that one is no longer a 'whole person' would result from construing the amputation as a loss. Once the nature of the threat has been decided a secondary appraisal then takes place. This is an appraisal of the resources available for dealing with the threat. Adjustment will depend on the person's view of his or her capacity to cope and the skill with which these coping strategies are applied.

Cancer as a Threat to Survival

When they are told of the diagnosis of cancer most patients' first thoughts are of death. They often go through a period of great turmoil in which they feel disbelief, confusion and a plethora of changing emotions. This initial distress gradually gives way to a more stable way of viewing the impact of the disease. The patients' conclusions about whether or not cancer will shorten their life is one of the most important factors in determining their adjustment. Greer and

Watson (1987) have identified five common adjustment styles: fighting spirit; helplessness/hopelessness; fatalism; anxious preoccupation, and avoidance. These styles do not necessarily correspond to the objective prognosis of the disease (a patient with terminal cancer does not necessarily have to be fatalistic or hopeless), but are more closely related to the patient's subjective idea of prognosis. For instance, someone who sees the diagnosis as a challenge, believes that they can exert some control over the situation, and has an optimistic view of prognosis, will develop a fighting spirit. Someone who sees the diagnosis as a death sentence, believes there is nothing anyone can do about it and sees the future as hopeless will develop a helpless/hopeless response.

Cancer as a Threat to the Self

The possibility of death is the most serious threat that any of us could face, but this is not the sole threat in cancer. For some patients the real or imagined effects of the disease or its treatment can prove more difficult to cope with than the fear of death. In the early stages of many cancers the disease itself does not cause pain or disability, but treatment can be very unpleasant. Surgery may be mutilating (for example, mastectomy), chemotherapy may cause hair loss, nausea and vomiting, and radiotherapy can produce tiredness and lethargy. The meaning of this for the individual's self-concept will again determine their ability to cope. Some patients find the change in their body image unacceptable; others find the treatments themselves frightening since they imply loss of control; while others find that the disability caused by treatment is a threat to their family role. The cognitive model predicts that such threats to appearance, physical and mental abilities and social role will affect individuals differently depending on the meaning they give to them.

Vulnerability to Psychological Disturbance

Given that personal meaning plays so vital a role in adjustment it is reasonable to ask whether there are any factors which predispose people to respond in a particular way to illness. In Beck's cognitive theory (Beck, 1976) certain attitudes and beliefs are said to act as vulnerability factors for emotional disturbance. Past experiences lead to the development of idiosyncratic, maladaptive assumptions which remain latent until activated by critical incidents which are related to the theme of the assumption. For instance, a woman who witnesses the death of several family members from cancer and nurses them through pain may conclude that all cancer is incurable and involves a painful, lingering death. If this woman develops a melanoma which is caught at an early stage and is potentially curable, it will be very difficult for her to believe that there is any hope. The assumption derived from her past experience is that she will inevitably die. Once the assumption is activated it acts as a 'schema' or template which filters and interprets information in a biased way. The woman's helpless/hopeless attitude to cancer will prevent her from attending to or trusting information from her doctors that she has a good prognosis. She may selectively attend to any negative information from other patients. This bias in the processing of information is observable in the contents of the patient's thoughts. She will experience negative automatic thoughts which rapidly come into mind unbidden and seem realistic and plausible (for example 'There's no hope'; 'I might as well give up'; 'I'm dead already'). She may also experience fleeting images of herself dying from cancer, or vivid memories of her relatives who died. Other underlying assumptions which might cause people to have difficulty in handling the threat of cancer to their survival include beliefs about their ability to cope with illness and adversity, fatalistic ideas about life and death being pre-ordained and rigid rules concerning the need to be in control at all times.

Assumptions which make patients vulnerable to threats to their self-image are often conditional in form. They derive from repeated learning experiences in which the person's self-esteem is linked with some external factor such as appearance, attractiveness, success and so on. For instance, a man whose father was a successful businessman might learn the rule that he could only be happy if he was a success at everything he did. He might be able to cope with the disease itself, but would become depressed at having to give up his job through ill health. One patient developed the belief that she could only be loved if she were sexually attractive. When breast cancer was diagnosed she refused even a lumpectomy because of the threat to her appearance. Local recurrence of the disease led to depression about her appearance and fears that her husband would leave her for another woman.

ADJUVANT PSYCHOLOGICAL THERAPY

APT is a brief, problem-focused therapy with two main aims:

(1) To reduce anxiety, depression and other psychiatric symptoms.
(2) To improve mental adjustment to cancer by inducing a positive fighting spirit.

Four broad strategies are used to achieve these aims:

(1) Encouraging open expression of feelings.
(2) Promoting in patients a sense of personal control over their lives and active participation in the treatment of their cancer.
(3) Helping patients to develop effective coping strategies for dealing with cancer-related problems.
(4) Improving communication between the patient and their partner or spouse.

Format of Therapy

To achieve these goals APT uses a structured framework based on Beck's cognitive therapy for emotional disorders (Beck *et al.*, 1979). The first one or two sessions may be less structured to allow the patient to tell their story and ventilate feelings. A list of problems is then drawn up with the patient, and subsequently an agenda is set at the beginning of each session to deal with one or more of the problems on the list. Homework assignments are used to give the patient the opportunity to practise the coping methods learned during each session. The therapeutic relationship is one of 'collaborative empiricism': therapist and patient work together to test the patient's maladaptive beliefs about cancer and its effect on their lives. Therapy is a joint problem-solving exercise, where the insights and suggestions of the patient and their partner can be as useful as those of the therapist. A course of therapy usually consists of 6 to 12 weekly sessions, each of which lasts 50 minutes.

Components of APT

1. Ventilation of feelings. Emotional expression often has an important part to play in the treatment of adjustment reactions. Researchers from various backgrounds have stressed the importance of a period of emotional processing of a traumatic event during which the full impact of the event is registered, and the consensus is that this processing can only take place when negative emotions are acknowledged and expressed (Rachman, 1980; Horowitz, 1979). With some patients, ventilation of feelings is needed before a problem-solving approach can be used. Many patients have not had the opportunity to discuss their feelings with professionals, relatives or friends. The reasons for this vary from lack of time, 'distancing' as a means of coping on the part of professionals and relatives, and a wish on the patient's part not to be a burden. APT encourages ventilation of feelings as part of the initial assessment and problem-definition phase of therapy. The techniques used are not unique to this therapy.

Listening skills, the use of open-ended questions, reflection, clarification and empathy are all part of the non-directive techniques used in all therapies. Burton's chapter in this volume describes these methods in more detail.

2. *Behavioural techniques*. Behavioural techniques are often used at the beginning of treatment because these techniques bring rapid symptom improvement and are easier to master early in therapy while the patient is training in cognitive techniques. Cancer robs people of control of their own bodies, and its treatment involves more passivity than the treatment of other conditions. Patients who develop a helpless/hopeless response tend to generalize this sense of loss of control to other areas. Their helpless feelings lead them to reduce the activities of which they are capable, and so get into a cycle of decreasing activity and increasing helplessness.

The therapist helps to break this cycle by the use of *activity scheduling*. The current level of activity is recorded by taking a detailed record of how the patient spends their time. From this information decisions can be taken about what further activities can be planned which might give the patient a sense of mastery or control over their life and environment. In addition to increasing self-efficacy, planning activities helps to structure the day and so distract the patient from negative thoughts. Many people with cancer spend so much of their time trying to live a normal life alongside their treatment that their days are filled with chores and little else. Scheduling pleasant activities as well as activities to promote self-efficacy can help to raise their spirits.

For more depressed patients it is useful to arrange *graded tasks* that encourage a gradual increase in activities. For instance, to improve their concentration patients might read for increasing lengths of time and watch television programmes for longer periods each day.

Relaxation training can be a helpful coping strategy for anxious patients. If they are avoiding fearful situations (for instance if a patient feels stigmatized and avoids social situations) they can be encouraged to construct a hierarchy of difficult situations, and use *graded exposure* to enter increasingly frightening situations.

All of these behavioural techniques are set up as experiments to test the patients' dysfunctional beliefs about the disease and their capacity to cope with it. These behavioural experiments are one of the most potent ways of changing beliefs. For instance, scheduling pleasant activities can be introduced as a way of establishing whether the patient really has lost the ability to enjoy anything now he or she has cancer.

3. Cognitive techniques

Monitoring automatic thoughts. Patients are taught the cognitive model of adjustment to cancer – it is not the cancer itself but the thoughts they have about it which is the main cause of their distress. An example can be given to illustrate this important link between thoughts and emotions. If you imagine that someone steps on your foot while you are getting into a lift how would you feel? If you felt angry and thought 'Why don't they take more care', imagine how you would feel if you then looked round to discover the person was blind. The pain in your foot is the same but your emotional reaction is different because you think differently about it.

During the session the therapist elicits automatic thoughts associated with the problems the patient is facing and demonstrates how the patient can identify their own negative thoughts. Once patients understand this link between negative thoughts and emotions they are encouraged to record mood and thoughts in a diary between sessions. Just recording thoughts produces some distance from them and can improve mood, but cognitive interventions are usually needed to produce lasting change.

Cognitive interventions. Cognitive coping strategies are techniques which patients can use to cope with negative thoughts. *Distraction* – attending to a particular task when troubled by negative thoughts – may be useful in certain situations, for example when undergoing an investigation or therapeutic procedure. *Self-instructions* such as statements like 'I've had this procedure before, I can cope with it' or 'This treatment is shrinking the lump, it is getting me well again' can also be helpful in these situations. These coping methods can be taught in the session while the patient imagines the feared event and practises how to cope with it (a form of *cognitive rehearsal*).

Cognitive restructuring goes beyond using cognitions to cope with or prepare for difficult situations. It attempts to alter the very meaning that cancer has for the person. The habitually negative style of thinking about cancer is challenged and modified to a more adaptive form. The therapist shows the patient how to challenge their negative automatic thoughts. Through the skilful use of questioning and guided discovery the therapist brings the patient to see how the thoughts are illogical or self-defeating. *Reality testing* (What's the evidence?) is the commonest method. Patients are taught to continually ask and look for evidence to support their beliefs rather than accept them immediately. A patient with a helpless/hopeless response was sure that she would never get well, and thought that she had to refrain from any strenuous activity during radiotherapy, which made her feel even more helpless. On discussion there appeared to be no clear reason for either of these assumptions, and the patient realized that she had not even asked her doctor what she could or could not do. She then decided to ask the radiotherapist and test her assumption.

Looking for alternatives is another method of challenging automatic thoughts. The same patient was only able to see the future as bleak and hopeless. The therapist asked her to assume for the sake of argument that the treatment was going to succeed, and list the goals she wanted to achieve in the future. At first this proved difficult because she even saw recovery as presenting tremendous problems, but with perseverance she identified some goals, such as finding a school for her daughter, doing creative writing, and changing her job. This exercise presented the patient with an alternative way of viewing her future which the therapist was then able to build on by getting her to start working right away on her goals, some of which could be addressed without waiting for a cure. Optimism about the future must always be encouraged within the framework of the reality of the disease. For patients with a poor prognosis more emphasis will be placed on maximizing their quality of life in the here and now.

Reattribution is a similar technique in which patients are taught to look for alternative causal explanations. For instance, an anxious patient may attribute aches and pains to a recurrence of cancer. A more realistic attribution might be that this particular pain had been present for many years and so was more likely to be arthritis.

Sometimes it is necessary to confront fears head-on using a technique known as *decatastrophizing*. The person is encouraged to consider the feared consequence which they may be avoiding. For instance patients who fear a recurrence can be encouraged to imagine the cancer coming back. They often find that they can imagine a number of ways in which they could cope with this event.

Patients apply these methods to the negative thoughts they record each day and replace them with more adaptive thoughts or rational responses. For instance, a patient may think:

Negative thoughts

'I have to sort out my family's problems. What am I going to do if I'm not well enough? They can't manage without me.'

The challenge to this might be:

Rational response

'I can't be responsible for my children's lives. They're grown up now and have to learn to cope for themselves. This is an opportunity for them to learn how to manage for themselves.'

Using the diary they are able to gradually overcome the habitual automatic reaction and so gain control over their emotions.

4. Working with couples.   Partners are involved in two main ways in APT. They can act as co-therapists, or they can be involved more directly as participants in the therapy. In marriages where the partner is not under too great a stress as a result of cancer, he or she often has the will and the emotional resources to be a support to the patient. APT utilizes this by engaging the partner as a co-therapist. Partners can remind patients of their strengths, and remember times when they have coped effectively in the past. Even if a depressed patient forgets what activities used to be pleasurable before they developed cancer, the partner can usually remember and help in the construction of activity schedules. Once homework assignments are set the partners can be used to prompt patients to carry out assignments, share assignments with them and give reinforcement for successful coping efforts. Not everyone has the resilience to do this: the stress of cancer may adversely influence the marital relationship and this will need to be addressed directly.

Patient and spouse are taught to monitor automatic thoughts about the partner and identify distorted thinking. Many couples do not talk about their feelings and so each partner jumps to conclusions about what the other is thinking and feeling: a distortion known as 'mind-reading'. For instance, a man with lung cancer may feel less of a man because he is weak and breathless. He becomes withdrawn and sullen. His wife may wrongly interpret this as anger against her, and, if she is threatened by conflict, may react by trying to placate him and look after him. The more she cares for him the more he feels useless and a vicious circle is set up. Often fairly simple interventions can help to correct misunderstandings and break into this circle. Just encouraging each partner to explain their perceptions and express their feelings reveals the problem and allows the couple to get back on the right track again. Sometimes the power balance of a relationship is upset by cancer. In this example once the problem was understood the husband might be encouraged to find some things he could do to help his wife and so feel more useful. Because the cancer patient is the primary patient in APT, the relationship cannot be the main focus of the whole therapy. If a relationship is very disturbed it may be more appropriate to work with the cancer patient individually or use more formal marital or family therapy.

Case history

Sarah was 31 years old, separated, and had cancer of the breast which was treated by lumpectomy and axillary clearance. Axillary lymph nodes were positive. For the first two weeks after diagnosis she was very distraught but she then switched herself off and threw herself into lots of social activities. Two months after diagnosis while receiving chemotherapy she became increasingly anxious, tense and depressed. She cried during an outpatient appointment and told the oncologist about her symptoms and the difficulty she had coping with cancer and other life stresses. At this point she was referred for a psychiatric assessment.

At interview it was clear that she had several real-life problems as well as symptoms of anxiety and depression. She was in the process of getting divorced when she got cancer; the cost of the divorce and loss of income because of her illness put her in financial difficulties. Her grandmother had been very ill and had died six weeks before the referral. Finally she was overweight and considered this to be a major problem. She was spending a good deal of her time ruminating about these problems, worrying over her finances and trying to make decisions regarding the divorce. She viewed cancer as something which had prevented her from solving these problems and getting on with her life. Other anxiety-related symptoms included excessive fear of chemotherapy, fear of cancer recurrence and a belief that her life was out of control. She felt depressed and guilty about being unable to cope, angry with herself for being unable to control her weight and generally hopeless about the future. She experienced difficulty getting off to sleep and was eating more than usual.

Sarah had no past history of psychiatric disorder. She came from a middle-class family, both parents were alive and she had an older brother and younger sister. Her sister-in-law had recently had a recurrence of breast cancer. She described a happy childhood, was intelligent but not academic and after leaving school had been very successful in various jobs, usually ending up as an essential member of the company. Her current job was as an estate agent. She worked very hard at this and found the 11 hours she put in every day very tiring. Her husband was Greek and came from a rich family. Their marriage started to go wrong when he began to gamble, overspend and take drugs. He was verbally abusive to her and she finally left him when he physically attacked her.

On the basis of this assessment the psychiatrist made a diagnosis of adjustment disorder with anxiety and depression. Scores on the Hospital Anxiety and Depression Scale (HAD) (Zigmond and Snaith, 1983) were in the clinical ranges for anxiety and depression (Anxiety 17, Depression 17).

Session 1. The first treatment session began the following week. Sarah had already derived some benefit from talking about her problems and felt a little less depressed. A problem list was constructed and the principles of the cognitive approach described to her. The main focus for the session was depression. She was continually criticizing herself for her shortcomings, expecting to be able to do everything she did before she was ill and berating herself for not coping. The therapist helped her to see that her depressed mood, together with the physical effects of chemotherapy, might be contributing to her inability to function at her usual high level. The idea that she was depressed about being depressed made some sense to her. As homework she recorded some of these negative automatic thoughts as well as recording what she did during the week on an activity schedule.

Session 2.   Sarah's mood had improved further; she said she was coping better through distraction. The activity schedule revealed that she was doing very little that gave her a sense of achievement or pleasure. She described a pervasive sense of helplessness. This became the focus for the session. Initially the therapist worked with Sarah to find some activities which might challenge these helpless feelings. She wanted to lose weight and also wanted to do something to improve her general health. She therefore had some motivation to carry out small activities which might help her physical state, such as going swimming once a week and walking her dogs every day. These were presented as the beginning of a graded process of returning to the sorts of thing she did before her illness.

Because she had few experiences of achievement and success she felt out of control. The therapist tried to decatastrophize some of the feared consequences of her financial situation. She felt she had to sell her house in order to obtain money to live on, but she was worried that if she did not sell it soon she would have to let it go for a much lower price than it was worth. Because the house market was at a standstill she felt trapped. Decatastrophizing allowed her to see that although it would be undesirable to lose money in this way it would not be the disaster she feared it would be. She was helped to reconstrue her idea that she was helpless by considering that in fact she was consciously *choosing* not to act at the moment. She was sensibly waiting for a few weeks to see what happened to the house market. This concept of not acting yet still being in control was completely new to her and had a certain liberating quality. As homework she now started challenging automatic thoughts using the daily record of automatic thoughts.

Session 3.   By this session her depressed mood had improved considerably, but she was feeling more anxious. She felt more in control of her financial situation, but was beginning to worry more openly about cancer and about chemotherapy in particular. The first part of the session focused on her fear of chemotherapy. She was taught a relaxation technique and the meaning of chemotherapy was then explored with her. It seemed that she thought of it as poison which would build up in her body and irreparably damage her. As well as challenging this idea verbally, the therapist helped Sarah to use imagery during relaxation to visualize her body removing the chemicals through its normal metabolic processes. Sarah was also beginning to admit that as well as needing to be in control, there were also times when she felt very lonely and wanted to be looked after. She talked about feelings of grief over the loss of her husband, and how although she knew he was bad for her she sometimes wished that he was still around. This ventilation of feelings helped to lift her mood in the session.

Sessions 4, 5 and 6. Sarah's mood was now much improved. She said she was feeling brighter and more in control. She was nearing the end of chemotherapy and was looking forward to getting back to a normal life. One of the problems she was now facing was a concern not to return to her old stressful lifestyle. She wanted to sell her house and give up work for a year or two. This seemed to be quite an extreme reaction. These two sessions explored some of the underlying assumptions which led to Sarah's difficulties in coping with cancer. She had two fundamental beliefs:

(1) I must be in control at all times or I am weak.
(2) I must be totally committed and successful at what I do or I will be letting people down.

These two beliefs had helped her to succeed at work but had caused problems when she got cancer. In particular, the normal distress she experienced as a result of all the negative life events she faced in such a short time was misinterpreted by Sarah as a sign of weakness. She was now trying to reassess her priorities, but the only alternative she could see to her old style of overwork was avoiding it altogether. Sarah learned ways to challenge and test these maladaptive beliefs and eventually went back to work, but made sure that she delegated more, kept to office hours and allowed herself more leisure activities.

At the end of therapy her scores on the HAD were now in the normal range (Anxiety 7, Depression 4). She was well at her two-month and six-month follow-ups, was continuing to work on some of the issues covered in therapy and was free from cancer. (At her six-month follow-up HAD scores were 1 and 1 respectively.)

Figure 1 shows the change in HAD scores over the course of therapy. Figure 2 shows the change in fighting spirit and helplessness/hopelessness over therapy as measured by the Mental Adjustment to Cancer Scale (Watson *et al.*, 1988).

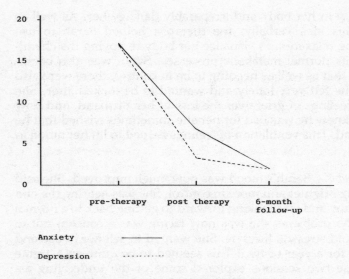

FIGURE 1   *Hospital Anxiety and Depression Scale scores*

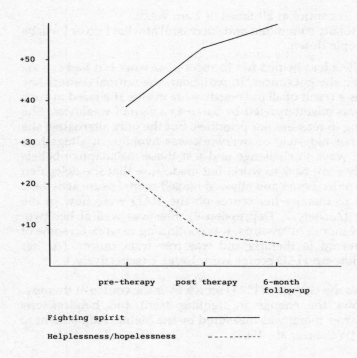

FIGURE 2   *Mental Adjustment to Cancer Scale scores*

EFFICACY OF COGNITIVE BEHAVIOUR THERAPY IN CANCER

There are relatively few studies to date which look at the effectiveness of a cognitive behavioural approach in cancer. Scott (1989) and Moorey and Greer (1989) have reported case studies. Tarrier and Maguire (1984) evaluated a form of cognitive behaviour therapy with depressed breast cancer patients who had undergone mastectomy. Ten patients received 2–4 sessions of a treatment which included relaxation and self-instructional training. Patients were randomly assigned to cognitive behaviour therapy alone, or in combination with an antidepressant (mianserin). Patients in both groups showed improvement but there was a tendency for those who received mianserin to do better.

Two other studies have used a group therapy format. Weisman and Worden (1980) screened patients with various cancers and allocated those who were considered to be at risk of emotional disturbance to group therapy. These were randomly assigned to four sessions of 'consultation therapy', which involved identifying problems, ventilating feelings and encouraging confrontation, or four sessions of 'cognitive skills training', which consisted of relaxation training and general processes of psychosocial problem solving. Both group therapies proved equally effective and superior to an untreated control group. Unfortunately the untreated control group was not strictly comparable since it was obtained from an earlier study and was not randomly allocated. Telch and Telch (1986) compared group coping skills training (six sessions of relaxation, stress management, assertive communication, cognitive restructuring and problem solving) and supportive group therapy (six sessions of non-directive therapy) in 41 patients with various stages and types of cancer. They found the coping skills training to be superior to supportive therapy and both groups showed more change than an untreated control group.

Adjuvant psychological therapy as described in this chapter has been reported to reduce anxiety and depression, increase fighting spirit and reduce helplessness in an uncontrolled series of 44 cancer patients (Greer *et al.*, 1990). A large study is currently underway at the Royal Marsden Hospital (see Moorey and Greer, 1989). In this study patients with various cancers who are within one to three months of diagnosis or first recurrence are randomly allocated to either six sessions of APT or to a no-treatment control in which they will receive the usual support of the hospital. This will probably be the largest study of its kind to be carried out with cancer patients.

APPLICATIONS OF APT IN ONCOLOGY UNITS

Our clinical work at the Royal Marsden Hospital suggests that APT is acceptable to patients and can be delivered as part of a consultation-liaison psychiatry service in a specialist cancer hospital. The therapy in its current format is a relatively complex package still employed as an experimental treatment. Two questions arise: which patients benefit from APT, and how well can its technique be generalized outside its present setting?

APT is suitable for a range of adjustment disorders, including depression and anxiety of clinical severity. In patients with more marked mood disturbance APT can be given alongside drug therapy. Patients who are so severely disturbed that they are intellectually impaired or deluded (i.e. those with functional or organic psychoses) are not suitable for this type of therapy. Anxiety and depression associated with marital and sexual problems respond well to APT. However, some marital problems involve a long-standing conflict and the cancer is of secondary importance. In these couples it may be more appropriate to employ formal marital therapy. Although APT was initially developed for patients with early disease it has been our experience that it can be effective in advanced disease. Stage of disease and performance status do not predict outcome of therapy (Greer *et al.*, 1990). The techniques used are not different from those used in early disease, but more emphasis is placed on quality of life, and living life to the full on a day-to-day basis. The structured form of cognitive therapy described here works best with outpatients who can attend for weekly sessions. Patients with advanced disease may be in hospital or too ill to attend this regularly. In these cases a less formal and less structured therapy may be helpful in which some of the cognitive and behavioural techniques can none the less still be applied.

APT consists of a set of techniques which are readily learned by mental health professionals working in general hospitals such as psychiatrists, psychologists, psychiatric nurses and social workers. Resources do not always allow patients with cancer who are in need of therapy to see a mental health professional, and it is hoped that APT can be taught to oncology nurses who perform a counselling role. Once its efficacy is established further work needs to be done on this.

In its current form, despite being a short-term therapy, APT still requires intensive therapist input of six to twelve hours. Another line of development is to explore even briefer therapy, or to look at how particular components of the package might be extracted for use by busy oncology counsellors. Our experience of teaching this therapy to counsellors has been that its emphasis on defining problems, and teaching specific self-help techniques is particularly attractive to people who come from a non-directive background. Until now counselling has been rather vague and ill-defined. Cognitive-behavioural therapy offers an empirically testable, prescriptive approach to the emotional distress of patients with cancer.

References

BECK, A.T. (1976) *Cognitive Therapy and the Emotional Disorders*. New York: International Universities Press Inc.

BECK, A.T., RUSH, A.J., SHAW, B.F. and EMERY, G. (1979) *The Cognitive Therapy of Depression*. New York: Guilford.

BECK, A.T. and EMERY, G. with GREENBERG, R.L. (1985) *Anxiety Disorders and Phobias: A cognitive perspective*. New York: Basic Books.

BLACKBURN, I.M., BISHOP, S., GLEN, A.I.M., WHALLEY, L.J. and CHRISTIE, J.E. (1981) The efficacy of cognitive therapy in depression: A treatment trial using cognitive therapy and pharmacotherapy, each alone and in combination. *British Journal of Psychiatry*, 139, 181–189.

BUTLER, G., CULLINGTON, A., HIBBERT, G., KLIMES, I. and GELDER, M. (1987) Anxiety management for persistent generalised anxiety. *British Journal of Psychiatry*, 151, 535–542.

DEROGATIS, L.R., MORROW, G.R., FETTING, J., PENMAN, D., PIASETSKY, S., SCHMALE, A.M., HENRICHS, M. and CARNICKE, C.L.M. (1983) The prevalence of psychiatric disorder among cancer patients. *Journal of the American Medical Association*, 249, 751–757.

DURHAM, R.C. and TURVEY, A.A. (1987) Cognitive therapy versus behaviour therapy in the treatment of chronic general anxiety. *Behaviour Research and Therapy*, 25, 229–234.

FARBER, J.M., WEINERMAN, B.H. and KUYPERS, J.A. (1984) Psychosocial distress in oncology outpatients. *Journal of Psychosocial Oncology*, 2, 109–118.

GREER, S. and WATSON, M. (1987) Mental adjustment to cancer: Its measurement and prognostic importance. *Cancer Surveys*, 6, 439–453.

GREER, S., MOOREY, S. and BARUCH, J. (1990) Evaluation of adjuvant psychological therapy for clinically referred cancer patients. (Manuscript submitted to *British Journal of Cancer*.)

HOROWITZ, M.J. (1979) Psychological response to serious life events. In V. Hamilton and D.M. Warburton (Eds) *Human Stress and Cognition: An information processing approach*. John Wiley & Sons.

LAZARUS, R.S. and FOLKMAN, S. (1984) *Stress, Appraisal and Coping*. New York: Springer.

MAGUIRE, G.P., LEE, E.G., BEVINGTON, D.J., KUCHERMAN, C., CRABTREE, R.J. and CORNELL, C.E. (1978) Psychiatric problems in the first year after mastectomy. *British Medical Journal*, i, 963–965.

MOOREY, S. and GREER, S. (1989) *Psychological Therapy for Patients with Cancer: A new approach*. Oxford: Heinemann Medical Books.

MORRIS, T., GREER, H.S. and WHITE, P. (1977) Psychological and social adjustment to mastectomy: A 2 year follow up study. *Cancer*, 40, 2381–2387.

MURPHY, G.E., SIMONS, A.D., WETZEL, R.D. and LUSTMAN, P.J. (1984) Cognitive therapy and pharmacotherapy singly and together in the treatment of depression. *Archives of General Psychiatry*, *41*, 33–41.

RACKMAN, S. (1980) Emotional processing. *Behaviour Research and Therapy*, *18*, 51–60.

RUSH, A.J., BECK, A.T., KOVACS, M. and HOLLON, S. (1977) Comparative efficacy of cognitive therapy and imipramine in the treatment of depressed outpatients. *Cognitive Therapy and Research 1*, 17–37.

SCOTT, J. (1989) Cancer patients. In J. Scott, J.M.G. Williams and A.T. Beck (Eds) *Cognitive Therapy in Clinical Practice: An illustrative casebook*. London: Routledge.

TARRIER, N. and MAGUIRE, G.P. (1984) Treatment of psychological distress following mastectomy: An initial report. *Behaviour Research and Therapy*, *22*, 81–84.

TEASDALE, J.D., FENNELL, M.J.V., HIBBERT, G.A. and ARMIES, P.L. (1984) Cognitive therapy for major depressive disorder in primary care. *British Journal of Psychiatry*, *144*, 400–406.

TELCH, C.F. and TELCH, M.J. (1986) Group coping skills instruction and supportive group therapy for cancer patients: A comparison of strategies. *Journal of Consulting and Clinical Psychology*, *54*, 802–808.

WATSON, M., GREER, S., YOUNG, J., INAYAT, Q., BURGESS, C. and ROBERTSON, B. (1988) Development of a questionnaire measure of adjustment to cancer: The MAC scale. *Psychological Medicine*, *18*, 203–209.

WEISMAN, A., WORDEN, J.W. and SOBEL, H.J. (1980) *Psychosocial Screening and Intervention with Cancer Patients*. Boston: Massachusetts General Hospital.

ZIGMOND, A.S. and SNAITH, R.P. (1983) The Hospital Anxiety and Depression Scale. *Acta Psychiatrica Scandinavica*, *67*, 361–370.

ANXIETY AND DEPRESSION: PSYCHOTROPIC MEDICATION

Jennifer Hughes

The epidemiology of depression and anxiety – mood disorders – among cancer patients has now been thoroughly researched, but the place of psychotropic drugs in their management has not. Much of the material in this chapter is therefore based on clinical experience rather than formal trials.

The antidepressants are the most suitable drugs for patients with formal mood disorder, whether depression or anxiety predominates. The benzodiazepines have a more limited role. Individual drugs will be discussed in detail in the second part of the chapter, the first part being concerned with the nature of mood disorders and identification of affected patients.

PATIENTS AT RISK

Surveys carried out on mixed populations of cancer patients indicate that between a quarter and a half of subjects suffer from anxiety and/or depression to a clinically significant degree (Bukberg *et al.*, 1984; Derogatis *et al.*, 1983; Plumb and Holland, 1977).

Mood disorders may develop in cancer patients of any age and either sex. Some kinds of cancer, such as carcinoma of the pancreas, some kinds of treatment, such as intensive chemotherapy regimes, and some stages of the illness, such as the time of first recurrence, are particularly associated with mood disorder. But anxiety and depression are not confined to these high-risk groups, and even patients whose cancer has been in prolonged remission are vulnerable.

The majority of mood disorders in an oncology setting are believed to represent an exaggerated psychological response to the stresses of having cancer: the threat of recurrence or death, the unpleasantness of the physical symptoms and the unwanted effects of treatment. Other factors also contribute. Some patients have an organic brain syndrome related to physical complications of their disease. Others have a mood disorder which is largely coincidental to their cancer, being of genetic origin or reactive to other social stress. Personality and circumstances are probably just as important as the cancer and its treatment in determining vulnerability to mood disorder. Socially isolated patients without close confiding relationships may be specially at risk.

EFFICACY OF PSYCHOTROPIC DRUGS

Little systematic research has examined the efficacy of psychotropic drugs in cancer patients, or indeed in physically-ill patients in general (Rodin and Voshart, 1986). The only widely-quoted controlled study of antidepressant treatment for cancer patients is the one by Costa *et al.* (1985), carried out in Romania on a group of 73 women, mostly inpatients receiving anticancer drugs or radiotherapy for breast or gynaecological cancers, and fulfilling research criteria for major depression. Patients were randomly allocated to receive either mianserin (a 'new' antidepressant) or placebo, and assessments carried out blind using various standard psychiatric rating instruments. Of 36 patients receiving mianserin, 28 (78 per cent) were considered to have a good response – a response rate at least as high as that to be expected in ordinary psychiatric practice. The mianserin group showed significantly greater improvement on all measures when compared to the placebo group. This benefit was apparent by the end of the first week, and maintained throughout the four-week follow-up period. Side-effects in the mianserin group were few, except for mild drowsiness; no adverse interactions with anticancer drugs were found, and drop-outs were significantly more common in the group receiving placebo.

A less rosy picture emerges from two American descriptive studies, one by Evans *et al.* (1988) on female cancer patients and the other by Popkin *et al.* (1985) on hospitalized medical patients including some with cancer. Both studies indicate that, although antidepressant drugs are effective for some cases of major depression coexisting with severe physical illness, a substantial number of patients are unable to tolerate therapeutic doses and others do not respond. This conclusion seems more in line with clinical experience.

There is a need for further research to clarify the place of antidepressants in the management of patients with cancer and other major physical illnesses, although placebo-controlled trials on such sick patients are likely to be hampered by ethical considerations. At present, these drugs are probably underused and the reasons for this will now be considered.

THE UNDERUSE OF PSYCHOTROPIC DRUGS

Psychotropic drugs, especially the antidepressants, are not widely prescribed for cancer patients in most centres. Local studies on lung cancer (Hughes, 1985) and on terminal care patients (Hughes and Lee, 1988) found that only about a third of patients with major depressive illness receive antidepressants and a study currently in progress in Southampton shows the same for patients with breast cancer. The reasons for not prescribing probably include the following:

• Under-recognition of symptoms likely to respond to drugs, due to the difficulties of diagnosing depression and anxiety in the physically ill, combined with lack of time for oncology staff to discuss psychological aspects.
• Reluctance on the part of both patients and staff to mention emotional problems, because of stigma, embarrassment or a sense of failure.
• The belief, common but illogical, that because anxiety and depression in cancer patients are 'understandable', they do not merit specific treatment.
• Concern about the side-effects of drugs, especially in frail patients who may already be taking large doses of other medication.
• Oncologists' unfamiliarity with the practicalities of choosing and using psychotropic drugs.
• Paucity of published evidence for the efficacy of psychotropic drugs in cancer patients.
• A belief that psychological treatments are more appropriate.

Some of these factors will be discussed in more detail below but first, identification of patients with mood disorders likely to respond to drugs will be considered.

SYMPTOMS OF MOOD DISORDER

Somatic Symptoms

These are just as common as psychological ones in patients with mood disorder, and often constitute the presenting complaints.

Somatic symptoms of depression include insomnia, loss of appetite, loss of weight, lack of energy, pain and general malaise. These are identical to the effects of malignant disease. Anxiety is also associated with multiple somatic symptoms, mostly those of sympathetic nervous system overactivity and/or overbreathing. They include shaking, muscle tension, fatigue, shortness of breath, palpitations, sweating, dry mouth, dizziness, nausea, diarrhoea, a 'lump in the throat' and flushing. These symptoms may occur episodically ('panic attacks') or be present continuously. Again, such anxiety-based complaints may be difficult to distinguish from cancer symptoms.

If somatic symptoms appear disproportionate to the severity of the cancer – for example if they develop in patients who have apparently had a successful excision of a localized tumour – there is a considerable likelihood that they are due to mood disorder. In other cases, there is no way of telling whether malignant disease or mood disorder is responsible. There will probably be an element of both, the mood disorder causing functional exacerbation of a symptom which has some biological basis.

Psychological Symptoms

Psychological symptoms can be equally difficult to evaluate in patients suffering from cancer, since they often have such obvious reason to feel misery, apprehension and despair.

Psychological features of anxiety are easy to recognize: worry, tension, dread, irritability, inability to relax. These feelings may be present all the time for no obvious reason, or may be centred on specific stimuli often related to the cancer: fear of recurrence, fear of dying, attending clinics, having injections.

Psychological features of depressive illness include:

- Sustained depressed mood, with or without tearfulness, especially if it is worse during the morning ('diurnal variation') and fails to lift in response to pleasant circumstances.
- Worthlessness and guilt, perceiving the physical illness as a punishment or stigma, and feeling a burden to others.
- Loss of interest. This symptom needs to be distinguished from the inevitable restriction of activities secondary to physical illness; for example the patient who claims to have lost interest in gardening may really mean that gardening is impossible because of his breathlessness.
- Poor concentration, for example inability to follow a newspaper or television programme. Again, this symptom is liable to misinterpretation if the patient is mentally confused, or distracted by severe physical symptoms.
- Inability to feel emotion, especially pleasurable emotion – for example loss of appreciation of the company of family and friends.
- Suicidal thoughts. Although many people might consider suicide to be a rational response to having cancer, suicide and suicide attempts are not common among patients with malignant dis-

ease, and the presence of suicidal thoughts – especially if the prognosis of the cancer itself is favourable – is highly suggestive of a treatable depressive illness.

Identifying Mood Disorder

Both depression and anxiety are universal human emotions, familiar even to psychologically healthy people at times of stress. Depression is the classic response to loss, and anxiety to danger. Though unpleasant, both mood states in moderation are believed to make a positive contribution to the process of coping and adaptation. Most cancer patients experience some degree of anxiety and depression at certain stages of their illness, and such reactions are perfectly appropriate, perhaps even desirable.

The 'normal' reactions imperceptibly shade into their 'pathological' equivalents. When anxiety and depression are somewhat more severe and prolonged than usual, yet still clearly understandable in terms of the stress of the physical illness and not interfering unduly with the patient's life, the term *adjustment disorder* may be applied. The next stage on, in which depression and/or anxiety are present to a degree which is out of proportion to any precipitating stress, no longer fulfil any adaptive function, take on a different and more unpleasant quality, and are accompanied by a characteristic pattern of both physical and mental symptoms, represents a fullblown psychiatric illness – here called *mood disorder*.

The distinction between 'normal' and 'pathological' mood is not clear cut, nor always easy to make, yet is important on clinical as well as academic grounds because of its relevance to management. Mood disorders are associated with sustained changes in physiology and in the activity of cerebral neurotransmitter systems, changes which can be modified by antidepressant drugs. Patients with true mood disorders often benefit greatly from drug treatment, whereas those who are merely showing a natural reaction to distressing circumstances do not.

There is no reliable laboratory test to identify cases which are likely to respond to physical treatments. The dexamethasone suppression test, which recently seemed to be a promising biological marker for depressive illness, has proved too nonspecific to be useful. Therefore it is necessary to make the diagnosis on clinical grounds.

DRUG TREATMENT AND PSYCHOLOGICAL TREATMENT

Various psychological interventions currently seem to be perceived as more appropriate than psychotropic drugs for the treatment of mood disorder in cancer patients. There is a trend to regard psychological treatment and drugs as incompatible, with psychological treatment being morally superior. If anxiety and depression are both inevitable and desirable stages in the process of accepting the cancer diagnosis, so the argument goes, it follows that their artificial suppression with drugs is inappropriate. This is a reasonable view so far as the milder, short-lived adjustment reactions are concerned, but when applied to severe sustained mood disorders it becomes inhumane. Witholding drugs from depressed patients because their depression is 'understandable' is no more logical than witholding analgesics from patients whose pain has an identifiable cause!

The two approaches – psychological and pharmacological – should be regarded as complementary, not mutually exclusive. Best results are probably obtained with a mixture of both. Drugs correct the underlying biological disturbance and relieve distressing symptoms. Psychological treatment aids the patient's adjustment by permitting the ventilation of feelings, ensuring an adequate level of information about the illness and access to practical help, and teaching specific techniques such as relaxation or cognitive restructuring.

Though most cancer patients are highly appreciative of psychological treatment from a skilled professional, and the balance of evidence shows that it does improve their quality of life (Greer, 1989), it is not without unwanted effects and, used alone, is seldom sufficient treatment for severe depression.

Ideally, both psychological treatment and drugs should be available. Even in the absence of facilities for formal professional psychological treatment the prescription of psychotropic drugs should always be accompanied by the type of interaction which goes to make up a good doctor–patient relationship: adequate explanation about the illness, discussion of what the drug is intended to do, and sympathetic listening to the patient's concerns.

The idea that resorting to drugs represents a cowardly second-best way of coping, which precludes effective self-help, is illogical and unconstructive. Drug treatment is also cheaper, easier and more widely available than counselling.

Having said all this, some patients nowadays are set against drugs and, unless they are so psychiatrically disturbed that drug treatment is judged essential, their wishes have to be respected.

There follows a description of the antidepressant and anxiolytic drugs in common use. A fuller account can be found in the book by Silverstone and Turner (1988).

DRUGS FOR DEPRESSION

Tricyclic antidepressants: these drugs are well-established as the standard treatment for depressive illness. They modify cerebral monoamine neurotransmitter systems involving 5-hydroxytryptamine (5-HT) and/or noradrenaline (NA). Many of their side-effects result from their anticholinergic properties. Common side-effects are dry mouth, constipation and dizziness due to postural hypotension. Drowsiness is sometimes a problem, but since most depressed patients suffer from insomnia, this can often be turned to advantage by giving the total dose at night. Confusion and various neuropsychiatric problems occasionally result from tricyclics, especially in patients with pre-existing metabolic disturbance or organic brain disease. In patients with cardiovascular disease, glaucoma or prostatic enlargement, tricyclics should be avoided because they can precipitate a worsening of their condition. Idiosyncratic reactions necessitating discontinuation of the drug include rashes, jaundice and agranulocytosis. Other unwanted effects include weight gain, blurred vision and sweating. Any side-effects are usually most prominent in the first few days of treatment, whereas the therapeutic effects may take several weeks to become evident. Overdose of tricyclics may well be fatal due to respiratory depression, cardiac arrythmias or status epilepticus.

Although this list of side-effects makes formidable reading, most patients with moderate or severe depression tolerate the tricyclics well. Long-term administration does not appear to carry any major hazards, nor does use of these drugs in pregnancy. Dependence on tricyclics is not a problem, although sudden cessation of large doses is occasionally followed by withdrawal symptoms.

The 'new' antidepressants. These drugs, in which the tricyclic structure of the older antidepressants has been modified, have been developed in an attempt to overcome the disadvantages of the tricyclic drugs, namely prominent side-effects, delayed onset of antidepressant action and toxicity in overdose. The attempt has been only partly successful. Although published trials do indicate that the new drugs are effective antidepressants with a low incidence of unwanted effects, they have not replaced the tricyclics, and it is the clinical impression of many psychiatrists that the new drugs are not such powerful antidepressants as the older ones when it comes to treating the more severe depressive states. The new drugs are also more expensive. Nevertheless, because of their relative freedom from anticholinergic effects they are in theory the obvious first choice in depressed patients with serious medical problems.

Monoamine oxidase inhibitors (MAOIs).   The MAOIs have an exaggerated reputation for being dangerous because they can cause hypertensive crises if combined with sympathomimetic drugs or tyramine-containing foods. They also potentiate a number of other drugs and anaesthetic agents. Because of these interactions they are not first choice antidepressants for cancer patients currently undergoing medical treatment, or likely to need surgical intervention. However, their use might be considered for patients whose physical disease is in remission. MAOIs are said to work best for 'atypical' depressive states, and for mixed anxiety/depression with a phobic element. Sometimes they are dramatically effective for cases of depression which have failed to respond to tricyclics. They tend to be stimulant rather than sedative, but like the tricyclics they can cause anticholinergic side-effects. Occasionally patients run into problems with tolerance and dependence.

In ordinary psychiatric practice, about 70 per cent of depressed patients respond well to antidepressants. These drugs are also effective for anxiety states and panic disorder. The response rate in patients with serious physical disorders such as cancer is unknown but on common-sense grounds seems likely to be rather less than this.

Examples of antidepressant drugs:

Amitriptyline, one of the longest-established and most widely-used tricyclic antidepressants, also appears to be one of the most powerful, although some patients cannot tolerate the side-effects. Its pronounced sedative properties can be advantageous for anxious patients, and the total daily dose can conveniently be given at night-time, often avoiding the need for a hypnotic as well. In cases where the patient has the classic depressive complaint of early-morning waking, amitriptyline is a good drug to choose.

Dothiepin is similar to amitriptyline but has less prominent side-effects, and is a popular well-established drug with sedative properties.

Amoxapine is a newly-introduced tricyclic whose fast action promises to be a big advantage, especially in cancer patients whose life expectancy is limited. Like other tricyclics, however, it has anticholinergic effects which may pose problems in the physically ill.

Mianserin is a 'new' compound which has been shown to be well-tolerated and efficacious in a cancer patient population, but is perhaps not the drug of first choice because it occasionally causes depression of the blood count.

Fluvoxamine and *Fluoxetine* are both recently-introduced antidepressants which act selectively on the 5-HT neurotransmitter systems and are free from anticholinergic side-effects but can cause nausea in the first few days of treatment.

Other members of group: clomipramine, dothiepin, imipramine, trimipramine (tricyclics); lofepramine, maprotiline, trazodone ('new' antidepressants); isocarboxazid, phenelzine, tranylcypromine (MAOIs).

Other drugs for depression. *Flupenthixol* is a neuroleptic drug which may be used in low dose for treating depression and anxiety, and has quite a rapid onset of action. *Lithium* in the form of the carbonate has its main use in long-term prophylaxis of recurrent major depression, and of manic-depression (unipolar and bipolar affective disorder). Various combinations of drugs can be used for cases of resistant depression. *Electroconvulsive therapy* (ECT), though not a drug, deserves mention here as the fastest-acting and most effective treatment for severe depressive states.

DRUGS FOR ANXIETY

Benzodiazepines: the popularity of these drugs, which were heralded as wonder compounds when they came into widespread use during the 1960s and 70s, has recently undergone a dramatic decline. Some authorities now believe they should never be prescribed; others, that they are useful compounds whose dangers have been exaggerated by the media. Used intermittently, or on a continuous basis for no more than a week or two at a time, they are highly effective anxiolytics and hypnotics which in most patients have no obvious side-effects, although in the sensitive or elderly person they may produce psychomotor impairment, and respiratory depression is a risk for patients with pulmonary disease. They are otherwise remarkably safe, even in overdose. The problem with the benzodiazepines, which has only been appreciated in the last few years, is their potential for causing both psychological and physical dependence with chronic use, so that although the therapeutic effect may have worn off, the patient cannot stop taking them without experiencing such symptoms as intense anxiety, nausea, shaking and fits. Because of the widespread publicity surrounding this problem, many patients nowadays are vehemently opposed to taking drugs of the benzodiazepine group, and many doctors are scared to prescribe them, especially in view of the prospect of litigation from dependent patients. Some psychiatrists believe the dangers of benzodiazepines have been greatly exaggerated, and that the adverse publicity has served to deprive many patients of effective treatment, when the alternative may be crippling anxiety or dependence on alcohol. Current guidelines recommend that prescription of benzodiazepines be restricted to short periods of three weeks or less and that counselling should be offered as an alternative.

The various benzodiazepines differ in their potency and duration of action, but the marketing of some as hypnotics and others as anxiolytics has little pharmacological basis. A long-acting one given at bedtime is best for patients who suffer from a combination of night-time insomnia and day-time anxiety. A short-acting one is better for patients whose problem is getting off to sleep, or who experience marked day-time anxiety confined to certain situations, for example before chemotherapy injections.

Examples include: *diazepam* (long-acting anxiolytic); *lorazepam* (short-acting anxiolytic); *nitrazepam* (long-acting hypnotic) and *triazolam* (short-acting hypnotic).

Other drugs for anxiety. The beta-blocking drug *propranolol* is useful for patients whose anxiety is primarily manifest through physical symptoms such as shaking, palpitations or muscle tension. *Buspirone* was recently introduced as a non-addictive alternative to the benzodiazepines; it has few side-effects but the delayed onset of action makes it only suitable for continuous treatment of chronic anxiety, as opposed to short-term or situation-specific anxiety. The *neuroleptics* or *major tranquillizers*, such as *chlorpromazine* and *haloperidol*, are mainly used in psychiatry for the treatment of psychotic illness, but are useful for calming acute disturbances in the physically ill and sometimes prescribed in terminal care settings, where their antiemetic properties are a useful bonus. *Barbiturates* are effective anxiolytics but seldom prescribed nowadays because of their potential for addiction.

CLINICAL ASPECTS OF PRESCRIBING PSYCHOTROPICS

Antidepressants: Antidepressant drugs are the compounds of choice for patients with a sustained mood disorder, whether depression or anxiety predominates. Many patients who take benzodiazepines on a chronic basis would probably gain more benefit from a course of antidepressants.

Antidepressant drugs work better for severe acute depressions than for mild chronic ones. The presence of 'somatic' depressive symptoms also tends to predict a good response, and antidepressant drugs may be successful in alleviating such symptoms even if there is doubt as to whether their origin is 'functional' or 'organic.' Antidepressants have hypnotic and analgesic effects which help to relieve insomnia and pain whatever their cause.

Though patients with mild disorders tend to respond less well to drug treatment, they have nothing to lose from a course of an antidepressant. Predictions of individual response are unreliable and there is no adequate substitute for an actual trial of the drug.

The presence of an 'organic' component to the mood disorder, for instance if the patient is known to have cerebral metastases or hyper-calcaemia, does not necessarily contraindicate the use of drugs. Although the ideal treatment strategy would involve correcting the physical abnormality, this is not always possible. Patients with organically-based mood disorders sometimes respond quite well to antidepressants, but there is a greater than usual risk of producing confusion and so a low dose should be used initially.

Over-cautious prescribing of these compounds, however, is a frequent error. Time and again, when depressed patients are referred to psychiatrists because they have allegedly failed to respond to drug treatment, it transpires that no adequate course of treatment has been prescribed, or that patient compliance has been poor. All that is necessary is to increase the dose of the antidepressant drug and continue therapy a few weeks longer.

The therapeutic dose range for the antidepressant drugs is wide. For amitriptyline, the 'standard' drug of this group, the smallest tablet available is a 10 mg one, and occasionally a dose as low as 10 mg daily does seem sufficient to give a therapeutic effect, especially in elderly or frail patients. The average depressed person, however, is likely to need 100 mg or 150 mg daily before a therapeutic response results. Some patients need higher doses still – 250 mg or even 300 mg daily.

Side-effects provide the best guide to individual dose requirements. The dose should start off low – say 25 mg at night in the case of a frail patient, or 50 mg for a fitter one – and be increased every few days, until either the depression is relieved, or the development of side-effects such as dry mouth, postural hypotension or drowsiness limit any further increase.

Many patients who are going to do well on a given drug report an improvement within the first week, but in other cases there is a delay of four to six weeks before the full benefits are apparent.

To encourage compliance, it is important to explain the need to persevere. Patients naturally become discouraged when the unpleasant side-effects of the drug occur well in advance of the therapeutic benefit, unless they have been warned about this possibility. Patients who complain of overwhelming side–effects from the start of treatment, however, are probably less likely to respond well.

If the antidepressant proves successful, another common mistake is premature discontinuation of therapy. Patients naturally want to 'manage' without drugs as soon as they feel over the worst of their depression. However, there is good evidence that relapse often occurs if the drug is stopped at this stage, whereas patients who continue their medication for another four to six months usually remain well. If a high dose has been used, or if side-effects continue to be a problem, then a lower dose may be used for maintenance therapy. When the time comes to reduce the dose, reduction should take place gradually. Some patients relapse when dose reduction is attempted, in which case the higher dose should be reinstated. There are no particular contraindications to long-term therapy with antidepressants, indeed some patients who are prone to recurrent mood disorder need to take these drugs indefinitely.

Benzodiazepines. With benzodiazepines, in contrast to antidepressants, short courses of treatment in the lowest effective dose are best. The much-publicized problem of dependence on benzodiazepines becomes a real risk after these drugs have been administered continuously for over a month. In cancer patients who have a limited life expectancy, dependence is perhaps not so important; a more cogent problem, however, is that long-term use of these drugs is associated with diminution of their effectiveness, and they cause a degree of emotional numbing and mild impairment of cognition which are usually seen as undesirable.

Benzodiazepines come into their own for managing points of crisis in the illness. The initial diagnosis of cancer, and presentation with recurrence, are times of great stress for patients because of the uncertainty and suspense – they tend to imagine the worst and, because the details of their diagnosis are not yet clear, it is impossible to provide informed counselling. Some patients become greatly distressed at such times, complaining of insomnia, preoccupation with illness and death, and showing uncontrolled displays of emotion. They are not suffering from a true mood disorder, and antidepressants may well make them feel worse, but a low dose of benzodiazepine prescribed for a period of a week or two will tide the patient over the crisis without producing dependence. Not all patients in this situation will want drugs – but it is kind to offer them, as opposed to enforcing a 'bite on the bullet' approach. Benzodiazepines are also useful for situation-specific anxiety, for example a single dose to be taken prior to a clinical procedure which the patient finds threatening.

SERVICE ORGANIZATION

Two questions require consideration: how to identify patients in need of drug treatment, and who should prescribe and monitor the drugs.

Identifying patients in need of drug treatment. Patients are often reluctant to volunteer emotional complaints of their own accord. This particularly applies to depressed patients, with their sense of guilt, shame, unworthiness and apathy. Though many affected patients are obviously anxious or tearful, some go undetected because they present a calm or smiling front.

The best way to pick up cases of mood disorder is probably by regular sympathetic inquiry, preferably from a member of staff who knows the patient well and has the time and interest to listen to any problems elicited by the inquiry. An alternative is screening with a self-rating questionnaire such as the HAD (Hospital Anxiety and Depression Scale), (Zigmund and Snaith, 1983), but this also takes time since some patients will require a detailed explanation of its purpose, and since those who score highly must be followed up by a personal interview if the procedure is to have any value. Screening needs repeating every few weeks; one-off assessment is not enough because mood disorders may arise at any stage of the course of the disease.

Unless an oncology unit has a member of staff – psychiatrist, psychologist or specialized nurse – with expertise in the emotional aspects of cancer, these suggestions are an unrealistic counsel of perfection. Many cases of mood disorder are likely to be missed completely in a busy ward or clinic, and others cannot be given the full assessment they require.

The actual *prescription of psychotropic drugs* must of course be carried out by a doctor. Although this need not be a psychiatrist, the correct use of these drugs does require some degree of skill and it is certainly not good practice for an oncologist with no psychiatric training to make a habit of prescribing psychotropics for any patients who turn up at the clinic looking rather anxious or miserable! If there is no doctor with suitable skills in the oncology unit, the best course may be to alert the general practitioner to the likelihood of mood disorder, and suggest a course of antidepressants. In any case, a phone call to the general practitioner is often a wise prelude to the prescription of psychotropic drugs by a hospital doctor. Besides being courteous, this consultation may add useful extra information, for example the patient may have withheld a past history of overdosing on drugs, or may already have been tried on a particular compound without success.

This review has focused on the use of antidepressants and anxiolytics to treat anxiety and depression. These and other psychotropic drugs have a broader application in oncology, for example in the management of nausea and vomiting, delirium and pain, and the reader is referred to Goldberg and Cullen (1986) for a wider discussion.

Summary and Conclusions

Psychotropic drugs, especially the antidepressants, are underused for treating mood disorders among patients with cancer and there have been few systematic studies of their value, although clinical experience suggests they do have a useful role. For patients with sustained depression and/or anxiety, a course of antidepressant drugs lasting several months is recommended, whereas the benzodiazepines are more suitable for short-lived or situation-specific anxiety. Drug treatment is not incompatible with a psychological approach, and a combination of drugs and counselling may work better than either method alone.

Case history

Mrs L had coped well with a diagnosis of breast cancer and a right mastectomy when she was 54 years old, but became depressed three years later when she developed bony metastases in the right hip. She was unable to continue her former active independent lifestyle, being forced to give up her favourite hobbies of playing golf and walking her dog, and to let her husband help her dress. Constant pain in the leg kept her awake all night and a succession of physical treatments, including a course of radiotherapy and regular medication with opiate analgesics, provided no pain relief at all. Although she 'kept up a good act' in front of others, she felt depressed all the time, cried when alone, and looked forward to death.

Despite a miserable childhood in an orphanage, Mrs L had achieved a happy marriage and family life of her own and had enjoyed her work as a fashion buyer. The suicide of her only sister ten years earlier, however, had been a devastating experience from which she had never recovered. The sister had had symptoms suggesting depressive illness prior to her death, and Mrs L herself experienced such symptoms for several months after the bereavement but did not seek medical treatment.

She was prescribed the antidepressant drug amitriptyline, starting dose 25 mg at night increasing by 25 mg weekly up to the maximum tolerated dose of 125 mg. She was seen for several discussion sessions, in which she expressed grief and anger about the losses in her life, and was given instruction in relaxation techniques. Six weeks later, her presenting symptoms had all improved, but were not entirely resolved.

This patient had a 'hardy' personality but was predisposed to mood disorder by a combination of genetic factors and adverse past life experiences. The pain in her leg, though primarily due to demonstrable pathology, was being magnified by her severe masked depression and the medication with tricyclics produced a real improvement in her plight.

References

BUKBERG, J., PENMAN, D. and HOLLAND, J.C. (1984) Depression in hospitalised cancer patients. *Psychosomatic Medicine*, *46*, 199–212.

COSTA, D., MOGOS, I., TOMA, T. (1985) Efficacy and safety of mianserin in the treatment of depression of women with cancer. *Acta Psychiatrica Scandinavica*, *72*, Suppl. 320, 85–92.

DEROGATIS, L.R., MORROW, G.R., FETTING, J., PENMAN, D., PIASETSKY, S., SCHMALE, A.M., HENRICHS, M. and CARNICKE, C.L.M. (1983) The prevalence of psychiatric disorders among cancer patients. *Journal of the American Medical Association*, *249*, 751–757.

EVANS, D.L., MCCARTNEY, C.F., HAGGERTY, J.J., NEMEROFF, C.B., GOLDEN, R.N., SIMON, J.B., QUADE, D., HOLMES, V., DROBA, M., MASON, G.A., FOWLER, W.C. and RAFT, D. (1988) Treatment of depression in cancer patients is associated with better life adaptation: A pilot study. *Psychosomatic Medicine*, *50*, 72–76.

GOLDBERG, R.J., CULLEN, L.O. (1986) Use of psychotropics in cancer patients. *Psychosomatics*, *27*, 687–700.

GREER, S. (1989) Can psychological therapy improve the quality of life of patients with cancer? *British Journal of Cancer*, *59*, 149–151.

HUGHES, J.E. (1985) Depressive illness and lung cancer (1 & 11). *European Journal of Surgical Oncology*, *11*, 15–20 & 21–24.

HUGHES, J.E. and LEE, D. (1988) Depression among cancer patients admitted for hospice care. In M. Watson, S. Greer and C. Thomas (Eds) *Psychosocial Oncology*. Oxford: Pergamon Press.

PLUMB, M.M. and HOLLAND, J. (1977) Comparative studies of psychological function in patients with advanced cancer – 1. Self-reported depressive symptoms. *Psychosomatic Medicine*, *39*, 264–276.

POPKIN, M.K., CALLIES, A.L. and MACKENSIE, J.D. (1985) The outcome of anti-depressant use in the medically ill. *Archives of General Psychiatry*, *42*, 1160–1163.

RODIN, G. and VOSHART, K. (1986) Depression in the medically ill: An overview. *American Journal of Psychiatry*, *143*, 696–705.

SILVERSTONE, T. and TURNER, P. (1988) *Drug Treatment in Psychiatry*, 4th ed. Routledge: London.

ZIGMUND, A.S. and SNAITH, R.P. (1983) The Hospital Anxiety and Depression Scale. *Acta Psychiatrica Scandinavica*, *67*, 361–370.

STEROIDS AND CHEMOTHERAPEUTIC AGENTS: NEUROPSYCHIATRIC ASPECTS

Gary Bell

The major advances of recent years in the early diagnosis and treatment of many cancers have not been without considerable cost to the quality of life of the patient. The side-effects of both chemotherapy and radiotherapy are major causes of physical and psychological distress. This chapter will focus primarily on the psychiatric side-effects of corticosteroids and their management, although a brief review of chemotherapeutic agents will also be included.

STEROID-INDUCED PSYCHIATRIC DISORDERS

The role of corticosteroids in the treatment and palliation of malignant disease is well established (see Table 1). Psychiatric side-effects of corticosteroids were reported shortly after their introduction into clinical use in the late 1940s (Hench et al., 1949). Over forty years later, no consensus exists as to the classification, diagnosis and management of steroid-induced psychiatric disorders (SIPDs). Variability in type and severity of presentation, delay in onset and the possible co-existence of disease-related and functional mental disorder account for much of this confusion.

Severe Psychiatric Reactions

A significant increase in the incidence of severe psychiatric reactions in association with corticosteroid use was reported in early controlled treatment studies of ulcerative colitis (Kirsner et al., 1959; Marx and Baker, 1967) and lupus nephritis (Cade et al., 1973). Little information is available concerning these reactions, which have been described as 'overt psychosis with schizophrenic characteristics' and 'agitated depression'. A meta-analysis of retrospective case reports by Lewis and Smith (1983) found severe psychiatric reactions in 5.7 per cent of steroid-treated patients, although the Boston Collaborative Drug Sur-

TABLE 1 *Indications for corticosteroids in malignant disease*

Treatment	
Reticuloses	– Hodgkin's disease
	– Non-Hodgkin's lymphoma
Leukaemias	
Multiple myeloma	

Symptom control

Raised intracranial pressure
Spinal cord or peripheral nerve compression
Superior vena caval obstruction
Lymphangitis carcinomatosis
Gastrointestinal obstruction
Anorexia
Liver capsule pain due to hepatomegaly

veillance Program (1972) reported only 21 cases in 718 subjects (3 per cent).

Clinical presentation was accounted for by either depression or mania in approximately 75 per cent of the cases in Lewis and Smith's meta-analysis (1983). Delirium was reported in 10 per cent, and 14 per cent had a non-affective psychosis. The Boston Collaborative Drug Surveillance Program (1972) classified 13 of 21 as psychotic, (six were manic and two were depressed) and the remaining eight as 'inappropriate euphoria'. Whilst an affective syndrome is the most common clinical presentation, this is often in the form of a 'mixed affective state' with considerable lability of mood rather than purely depressive or manic features. Behaviour is often unpredictable and varies from extreme overactivity and restlessness to marked psychomotor retardation. More recently, a reversible dementia-like syndrome, characterized by memory impairment, occupational dysfunction and psychomotor retardation, has been reported (Varney *et al.*, 1984). This may, in fact, represent a depressive pseudodementia.

The onset of severe psychiatric reactions is usually abrupt and occurs within the first two weeks of starting high dose corticosteroids, although a delay in onset of up to three months has been reported (Glaser, 1953). Thus delay in onset is often responsible for the diagnosis of a SIPD not being considered and failing to initiate an appropriate course of management.

Minor Mood Changes

Euphoria, depression, insomnia, irritability and restlessness have frequently been reported in association with corticosteroid usage, although the exact nature of this relationship has been questioned (Mitchell and Collins, 1984). Such mood changes may simply reflect fluctuations in the patient's physical state. Three studies have examined this question. Lewis and Fleminger (1954) studied 12 patients, all with a past history of mental illness. Mean doses of approximately 21 mg of Prednisolone equivalent per day were prescribed in patients with rheumatoid arthritis for 52 days. Transient euphoria, 'out of proportion to any physical improvement', and irritability were described in five and three patients respectively. Surprisingly, the authors concluded however that such symptoms were 'psychological reactions to the welcome change they perceived in their physical condition'.

Mitchell *et al.* (1984) studied psychological changes in 21 patients with chronic airflow limitation. A double blind randomized crossover trial compared the effect of oral Prednisolone (40 mg/day) and placebo for 14 days. Whilst psychological improvement was seen in both groups, no difference between groups was demonstrated. The lack of standardized psychological measures and the timing of measurements make the results difficult to interpret. In contrast, a recent single blind study by Swinburn *et al.* (1988) of 20 patients with chronic obstructive airways disease demonstrated a statistically significant improvement in mood state after three days of 30 mg Prednisolone following three days of placebo. This occurred before changes in lung spirometry and arterial saturation were evident. Unfortunately, the assessment of euphoria was indirect, relying on improvement in scores of anxiety and depression. No assessment of other recognized minor symptoms was made. These apparently contradictory findings may reflect the lack of adequate rating scales for repeated assessments of subtle mood changes.

Vulnerability and Aetiological Factors

Likely factors that have been identified in severe psychiatric reactions appear to be female sex (Lewis and Smith, 1983) and steroid dosage (The Boston Collaborative Drug Surveillance Program, 1972). There is no evidence that age and only weak evidence that a past psychiatric history or abnormal premorbid personality confer a higher risk (Lewis and Fleminger, 1954; Lewis and Smith, 1983). Both Lewis and Smith (1983) and The Boston Collaborative Drug Surveillance Program (1972) have shown a statistically significant dose–response relationship. In the Boston Collaborative Drug Surveillance Program, psychiatric reactions were recorded in 1.3 per cent of 463 patients receiving Prednisolone at a dosage of 40 mg or less per day, 4.6 per cent of the 175 patients taking 40–80 mg and 18.4 per cent of the 38 patients in excess of 80 mg daily. Lewis *et al.* (1971) demonstrated serum albumin levels lower than 25 gm/1 to be associated with a two-fold increase in all Prednisolone side-effects. Uribe and Go (1979) showed the frequency of side-effects of long-term Prednisolone administration to be increased if albumin levels are low or bilirubin levels raised. These findings suggest that the concentration of circulating unbound Prednisolone may be significant in the production of a SIPD.

The peak plasma Prednisolone level may also be significant, as single daily doses may confer a higher risk than divided doses (Glynne-Jones *et al.*, 1986). There are no reports to date of psychiatric morbidity associated with the use of enteric-coated Prednisolone, which results in a lower peak. Absorption of both standard and enteric-coated Prednisolone is variable within and between individuals (Morrison *et al.*, 1977; Wilson *et al.*, 1977; Henderson *et al.*, 1979), and may explain the difficulty in predicting individual risk. Centeno *et al.* (1978) proposed a nomogram to adjust Prednisolone dose according to serum albumin level, although this has not been incorporated into clinical practice.

The pathogenesis of SIPDs is poorly understood, although there is increasing evidence to implicate disruption of catecholamine neuro-transmission. Glucocorticoids have been suggested as mediators of enhanced catecholamine turnover by increasing tyrosine hydroxylase (the rate-limiting enzyme in catecholamine synthesis) activity (Black, 1982). Decreased catecholamine levels have been implicated in the pathogenesis of both Alzheimer's disease (Bondareff *et al.*, 1981) and affective disorders (Schildkraut, 1965). This is consistent with the finding that depression is a well-recognized complication of both Cushing's disease and Addison's disease. Catecholamines may also have a role in the provocation of psychosis since amphetamines, which enhance catecholamine neuro-transmission, are known to produce a psychosis phenomenologically similar to paranoid schizophrenia, and dexamethasone has been shown to produce electroencephalographic changes similar to those induced by amphetamines (Itil and Herrman, 1978).

MANAGEMENT

The ill-defined and diverse nature of SIPDs has invariably made it difficult to formulate specific treatment strategies, although general principles of management apply.

Assessment. Acute psychiatric disturbance in patients with malignant disease is not uncommon, often begins abruptly and usually requires urgent intervention. It demands a detailed history, especially from relatives, and, if an inpatient, a thorough physical and mental state examination by ward staff and a careful review of all investigations and treatments to date. Wherever possible, a period of observation forms an essential but often neglected component of any assessment.

Differential diagnosis. In view of the fact there are no specific diagnostic tests, a broad differential diagnosis, in particular disease progression, hypercalcaemia and other drugs, needs to be considered (see Table 2). Cerebral metastases usually present with signs of raised intracranial pressure or focal neurological signs or seizures. Most patients experience a swift and dramatic improvement in their neurological function on starting corticosteroid treatment. Subsequent deterioration in neurological or psychological function is usually interpreted as disease progression. In this event, it is common practice to reintroduce or increase the dose of corticosteroids without recourse to diagnostic procedures. It is therefore essential to consider the possibility that such symptoms are corticosteroid-induced if further deterioration is to be prevented (Bell *et al.*, 1987). A major distinguishing feature of most acute confusional states is that neither disorientation nor fluctuating levels of consciousness are prominent.

Functional causes of acute psychiatric disturbance should not be ignored. Psychological reactions to a diagnosis of cancer and the physical and emotional losses it brings are common and occasionally extreme. Whilst the diagnosis of a SIPD is very much a diagnosis of exclusion, it is usually made on the basis of a temporal association with initial exposure to corticosteroids, and is supported when symptomatic improvement follows dose adjustment (either division or reduction).

Treatment. Initial treatment strategies include division of the daily dose of corticosteroids into three or four aliquots (Glynne-Jones *et al.*, 1986) or dose reduction. If psychiatric symptoms are severe or persist, or if there is marked disturbance of behaviour, neuroleptic medication should be prescribed. Haloperidol is very effective and tends to be calming rather than sedating. If sedation is a priority, Chlorpromazine should be used, although care should be taken in patients with cerebral metastases because of its epileptogenic properties. It is important that adequate doses of neuroleptic are used, particularly if there is marked behavioural disturbance. On rare occasions, it may be necessary to detain patients in hospital under the Mental Health Act.

In cases of depression, electroconvulsive therapy (ECT) has been reported to be effective if symptomatic improvement does not follow

TABLE 2   *Differential diagnosis of acute psychiatric disturbance in malignant disease*

Primary cerebral causes	– Tumours (1° and 2°) – Infections e.g. meningitis – Abscess (esp. listeria) – Subdural haematoma

Systemic causes	– Infection (esp. chest and UTI)
	– Metabolic hypo/hypernatraemia
	      uraemia
	      hypoxia
	      hypercalcaemia
	      hypo/hyperglycaemia
	      hepatic dysfunction

Functional causes	– Mood disorders hypomania depression – Paranoid disorders

Therapeutic drugs	– CNS depressants hypnotics
	      antidepressants
	      antihistamines
	      neuroleptics
	– Narcotic analgesics
	– Dopaminergics levodopa
	      bromocryptine
	– Anticholinergics
	– Beta blockers esp. propranolol
	– Digoxin
	– Cimetidine
	– Isoniazid
	– Non-steroidal anti-inflammatories
	– Corticosteroids

Drug withdrawal	– Benzodiazepines esp. lorazepam

steroid reduction (Peterson, 1975; Lewis and Smith, 1983). Tricyclic antidepressants are contraindicated as they usually exacerbate SIPDs (Hall *et al.*, 1979). Where long-term or repeated use of corticosteroids is essential, lithium prophylaxis should be considered (Falk *et al.*, 1979), but instituted only after psychiatric consultation.

Patients should, wherever possible, be nursed on the radiotherapy/ oncology unit. This may require additional specialist nursing staff but is preferable to transferring a physically ill patient to a psychiatric unit, particularly when the majority of acute disturbances settle rapidly with appropriate treatment.

Prognosis.   A review of the literature suggests 93 per cent of patients who suffer from SIPDs achieve a full recovery, 4 per cent have continuing or recurrent psychiatric symptoms and 3 per cent commit suicide (Lewis and Smith, 1983). There are no clearly defined adverse factors, but in terms of management depressive features or a dementia-like syndrome may be more difficult to treat.

Conclusions

SIPDs should be seen as a spectrum of disorders, both in terms of type and severity, ranging from minor symptoms such as insomnia, restlessness, irritability and euphoria to the more severe 'steroid psychoses' which may present as a disturbance of mood, belief, cognition or behaviour or any combination of these symptom groups. Their aetiology remains largely unresolved; future studies using standardized rating scales in clearly-defined patient groups are needed to refine our understanding both of the range of symptoms involved and the mechanisms whereby corticosteroids induce them. This may, in turn, not only lead to better recognition and management of this relatively common group of disorders, but also shed light on the pathogenesis of the functional psychoses.

CHEMOTHERAPEUTIC AGENTS

Chemotherapeutic agents are used extensively in combination with each other and/or with steroids in the treatment and palliation of a wide range of malignancies (see Table 3). Psychiatric side-effects of chemotherapeutic agents are common but fortunately mild in nature. Severe psychiatric reactions are rare. Incidence of reported central nervous system complications ranges from 5 per cent to 86 per cent depending on the class of chemotherapeutic agent. Psychiatric sequelae are rarely seen in the absence of neurological complications. The most common forms of psychiatric disorder are organic mental disorders, reported in association with alkylating agents, anti-metabolities, L-Asparaginase and miscellaneous agents (Silberfarb *et al.*, 1980), and depression, which is associated with alkylating agents, vinca alkaloids, especially vincristine (Silberfarb *et al.*, 1983) and L-Asparaginase. Agitation is commonly observed with Mithramycin. The majority of symptoms occur shortly after administration of the chemotherapeutic agent, although a delay of several days or weeks may occur with some alkylating agents, L-Asparaginase and methotrexate. Most psychiatric symptoms are reversible, and appear to be dose related. A degree of irreversibility has been reported with methotrexate-induced behavioural disturbance. Persisting cognitive deficits have been reported and are more likely with inpatients who have received a number of chemotherapeutic agents.

TABLE 3   Chemotherapeutic agents

Alkylating agents –cyclophosphamide, chlorambucil, mustine
Cytotoxic antibiotics –adriamycin, epirubicin, bleomycin, mitomycin
Antimetabolities –methotrexate, fluorouracil
Vinca alkaloids and etoposide –vinblastine, vincristine, vindesine
Enzymes –L-Asparaginase
Miscellaneous agents –carboplatin, cisplatin, mitozantrone, procarbazine

Interferon, which is an immune modulator, and which is being used increasingly in conjunction with chemotherapeutic agents, has been associated with both neurological and psychiatric side-effects. These include 'organic personality syndrome', 'organic affective syndrome' and a delirium. The onset is usually within one to three months of starting treatment and appears to be dose related. Symptomatic improvement is usually three to four days after dose reduction with complete resolution after cessation of interferon (Renault et al., 1987).

There are no specific treatment strategies for psychiatric syndromes caused by chemotherapeutic agents apart from withdrawal of the specific agent. In the rare event of a severe psychiatric reaction, the general principles of managing an acute psychiatric disturbance, as outlined above, apply.

Conclusions

The relatively minor nature of psychiatric symptoms reported in association with chemotherapeutic agents has received little attention despite being commonplace. Systematic evaluation using standardized assessments is essential to our understanding of these reactions and the development of appropriate treatment strategies. In common with the corticosteroid-induced minor mood disturbance, much of this morbidity goes largely undetected by medical staff. The assumption is that these symptoms are indeed 'minor'. Specific questioning, however, often reveals considerable distress which cannot be solely attributed to the emotional impact of the disease. The distressing nature of cancer treatments and their psychiatric sequelae highlight the need for adequate provision of consultation liaison psychiatric services to radiotherapy and oncology units. This is essential if staff in such units are to develop the necessary clinical skills for the detection and management of their patients' psychological distress.

References

BELL, G., GLYNNE-JONES, R. and VERNON, C.C. (1987) Cerebral metastases and dexamethasone: Psychiatric aspects. *Palliative Medicine, 1,* 132–135.

BLACK, A.C. (1982) Biochemical mechanisms of steroid-induced psychosis. *New York State Journal of Medicine, 82(7),* 1024.

BONDAREFF, W., MOUNTJOY, C.Q. and ROTH, M. (1981) Selective loss of neurones of adrenergic projection to cerebral cortex (nucleus locus coeruleus) in senile dementia. *Lancet, i,* 783–784.

THE BOSTON COLLABORATIVE DRUG SURVEILLANCE PROGRAM (1972) Acute reactions to prednisolone in relation to dosage. *Clinical Pharmacology and Therapeutics, 13,* 694–698.

CADE, R., SPOONER, G., SCHLEIN, E., PICKERING, M., DE QUESADA, A., HOLCOMB, A., JUNCOS, L., RICHARD, G., SHIRES, D., LEVIN, D., HACKETT, R., FREE, J., HUNT, R. and FREGLY, M. (1973) Comparison of azothiaprine, prednisone and heparin alone or combined in treating lupus nephritis. *Nephron, 19,* 37–56.

CENTENO, F., ROBLES, G., URIBE, M., GIL-LOZADA, S. and SUAREZ, G.I. (1978) Nomogram for prednisone-prednisolone adjustment dose in patients with hypoalbuminaemia. *Rev. Investigacion Clinica (Mexico), 32,* 35–39.

FALK, W.E., MAHNKE, M.W. and POSKANZER, D.C. (1979) Lithium prophylaxis of corticotropin-induced psychosis. *Journal of the American Medical Association, 241,* 1011–1012.

GLASER, G.H. (1953) Psychotic reactions induced by corticotropin (ACTH) and cortisone. *Psychosomatic Medicine, 15,* 280–291.

GLYNNE-JONES, R., VERNON, C.C. and BELL, G. (1986) Is steroid psychosis preventable by divided doses? *Lancet, ii,* 1404.

HALL, R.W.C., POPKIN, M.K., STICKNEY, S.K. and GARDNER, E.R. (1979) Presentation of the steroid psychoses. *Journal of Nervous and Mental Disease, 167,* 229–236.

HENCH, P.S., KENDALL, E.C., SLOCUMB, C.H. and POLLEY, H.F. (1949) Effect of hormone adrenal cortex (17-hydroxy-11-dehydroxycorticosterone; compound E) and of pituitary adrenocorticotropic hormone on rheumatoid arthritis; preliminary report. *Proceedings, Staff Meetings Mayo Clinic, 24,* 181–197.

HENDERSON, R.G., WHEATLEY, T., ENGLISH, J., CHAKRABORTY, J. and MARKS, V. (1979) Variation in plasma prednisolone concentration in the renal transplant recipients given enteric-coated prednisolone. *British Medical Journal, i,* 1534–1536.

ITIL, T.M. and HERRMAN, W.M. (1978) Effects of hormones on computer-analyzed human electroencephalogram. In M.A. Lipton, A. Di Mascio and K.F. Killiam (Eds), *Psychopharmacology: A generation of progress.* New York: Raven Press.

KIRSNER, J.B., PALMER, W.L., SPENCER, J.A., BICKS, R.O. and JOHNSON, C.F. (1959) Corticotropin (ACTH) and the adrenal steroids in the management of ulcerative colitis. Observations in 240 patients. *Annals of Internal Medicine,* 50, 891–927.

LEWIS, A. and FLEMINGER, J.J. (1954) The psychiatric risk from corticotrophin and cortisone. *Lancet, i,* 383–386.

LEWIS, D.A. and SMITH, R.E. (1983) Steroid-induced psychiatric syndromes: A report of 14 cases and a review of the literature. *Journal of Affective Disorders,* 5, 319–332.

LEWIS, G.P., JUSKO, W.J., BURKE, C.W. and GRAVES, L. (1971) Prednisone side effects and serum albumin levels: A collaborative study. *Lancet, ii,* 778–780.

MARX, F.W. and BAKER, W.F. (1967) Surgical results in patients with ulcerative colitis treated with and without corticosteroids. *American Journal of Surgery,* 113, 157–163.

MITCHELL, D.M. and COLLINS, J.V. (1984) Do corticosteroids really alter mood? *Postgraduate Medical Journal,* 60(705), 467–470.

MITCHELL, D.M., GILDEH, P., REHAHN, M., DIMOND, A.H. and COLLINS, J.V. (1984) Psychological changes and improvement in chronic airflow limitation after corticosteroid treatment. *Thorax,* 39, 924–927.

MORRISON, P.J., BRADBROOK, I.D. and ROGERS, H.J. (1977) Plasma prednisolone levels from enteric and non-enteric coated tablets estimated by an original technique. *British Journal of Clinical Pharmacology,* 4, 597–603.

PETERSON, G. (1975) Organic mental disorders induced by drugs or poisons. In A.M. Freedman, H.I. Kaplan and J.B. Sadock (Eds) *Comprehensive Textbook of Psychiatry, vol. 1.,* 2nd ed. Baltimore: Williams & Wilkins.

RENAULT, P.F., HOOFNAGLE, J.H., PARK, Y., MULLEN, K.D., PETERS, M., JONES, D.B., RUSTGI, V. and JONES, E.A. (1987) Psychiatric complications of longterm interferon-alpha therapy. *Archives of Internal Medicine,* 147(9), 1577–1580.

SCHILDKRAUT, J.J. (1965) The catecholamine hypothesis of affective disorders: A review of supporting evidence. *American Journal of Psychiatry,* 122, 509–522.

SILBERFARB, P.M., PHILIBERT, D. and LEVINE, P.M. (1980) Psychosocial aspects of neoplastic disease: II affective and cognitive effects of chemotherapy in cancer patients. *American Journal of Psychiatry,* 137, 597–601.

SILBERFARB, P.M., HOLLAND, J.C.B., ANBAR, D., BAHRA, G., MAURER, H., CHAHINIAN, A.P. and COMIS, R. (1983) Psychological response of patients receiving 2 drug regimens for lung carcinoma. *American Journal of Psychiatry,* 140, 110–111.

SWINBURN, C.R., WAKEFIELD, J.M., NEWMAN, S.P. and JONES, P.W. (1988) Evidence of prednisolone induced mood change ('steroid euphoria') in patients with chronic obstructive airways disease. *British Journal of Clinical Pharmacology,* 26, 709–713.

URIBE, M. and GO, V.L.W. (1979) Corticosteroid pharmacokinetics in liver disease. *Clinical Pharmacokinetics,* 4, 233–240.

VARNEY, N.R., ALEXANDER, B. and MACINDOE, J.H. (1984) Reversible steroid dementia in patients without steroid psychosis. *American Journal of Psychiatry,* 141, 369–372.

WILSON, C.G., MAY, C.S. and PATERSON, J.W. (1977) Plasma prednisolone levels in man following administration in plain and enteric-coated forms. *British Journal of Clinical Pharmacology,* 4, 351–355.

TERMINAL CARE

Sheila Cassidy

Terminal care is as old as humankind itself and has long been equated with TLC – tender loving care – for those for whom medicine had nothing more to offer. The past 20 years however have seen the emergence of the new speciality of palliative medicine whose *raison d'être* is neither cure nor prolongation of life, nor even the often quoted 'death with dignity', but the achieving of the maximum fullness of living for men, women and children with far-advanced incurable disease.

Specialists in palliative medicine work with patients of widely differing ages and cultural backgrounds but with a limited range of diseases: cancer, AIDS and degenerative neurological diseases such as motor neurone disease and occasionally multiple sclerosis. The *principles* of care, however, have a much wider application, often to the whole of medicine.

With cure no longer an option, these specialists are forced to explore new ways of caring and in this exploration discover the painful gap between the needs of patients and the way in which those needs are being met in our hospitals and the community. Working very often outside the system (for example in non-NHS units), they are freed from the constraints of hospital bureaucracy and thus able to respond with immediacy and creativity to people's needs in a way that would be quite impossible in an ordinary hospital.

For example, for the past five weeks in the hospice where I work, my team and I have cared for a 20-year-old young man with a brain tumour. After a few days it became apparent that he was desperately unhappy because he was separated from his dog, so we sent for it. For the next eight weeks the patient, his mother and the dog lived together in one large room, joined from time to time by his 13-year-old brother. I shall not easily forget the day when I looked in the room to find my patient peacefully asleep guarded by a gently growling red setter on the other bed! The best memory however is of the day David said to his mother, 'Maybe I'm not dying after all – but it's so lovely here, let's pretend I am, so we can stay.'

Terminal care services, like all good services, are designed to be needs driven. They strive to make a living reality of the ideal of caring for the patient and their family by providing an individually-tailored, holistic system of care to meet the patient's emotional, spiritual and social needs as well as their physical ones. A care of this depth and breadth demands not only a multi-disciplinary approach but a cohesive team whose members communicate freely and can work happily together, enjoying and valuing what they do and supporting each other. Such a team needs not only clear and strong leadership but also a mutual respect between the different members, whatever their age or status.

Before I go any further I would like to lay my credentials (and lack of them) clearly on the table. I write as a palliative care physician with ten years' experience in terminal care but no formal training in psychiatry or psychology. Whilst I have a particular interest in the psychological care of the dying, that interest is more practical than academic, and my psychological work is inextricably interwoven with physical doctoring, teaching and administration in a busy hospice. It is important to understand that the psychological care to be described is carried out, almost in its entirety, by 'ordinary' doctors and nurses, not by those with specialist psychological or even counselling training. The majority of patients we see are suffering from emotional distress rather than psychological pathology.

Chapter outline. The psychological care of the terminally ill will be discussed under the following headings:

> *The patients*
> *The setting*
> *The practitioners*
> *Aims of care*
> *Problems and their management*
> *Special techniques*
> *Service description.*

THE PATIENTS

In my service, we work almost exclusively with adult men and women with advanced incurable malignant disease. These patients range in age from 12 to over 90 years, with the majority between 40 and 80. The range of malignancies seen is wide, but the commonest are cancer of the breast, lung, gastrointestinal tract, ovary, cervix, prostate and brain. Of particular psychological interest are the less common tumours of head and neck or genital region which lead to severe tissue destruction and mutilation.

THE SETTING

The way in which we work with patients is influenced, to some degree, by the setting in which they are seen, be it an outpatient department, the patient's own home or the hospice.

Hospital ward. Ward consultations tend to be made by senior medical members of the team on a one-off basis. These visits are usually either for assessment of patients' suitability for transfer to the hospice or for advice on physical or psychological distress. Such visits tend to be lengthy (one hour or more) and frequently involve the breaking of bad news and a discussion of prognosis (this situation is discussed later in the chapter).

Hospital outpatient department. I do a weekly outpatient session at the hospital in which I see patients both with a radiotherapist colleague and on my own. This clinic is a useful forum for ongoing psychological support.

Patient's own home. In our service, senior members of the medical staff visit patients at home only at the request of their general practitioner or the home care nurse. As with hospital visits, this is normally to assess the patient for admission to the hospice or for specific advice on physical or psychological problems. The home care sisters, on the other hand, see patients regularly in their own homes over a period of weeks or months, providing advice on symptom control and psychological support to patient and family.

The hospice. Psychological care within the hospice is very much a team affair and may be divided into (a) *general support* by all members of staff and (b) *'counselling'* by trained medical and nursing staff. (By 'counselling' we mean one-to-one conversations with the patient involving listening, informational and emotional care, active screening for psychological distress and the giving of advice where appropriate.)

THE PRACTITIONERS

The practitioners in our unit may be divided into:
(a) senior medical staff
(b) trainee doctors (senior house officers on a four-month placement)
(c) trained nurses
(d) auxilliary nurses

(e) home care sisters
(f) social workers

Patients may have contact with any or all of these practitioners, although they will usually develop a closer relationship with one particular member of staff. It is quite common, however, for some patients to unburden themselves to a number of different members of staff according to when they feel the need to talk and who is readily available. In the inpatient situation therefore, a degree of pooling of information between staff is necessary. A more detailed description of the hospice where I work and its different practitioners is given at the end of the chapter.

AIMS OF CARE

The aims of those involved in terminal care can best be described as the providing of a covenant relationship. By this I mean that the caring team covenants or promises to accompany the patient and their family throughout their illness until they die. The psychological care offered in this situation is, therefore, different from the usual 'contract' of psychotherapy offered to other patients in which treatment is for a limited period. Nor is our treatment dependent upon the compliance and cooperation of the client; it is accepted that the distress involved in a terminal illness may from time to time cause the patient to experience such anger or confusion that they either behave 'badly' or distance themselves from the team.

The care provided may be divided into the following categories:

(a) informational care
(b) emotional care
(c) monitoring psychological state
(d) referral on to appropriate specialists.

The exact nature of this care will be discussed in detail later.

PROBLEMS ENCOUNTERED IN THE CARE OF THE TERMINALLY ILL AND THEIR MANAGEMENT

For practical purposes I will divide psychological problems into the following categories: fear; loss; anger; alienation; depression, and weariness of living.

Fear

I believe that fear is universally experienced, at some stage, by those facing death. It may not be articulated and it may well not manifest itself in anxious behaviour, but it is there, at some level. This fear is both understandable and inevitable because someone who is dying is facing the destruction, the annihilation of all that they know and love and is moving towards an unknown future, whether that future be total oblivion or a new form of life and being.

What then, can the carer do to help those possessed of this existential dread? Is there anything we can do? The answer is both yes and no, for while many fears may be removed with appropriate counselling, the dread of the unknown usually remains. That is why we speak so frequently of 'accompanying' the dying, of being alongside them, sharing their grief and fear, even when we cannot take it away.

From a practical point of view, the management of fear consists of:

(a) diagnosing fear;
(b) eliciting *what* the patient is afraid of;
(c) working through and if possible removing irrational fears;
(d) acknowledging reasonable fears and providing *truthful* reassurance where possible;
(e) human comforting, and
(f) providing a 'safe' environment.

Diagnosing fear.   Fear is diagnosed by a combination of observation, intuition and direct questioning. Sometimes it is quite obvious from a patient's haunted look or the way he or she literally shakes that they are quite terrified. Others may appear to be quite at ease and their fear emerges late in a conversation.

It is important not only to diagnose the existence of fear but to unravel its various elements because existential dread and justifiable fears of impending weakness and death are frequently mixed up with fears of all sorts of things which are very unlikely to happen. One of the commonest fears is that of *unbearable pain*. Most people associate cancer with pain and whilst it is true that some malignant processes *do* cause severe pain, it is equally true that many patients suffer no pain at all. If it is unlikely that the patient will experience much pain one can happily reassure them; if moderate pain is likely one can explain that most pain can be controlled and all pain alleviated at least in part.

More difficult are fears of *choking*. A patient with a tumour of the mouth or upper airways may be very fearful of suddenly being unable to breathe. For example, Mrs A. has a tumour of the trachea which from time to time obstructs her airway. If she is not rapidly sucked out she will die. She knows this, and we know it, and there is no point in pretending it could not happen. We manage the situation by having the suction equipment to hand, by giving her a bell (she cannot call out) and by nursing her in an open ward so that she is never alone. In this way, her fear is reduced to manageable proportions. The safety of being in the hospice overrides her very strong desire to be at home.

If a patient suffocates, and we cannot relieve the obstruction we would hold them in our arms for comfort and sedate them as quickly as possible with an injection of Diazepam 10 mg., Diamorphine 10 mg. and Hyocine 0.4 mg.

The same procedure holds true for patients at risk of *sudden haemorrhage* (for example patients with destructive disease overlying a major vessel in the neck or groin). If the patient does not realize that they are at risk of bleeding, we would not tell them; if they *do* realize it and it *is* likely we would not deny it, but explain that we would be with them and have means to relieve their distress. In fact, threatened haemorrhage frequently does *not* occur because the slow progress of the disease causes thrombosis. If it does happen, we hold the person close and sedate them deeply.

Another common fear is of *losing control* – of independence, mind or sphincters. Opioid analgesia, inexpertly used, causes hallucinations and confusion and many patients have seen elderly relatives very confused during their last illness. Once again the same principles hold true: if confusion or incontinence is unlikely, we reassure; if it is almost inevitable we promise to support. The journey from full control over one's mental and bodily functions through to complete dependence upon others is a very painful one and patients require much sensitive support during each progressive loss. It is often worth articulating what most of us know but tend to forget: that nurses and doctors have actually *chosen* to care for those who cannot do so for themselves and that the intrinsic worth of human beings is not dependent upon their strength, their beauty, their intelligence or their productivity, but upon the fact that they are human.

It is important to differentiate between a patient's fear of the *process* of dying and of actually *being dead*. Most people are afraid of the process but are quite at ease about death itself which they see either as peaceful oblivion or a life of happiness with God. A few patients, however, are afraid of what will happen *after* death. This fear is less easy to handle and there is no right way for each patient or each carer.

Case history

Peter was 17 and dying of leukaemia when I was asked to see him on the ward because he was becoming incommunicative and apathetic. Speaking to him alone, I discovered he had no faith in God or an afterlife but had a vision of a terrifying void. There was no way I could confirm or disprove Peter's fears. What I did, in fact, was bring him to the hospice where, little by little he became reconciled to his impending death and was able to live his days more fully. I said to him, as I have said to many people: 'I don't know if there is a God, nobody knows – but I believe there is, if that is any help to you'. Sometimes the faith of a trusted carer can comfort the fearful – providing the carer remains sufficiently sensitive and respectful of the patient's space and individuality. To proselytize or force one's own faith on to a patient is quite unpardonable.

Case history

Mary was a lady in her late 70s who one day admitted she was afraid that God could not love her because she had been so wicked. Intrigued, we enquired further and found that at the height of her youth and beauty she had seduced the husbands of several of her friends. This transgression required a more formal forgiveness than I could offer her and we asked if she would like to see a priest. Duly absolved she pronounced herself at peace with God and man and died the next day!

Fear of God is something which must be carefully elicited, especially if the patient is troubled by a childish vision of a vengeful judgemental God. It is in circumstances such as these that a good chaplain can be invaluable – but he like other carers must hone his communication skills so that he can actively screen for such fears. It is not enough to say a few prayers or talk about cricket.

The *fear of being a burden* on one's family is very common and must be faced head-on because, in truth, the sick *are* a burden. Families' ability to care for their sick varies enormously and sometimes seems to bear little relationship to their apparent resources. It is the job of the professional to enable those who wish to care to do so and to avoid, in so far as is possible, standing in judgement on those who clearly can't or won't care. Sometimes one has to give carers permission to abdicate their responsibility for a while and at other times encourage the unwilling. The hardest task of all is comforting those patients who have been rejected by their partner or children.

Loss

The universal experience of the terminally ill is that of loss: of a multitude of losses which are mostly unvoiced by the loser and barely acknowledged by family or carers. The first thing to be lost is the *sense of invulnerability* which seems to be a universal coping strategy of those who are well. At an intellectual level you and I know we are just as much at risk of getting cancer or being involved in a major car accident as the next person – but as a framework for living we assume this kind of disaster will happen to other people, not to us. Once it has happened, however, one knows deep in one's guts that disasters *can* happen, and one is robbed forever of the carefree insouciance of the unblemished.

Next there comes the loss of that indefinable quality of *well being*, that sense of wholeness and vitality when one's body obeys the merest whisper of command and one has energy for living and loving and for conquering the world. It is difficult to put oneself inside the shoes of those who have not felt really *well* for months or even years. The psychological spin-offs of sadness, irritability and general loss of *joie de vivre* affect all the person's relationships. It is worth remembering how readily we respond to care for someone who is sick – but how rapidly the novelty wears off, especially when it interferes with our freedom to work and play as we would wish. It follows that any medical effort to make people *feel* better, even if they cannot be cured, is time well spent.

Loss of physical beauty is another almost universal sadness of the dying. This loss may come by way of mutilating surgery of their face, breast or belly or by the loss of hair caused by chemotherapy or cranial radiation. A more insidious loss is that of gradually increasing cachexia and it is both salutary and disturbing to the carer to look at the shyly proffered photographs of the patient when well. The sicker people *look*, the more we feel they are 'different' from us and, therefore, the less they threaten our sense of immortality. It is always more disturbing to work with someone who looks well despite the fact that they are dying: it is harder for them and harder for their carers to accept that they have a mortal disease. One feels somehow that they have a time bomb planted inside them and, in some quite irrational way, that one is in part responsible for the planting of it.

With loss of physical beauty goes loss of the *sense of self-worth*. A person's identity is intimately caught up in the way they look and in particular with their physical integrity. Patients with mutilating disease of face or breast or genitalia inevitably feel diminished as people and they need much sensitive reassurance from their carers and family. From time to time these patients are rejected by their families.

Case history

Albert had a slow-growing malignancy of his face. He was so terrified of doctors that he refused to go to see his general practitioner, staying in his house and covering his face. By the time he sought medical help he had lost his nose, one eye and half of his mouth and was beyond cure. His wife was so angry with him and so disgusted by his disease that she felt unable to care for him and, though fully ambulant and self-caring he remained in the hospice for the six months prior to his death. He retained his sense of usefulness by working in our garden, planting for us the gladioli from his own greenhouse.

Another patient, Mary, had a similar condition and she lived with us for about nine months, until she was quite blind and her face was replaced by a gaping hole. She was a particularly enchanting little Irish lady, much loved by the nurses who would sit with her to write their report in the evening. From time to time I would say to her, Mary, do you know how much we love you?' and she would flush with pride. The day she died I nearly caused a mutiny among the staff by admitting another (desperately needy) patient to her bed before 24 hours had elapsed.

Such horrific losses are best managed in a quite unselfconscious way by treating people normally and, when appropriate, spelling out to them how much they mean to those who come into contact with them. It is worth recounting yet another case history.

Catherine was a woman of sixty whose carcinoma of the maxilliary sinus had spread to involve the whole of her face; her nose, cheek and one eye were completely gone and the other eye disappeared under a massively swollen eyelid. She looked a monster and smelt quite disgusting – the sort of travesty of a person that makes relatives mutter 'if it was a dog you'd have it put down'. So distressed were we by her mutilation that we decided that she would be better quietly sleeping and sedated her. To our chagrin, however, she fought the drugs and when we asked her if she wanted to be sleeping, said a firm 'no'. Escaping from her Valium-induced haze she demanded to be taken to the hospice lounge where she sat at the piano and sang with her sister! It was a salutary reminder to us that while it is permissable to sedate a patient because of their own distress it is not acceptable to sedate them because either their relatives or the staff feel that they can't take any more.

Another particularly difficult loss for all concerned is the *ability to communicate*. This happens to patients with cancer of the larynx, mouth or tongue or those with strokes or some brain tumours. The patient experiences a terrible frustration at not being able to express their thoughts, feelings or needs and this is especially bitter if they are too weak to write. A particularly difficult scenario is when the patient can talk but what they say is virtually incomprehensible. One says 'I'm sorry, I didn't catch that', and they repeat it, and still one does not understand. The temptation to make some vague remark and run becomes almost overwhelming and produces a deep guilt and sadness in the carer. If patients can write, then carers must have the patience to communicate in this way. Sometimes speech therapists can help, but more often than not that there is little that can be done. In this situation it is important for the staff to be open amongst each other about how painful they find things because there is support when distress is shared.

Loss of *mobility and independence* which comes inevitably to all who do not die suddenly is hard for everyone but especially so for the young. Much care must be taken to be sensitive to people's needs for toileting and so on, and simple details such as taking people to the lavatory on a wheeled commode rather than leaving them humiliated behind inadequately drawn curtains are important. Many patients suffer bitterly at having to give up their homes. For those who live alone risks must sometimes be taken, for people have the right to wager their freedom against the chance of falling in the night and being found dead in the morning. More difficult to help are those patients who try to manipulate their exhausted partner or children into taking them home, and sometimes one must be firm and say no because a relative has reached the end of their tether. Sometimes it is necessary for a patient to see for themselves that they cannot cope and we frequently send people home for a trial visit. Usually they return sadder and wiser but sometimes they prove us wrong and cope against all odds.

Another loss which causes deep sadness but is rarely referred to is that of *sexual or ordinary physical closeness*. If a couple wish for intimacy it is good to be able to give them the necessary privacy. In other cases it is well to be conscious of people's need for warmth and human touch. The daily baths possible in a hospice are a source of affirmation and sensual pleasure as is aromatherapy and massage. I am now quite comfortable with hugging and being hugged by my patients and their relatives: I well recall arriving in the intensive care unit as part of the radiotherapy consultant's ward round, to find that one of our younger patients was quietly exsanguinating. His distraught wife flung herself sobbing into my arms while the rest of the ward round quietly evaporated. One very frightened seventy-year-old lady demanded a massive hug of nearly every doctor or nurse who came within grabbing distance: it was her way of coping with the terror she could not articulate. I have some sympathy with the prescription offered in *The Second Little Book of Hugs* (Keating, 1988): 'Four hugs a day for survival, eight for maintenance and twelve for growth'. If we extend the concept of hugging to verbal affirmation, I think there's a lot of truth in it.

Perhaps the most painful loss of all is the loss of *role* because that, like physical integrity, is intimately connected with our sense of personal worth. When a man can no longer work and care for his wife, or a woman no longer cooks for her husband and children they are at risk of feeling gravely diminished. It is important, therefore, to help people to stay at work as long as they wish and feel able, and to replace their lost role with another one. One must be alert, for example, to the pain caused by the over-zealous mother-in-law who moves in to take over the running of her son's house and family from his ailing wife. A little gentle explanation to husband and carers should help them to include the sick wife as much as possible in the running of her house so that she is not forced to abdicate her role before it is necessary. Sometimes in the hospice we are able to reveal to a particularly disabled patient that they have an unexpected and vital role in their new community. I remember Joan, a lady of 50 with multiple fractures who could not so much as turn over in bed, but who was a haven of comfort for any nurse who was tired or fed up. Such patients are common and it is worth spelling out clearly to them how much they are valued – for otherwise, how can they know?

The principles of managing loss, therefore, are to try to mitigate it wherever possible and to acknowledge it by empathic understanding.

Anger

Anger is an important issue in the care of the dying and one which needs careful handling if misunderstanding and hurt are to be avoided. Anger may be divided into:
(a) existential – anger against fate or God;
(b) anger against carers, and
(c) projected anger.

Existential anger is common but rarely presents a problem. Most people are sad rather than heatedly angry, asking the inevitable questions: 'Why me? What have I done to deserve this? I've lived a good life; I've never done anyone any harm'. The management of this kind of anger consists largely in listening, for most people's questions are in fact rhetorical – a sort of howl of anguish and despair. Carers often feel ill at ease in the face of these questions but they need have no fear. Even if the patient *does* demand an answer (and mostly they don't) the cleverest philosopher or theologian can only say – 'Truly, I don't know. I don't know why Jane aged 29 is struck down with ovarian cancer, or David the talented musician must die of a brain tumour two weeks before his 21st birthday'. Of one thing, however, I am sure: those who *do* have slick religious answers to such questions are pastorally dangerous and theologically naive.

Anger against carers, especially doctors, is common and must be actively screened for and taken seriously. There are two important principles in the management of anger against oneself or one's colleagues: the first is: give the person all the space they need to ventilate their anger, and the second is: don't cover up. Patients' anger may be justifiable anger or unjustifiable anger.

Justifiable anger is often expressed against the general practitioner for the way in which he or she dismissed the patient's initial complaints of the cancer. 'I *told* him my belly was swelling' a woman sobs, 'and he said it was just the middle-aged spread. I told him I was bleeding and he said it was piles. I went again and again but it wasn't until there was a locum there that I was examined. He got me into the hospital the next day, but it was TOO LATE.'

It is very painful for doctors to listen to this kind of talk. One is torn apart by a self-righteous fury, but also by a sneaking fear that perhaps one might also have missed the diagnosis. Mercifully most patients ask only that you hear them out. Sometimes it can be helpful to explain, very gently, that an earlier diagnosis would probably have made no difference. If it *would* have made all the difference one can only be silent or, if pressed, gently and sadly truthful. Sometimes I try to explain how difficult it is for general practitioners who are faced with so many problems which *could* be malignant but probably are not – but I'm not sure that this is particularly helpful.

Unjustifiable anger. Sometimes anger is quite unjustifiable and one longs to lash back, but again one must sit and listen patiently, giving the person space to ventilate their fury. Such anger usually burns itself out if adequate space is given; sometimes careful explanation clears up misunderstandings. Sometimes, alas, it festers on to become a manifestation of intense grief.

Projected anger. The phenomenon of projected anger is common amongst the dying and their relatives and it is important that carers are aware of it. It is always hard for nurses who have done all they can think of for a particular patient to be faced not with gratitude but complaints. In the same way it is hard for partners to be on the receiving end of a constant stream of irritation and complaint from the person they love. Explanation here is imperative if people are not to be badly hurt. I would try to help the person on the receiving end of the anger to empathize with the patient's frustration and distress and to understand that by patiently receiving this pent-up anger they are relieving distress.

Alienation

By alienation I mean the painful distancing of patients from their relatives, friends and carers because of inept or inadequate communication or lies. The essence of the problem is this: families and/or carers decide, unilaterally, that either the patient would not be able to 'cope' with the truth about their condition or that it would be kinder not to tell them. They therefore restrict the flow of information to the patient by use of half-truths or simply lie outright. The patients, however, knowing themselves ill and sensing that people are holding out on them feel increasingly isolated. Realizing that something is terribly wrong they can neither verify nor disprove their suspicions. Some patients take active steps to clarify their position but many find the effort too painful and withdraw more and more into themselves, cut off from support at precisely the moment that they are most in need of it. This *conspiracy of silence* is the cause of much pain and misunderstanding and one of the prime tasks of those who care for the terminally ill and their families is to assess the degree of such a conspiracy and work out how best to unravel it. Carers may feel trapped into lying and unable to extricate themselves with honour, but once one knows how to go about it the situation can usually be resolved without bitterness. Before one enters into battle, certain principles must be borne in mind:

(1) The carer's first duty is to the patient, not to the relatives.
(2) The relatives do not have the right to forbid a carer to tell their patient the diagnosis, however much they may be convinced of the right.
(3) There is a deep-seated myth in ordinary people that if you tell a patient that their disease is incurable they will 'give-up' and die.
(4) The principle of breaking bad news is to find out first what the patient *knows* and secondly, what they *want* to know, and then answer their questions gently and truthfully.
(5) It is never acceptable to lie outright in answer to a straight question about diagnosis or prognosis, *but*
(6) It is equally wrong to force painful information on a patient who does not wish to receive it.
(7) Elicit the patient's *coping strategy* and respect it.

Once the patient's questions have been answered the carer has the task of explaining to the relatives what he or she has done. This is not always easy, but most people understand that it is wrong to lie outright and are grateful for the opportunity for open communication. The technique of breaking bad news will be discussed in detail later. The improvement in communication and mutual support between people who love each other after such a facilitation manoeuvre is one of the great rewards of those working in terminal care.

Depression

The diagnosis of depression in patients with far-advanced cancer is notoriously difficult because these patients commonly have every reason to be sad, anorexic and lethargic. Whilst one cannot cure the inevitable grief of loss with antidepressants, many terminally ill patients do become clinically depressed and do respond to anti-depressant medication. In our unit we have a high index of suspicion for depression and enlist the help of our liaison psychiatrist in making the diagnosis. Persistently low mood, frequent tears, early-morning wakening and a low self-image are the most useful diagnostic indicators and we readily substitute a drug such as Prothiaden for the patients nocturnal Temazepam.

Our drug usage pattern tends to vary and we have, over the years moved from Mianserin as our anti-depressant of choice through Lofepramine, Prothiaden and currently, Trazodone. As in other branches of medicine we are always searching for rapid improvement of mood without confusion, drowsiness or systemic side-effects. Quite commonly, the dying are just plain sad at their loss and impending death and one must simply be present to them in their grief. This is one of the really hard things about hospice care: standing one's ground impotently while a patient speaks of the nigh intolerable sadness of leaving partner or children behind. Here the carer can only hold on to the knowledge that the simple fact of sharing another's grief makes it just a little easier to bear and that such giving *must* be counterbalanced by joy and respite in one's own life. There is a limit to the amount of other people's grief that any of us can bear and taking adequate time out is a necessary part of a carer's discipline.

Weariness with Living

One of the hardest conditions to treat in the dying is what I call the weariness of being ill. There frequently comes a time, during the last stages of a fatal illness, when patients are so weary of malaise, discomfort and dependence that they long for death. It is not really a question of inadequate symptom control or of lack of loving supportive care, but of a simple weariness of a life in which they are suffering constant discomfort and their bodily functions are daily less satisfactory. I remember so well Maggie, a lady in her 50s who had a carcinoma of the kidney with multiple bone metastases. For many weeks she remained wonderfully cheerful and resilient despite fractures of spine, femur and both arms. Little by little, however she ran out of energy and the days dragged sadly by. Her bowels were difficult to control and she was humiliated by a faecal leak or hurt by frequent manual evacuations. The time came when she had said her goodbyes but still the days dragged by. Such weariness and sadness is difficult for all, especially when patients who hitherto were dignified and cheerful become querulous and complaining.

Sometimes such patients long for death and ask their carers for euthanasia. This is always difficult to handle but must be faced openly for it would be a fearful insult and betrayal of trust to try to 'jolly' such a person along. Sometimes one finds there is some specific issue worrying the patient and this can be resolved, but more often one is left with this intolerable greyness of spirit. In such a situation I might offer to the patient to sedate them a little. It is important to offer this, not to impose it because of one's own distress. I would say 'would you rather be a bit sleepy – would that make things easier to bear?'. If the answer is 'yes' we would probably use a small dose of Methotrimeprazine (25–75 mg.) daily via a syringe driver. Sometimes we use small and intermittent doses of Diazepam (5–10 mg.) orally or rectally so that people can sleep away a painful mood.

It is worth saying a word about Diazepam: we find it a very useful drug used as a one-off to control episodes of severe agitation and as sedation in the last 24 hours of life. We have *not* found it useful administered on a regular basis and find it makes patients lethargic and depressed.

Hard as this state of weariness of life is to bear for patient, relatives and staff alike, it has its compensation for when such a patient finally dies, family and carers often experience a profound sense of relief. Outsiders often imagine that each death must cause nursing and medical staff grief and a sense of loss, while the reality is that the sense of relief is normally much stronger than the sadness. By far the hardest thing to bear is the period of emptiness and desolation where one feels too impotent to help or even comfort.

Staff *do* experience grief of course and those in a leadership role must be sensitive to this. Sometimes sadness is overt and people can share it. This is most common when the patient is young or has been in the hospice a long time. Patients with severe destructive disease who live a long time and require hours of intimate nursing attention often become very close to the nurses and one must be wary of filling their beds too rapidly. There is another more subtle form of unnamed grief that can sometimes surface quite awkwardly and unexpectedly. I remember that during the theatre production of C.S. Lewis's play *The Shadowlands* that I was suddenly overcome by grief. The stage portrayal of a death-bed scene somehow triggered months of suppressed sadness and I found myself racked by the most awful sobs (mercifully silent) with the tears pouring down my cheeks. I'm sure that such discharge of grief is healthy and I find it strangely reassuring that I personally still have the capacity to mourn when I have become so terribly at ease with death.

SPECIALIST TECHNIQUES

On reflection, I find we in terminal care have few specialist psychological techniques. We do not practise in-depth psychotherapy nor do we utilize many of the behavioural or cognitive methods of clinical psychologists. Relaxation techniques prove helpful from time to time but they have not become an integral part of our work (perhaps they should). There are a number of factors which make work with the dying subtly different from routine psychology. One of these is the extreme variability of the patient's attention span and sense of well-being. There are times when the dying want to talk in depth – and there are times when they have no strength and want only to sleep or chat or watch television. Carers working in a hospice find that their psychological work is done very much on the hoof – five minutes here, fifteen minutes there, on patient demand rather than physician's choice. The talking therapy is shared between all sorts of people: the liaison psychiatrist, the auxilliary night nurse, the medical director and so on – all these have their part to play in listening and sharing joys and sadness.

Facilitating Acceptance

In our unit, the more difficult work of helping patients from denial through to acceptance tends to be initiated by senior medical staff. We would only set out to confront a patient if it seemed that their chosen coping strategy was not serving them well. If denial is working for a patient we would not interfere. An example of change of strategy was the case of Daisy, an elderly lady with lung cancer. When I first visited her in the hospital she cried out as I approached: 'Don't tell me, don't tell me'. I took her hand and asked what it was I shouldn't tell her and it was clear she couldn't face being told she was going to die. The secret was so open between us that it was quite funny, but I agreed not to tell her and she came to the hospice, saying firmly 'I'm going to get well.'. After about six weeks, when she was clearly failing, she grasped my hand (after I had extricated myself from yet another of her massive bear hugs) and asked 'Why aren't I getting better?'.

Now this was a brave, clear question and I told her that the tumour in her lung was growing. That was enough. There was no need to spell out that she was going to get worse and die – there rarely is. After more tears and hugs we parted and she asked no more questions. Breaking bad news within the hospice setting frequently happens this way. People suddenly pluck up the courage to ask in the middle of a ward round – like Lizzie, aged 31, with a sarcoma of her leg who, while I was standing behind her examining her chest asked 'Am I going to die?'. The fact that I had three nurses with me, two of them visitors, did not deter her – maybe she felt safer with an audience. That was *her* chosen moment and it was up to me to respond as best I could. As it happens the conversation went well and proved a good teaching opportunity for the visitors.

Although this kind of interaction is reasonably common in a hospice setting some patients simply do not have the courage to ask and we like to give them an opportunity to discuss their diagnosis if they wish. The whole question of breaking bad news remains a very loaded one because the majority of doctors and nurses see the options only in black or white. In reality, however, the issue is not 'to tell or not to tell', but how to communicate with patients in a way which makes it easy for them to request information if they want it. More than anything, breaking bad news is a *process* rather than an event.

Breaking Bad News

The following is a description of the technique I use and teach for imparting information in the ordinary clinical setting. It works well for me and is, I believe suitable for other doctors and for those specialist nurses who have a long-term in-depth relationship with their patients. The key to this manoeuvre is the modification of the ordinary technique of history taking so that not only the patient's physical problems are elicited but also what they *know* and *feel* about their illness. By tracing the story of their illness step by step with the patient, the carer can not only elicit what the patient knows but get a reasonably clear idea of their preferred coping strategy. By attentive listening and empathic understanding the carer not only gains the patient's confidence but begins a process of simple counselling which will help them to ventilate their emotions and, in the fullness of time, come to terms with their situation.

I use this technique routinely at new consultations, either in the hospice, on the ward or in outpatients. For a new patient, it is prudent to allow an hour, although it may well take a good deal less. The process may be summarized as follows:

(1) *Clarify the patient's story* in your own mind as far as possible. Read the notes. Talk to ward staff. In particular be sure of your facts

about the diagnosis. Read the operation notes and the histology carefully.

(2) See the patient alone (or if a trainee needs to come instruct them to sit out of the patient's direct line of vision and not to join in the conversation). If relatives are at the bedside I would ask them to wait outside, promising to speak to them later.

(3) See the patient in privacy, in a side ward, office, bathroom or wherever, *not* just behind closed curtains. (I have caused havoc in a radiotherapy ward by having a conversation about dying in the hearing of six other patients!)

(4) Introduce yourself: who you are, who sent you and why you have come. Make the link with their known carers: 'Dr Jones asked me to come...'.

(5) Explain that you know about their case (ill patients are frequently dismayed at yet another new face and another history taken), but that you'd like to hear it 'in your own words' – how it was for you'.

(6) Taking the history. Begin at the beginning. 'How long have you been poorly? What's the first thing that went wrong...?' One explores the patient's story in an orderly sequence, beginning with the first suspicion that something was wrong. The key questions here are: 'What did you think?' and 'What did you feel?'. By this means one often finds that the patient has suspected that he or she had cancer right from the outset. The question 'whom did you tell?' will elicit whether or not the patient has a confiding tie and therefore how in need of support they are.

The next step is to enquire about the visit to their general practitioner. What did he or she tell the patient about their illness? What did the patient *think*, what did they *feel*? By enquiring into this stage of the story the carer can elicit whether or not the general practitioner has a supportive relationship with the patient and whether he or she has been working truthfully.

The same enquiry procedure holds good for the hospital visit and any further operations or treatment. Slowly one elicits not just what the patient has been told but what they have *understood* and what emotional impact this information has had upon them. The story is frequently a sad one, fraught with fear, misunderstandings and anger and the patient frequently weeps. Being gently present to someone in this situation, listening to their anger and fear is a powerful act of affirmation and can be of enormous support to the patient. 'No one's ever listened to me like this before' is a not infrequent comment.

(7) Discovering what the patient wants to know. It may well become obvious that the patient suspects they have cancer and they ask for confirmation of the diagnosis. At other times, however, one needs to be more active. Having heard the patient's story so far, I would ask an open question about their present state. 'And how are you *now*?' Sometimes this will elicit a question: 'I don't seem to be getting any better... What's happening?'. If this does not happen, I would ask clearly: 'Tell me, how much do you *understand* about your illness?'. This frequently triggers the question 'It's cancer, isn't it?', in which case one confirms it, gently. They may, however, say 'Not much', in which case one must pause a while and give them space to ask. If no question is forthcoming one must be alert to the fact that they may wish to cope by denial. I would then ask, very gently 'Would you like me to explain things to you?'. Many patients answer readily 'Yes please, I want to know.'. If this happens, one can be quite confident and begin the process. They may, however, meet the question with silence, in which case I would say 'Or would you rather take things one day at a time?'. The patient who wishes to cope by denial will probably be swift to accept this offer and one must respect their decision. It is wrong to dynamite someone's coping strategy by forcing unacceptable information upon them.

(8) Explaining about the illness. If the patient *does* wish to know what is wrong, I would begin the process of telling by what Buckman and Maguire (1985) calls 'the warning shot' with a remark such as 'I'm afraid things are not as straightforward as we'd hoped.'. One then pauses and the patient may ask a direct question. If not, one continues, anchoring their attention on some familiar episode, for example, You remember the doctors took a little piece of tissue out of that gland in your neck...? Well, they looked at it under the microscope and found that it was the same sort of tissue as the cancer you had five years ago.' Sometimes patients need only to know that they cannot be cured. At other times they wish to understand exactly what is going on. If the latter is the case I would explain the processes of metastasis or tissue invasion by means of diagrams and familiar images. It is important to tailor our language to fit our patients and to monitor their understanding continually. For example Jane (aged 39) had a cancer of the cervix, recurrent after major surgery five years previously. She was bitterly angry and could not understand why the tumour could not be cut out. In such situations I often use the image of Polyfilla which has hardened in a cup: one cannot get it out without breaking the cup. Eventually, she understood and her anger turned to a terrible grief.

(9) Prognosis. After such conversations one comes inevitably to the question of *prognosis*. I would never volunteer a prognosis but if it is asked for try to be reasonably truthful. It is important to move slowly because some patients have no conception of how short their life expectancy is and to be totally truthful at the outset could be overwhelming. I would start off vaguely: 'I think we're looking at months, rather than years', and move towards the most accurate prediction that I think the patient can take.

(10) Closing the interview. In such a situation one must give warning that one is drawing the interview to a close and give the patient the opportunity to formulate any last questions. 'I'm afraid I'm going to have to go in a minute. Is there anything more you'd like to ask me?'

When the patient has asked all the questions they wish to, one offers to speak to their relatives. I would by choice then go and see the relatives on their own and after I have explained the situation to them, return with them to the patient and leave them to speak or weep together. I would also offer to speak to their family doctor and to send in a home care nurse if they are going home. It is important to make clear what support you have to offer and what your availability is. It is at this point that we would make clear the 'covenant' nature of our relationship with the patient. 'I'm sorry – we cannot make you better, but I promise you that we will look after you and be with you.' I would then give the patient a further appointment and tell them how to contact a member of my team urgently.

This is the only structured interview technique that I use and it is not uncommon to be able to bypass the first stages of it. It sometimes happens that I walk into a new patient's room and they greet me by name and say 'I'm so glad you've come.'. My behaviour then would be very intuitive, often moving rapidly into a close empathic relationship. Sometimes people are very ill and weak when I see them and there is no place for interrogation. Then I might first hold their hand and say 'Would you like to come to the hospice for a while and let us look after you?'. The words are always tailored to the patient and their situation. I believe the Rogerian model is the closest to the way we work. Rogers' conditions for growth in the therapeutic relationship (Rogers, 1961) are listed below and they represent the unarticulated basis to the way we relate to our patients.

(1) Congruence
(2) Empathy
(3) Unconditional positive regard
(4) Revealing those qualities to the client

In particular we would be ill at ease with the formality which is the norm in some doctor–patient relationships. Because we are referred patients whom other doctors have said 'there is nothing more to be done', we are often working with our hands empty (in other words, there may be no further physical treatment available and symptom control may be as good as is possible). This empty-handed approach has led to a way of using resources of personality and human warmth which many carers reserve for their friends and families. Perhaps it is the short-term nature of our relationships with our patients that makes it 'safe' to give more of ourselves than we would give to someone who might live long enough to abuse our trust. More than anything, however, it is being a member of a *team* that makes this way of working possible. The dying are frightened, lonely people whose needs cannot be confined to office hours.

SERVICE DESCRIPTION

The unit in which I work is typical in organizational terms of many terminal care services in the UK, and consists of the following:

(a) An inpatient unit with 20 beds
(b) A domicilliary nursing service caring for around 120 patients
(c) A daycare unit
(d) A bereavement counselling service
(e) A team of community volunteers
(f) A small group of specialists who visit on a sessional basis.

The staffing of these various units is as follows:

(a) Inpatient unit. This is a busy unit averaging 24 admissions and 18 deaths per month. Patients are admitted from home or hospital according to their need and bed availability. Priority is given to the young, those requiring pain or symptom control, those with severe destructive disease, emotional distress, those near to death and those who live alone. The unit is managed by a ward sister who, under the supervision of the matron, co-ordinates a team of 18 staff and state-enrolled nurses and 22 auxilliary nurses.

The medical cover is co-ordinated by the medical director who works with three other doctors, two clinical assistants (who together constitute the equivalent of one full-time post) and a senior house officer who is part of the general practitioner vocational training scheme.

(b) The domicilliary nursing team consists of six specialist nurses each caring for 20–25 patients. They are based at the hospice and have free access to the senior medical staff for both advice and home visits but we no longer meet formally to discuss their patients.

(c) The day care unit is run by a nursing sister who co-ordinates her own volunteers who pick up the patients from their homes in the

hospice ambulance and take them home again in the afternoon. The numbers vary between 12 and 15, some patients coming weekly, others up to three times a week. Day care is designed with social support as its primary objective; medical supervision is secondary, with dressings and treatments done as needed. We find this works well and the service is popular; the patients pass the time talking to each other and the volunteers, but also enjoy services such as bathing, hair dressing, aromatherapy and chiropody. We hope to start more organized diversional therapy when we have more space.

(d) The bereavement visiting service consists of volunteers trained and co-ordinated by the senior social worker. They meet monthly for supervision and allocations of new cases and visit bereaved clients in their own homes. There is a monthly social evening for clients and volunteers which is well attended.

(e) The community volunteers are a group of helpers who will befriend or assist patients in their own homes. They are co-ordinated by the junior social worker.

(f) Visiting staff:

(i)   A pain clinic anaesthetist one session weekly;
(ii)   A liaison psychiatrist, a senior registrar attends the weekly case conference and sees patients as requested – usually for patients thought to be anxious, depressed or possibly demented.
(iii) Chaplaincy: We have a lay 'pastoral co-ordinator', whose mandate is to assess the patient's religious and/or spiritual needs and organize the appropriate pastor to visit. We have recently appointed a chaplain.

Organization and Communication

Efficiency, team cohesion and morale are heavily dependent upon communication within the team and this is deliberately built into the working day. Apart from the normal nursing report sessions, each morning there is a 30-minute review of all the inpatients which is attended by the sister, and all available medical staff. We have maintained this pattern of work for the past nine years and see it as crucial to the smooth running of the unit. It serves additionally as a teaching forum and as a means of staff support. There is a weekly multidisciplinary case conference chaired by the senior doctor present and attended by doctors, nurses, social workers, the pastoral co-ordinator, counsellor and the liaison psychiatrist. All patients are discussed and their physical, emotional, psychosocial and spiritual needs monitored.

There is also a newly instituted audit/morbidity meeting attended by as many staff as possible. The patients dying during the previous week are mentioned by name and briefly prayed for, mainly in silence. (This gives a token space for staff to acknowledge their own sadness.) These cases are then discussed in detail under the headings of physical care, emotional, spiritual and social care, the question being asked each time: How satisfactory was our care? How far did we go towards meeting that person or their family's needs? What did we do well, where did we fail and how can we do better another time?

It is impossible in such a brief and bare description to convey the spirit of the hospice. I believe that the most powerful psychological treatment we provide for our patients is the opportunity of belonging to a caring community. Clearly it does not work for everyone, but for many patients the sense of safety and acceptance that they experience provides an unimaginable dimension of joy in the midst of the devastation of their last weeks.

> No revolution will come in time
> to alter this man's life except
> the one surprise of being loved.
>
> Sydney Carter

References

BUCKMAN, R. and MAGUIRE, P. (1985) *Why Won't They Talk to Me?* [video] Shepperton: Linkward Productions.
KEATING, K. (1988) *The Second Little Book of Hugs*. London: Angus & Robertson.
ROGERS, C. (1961) *On Becoming a Person*. Boston, MA: Houghton Mifflin Co.

CARE OF THE CANCER PATIENT'S FAMILY

Kerry Bluglass

The development of treatment for physical and psychological distress in cancer patients is now beginning to have a major impact on their care. Thoughtful professionals have also now begun to perceive the stress and distress which can also affect the surrounding family members and care givers. In the past some of this distress has undoubtedly arisen from, or has been exacerbated by, the lack of appropriate symptom relief for cancer, particularly in the terminal phases of the disease, and has complicated the bereavement outcome for many relatives. Some of the undeniable difficulties in the care of the patient of any stage of the illness undoubtedly arise from mis-understandings of the place of the patient in his or her whole family setting, of the nature of the role they play in the family system, and the changes which the threat of their illness, disfigurement, inca-pacity or death poses to the family as a whole as well as to its individual members. As we have come to realize in the last few years of intensive study into psychosocial aspects of cancer care, the treat-ment of the patient in fact involves treatment of the whole family unit. Detailed attention to the specific as well as general needs of individual family members is important.

DEFINING THE FAMILY

At the same time as we have come to realize that the patient is frequently the sum of the close and sometimes extended members of what we call the family, there has been a similar recognition that rapid social change (including on-going changes in relationships, kinships and marriage patterns, geographical mobility, divorce legis-lation and employment) requires us to accept a much wider view of the family unit than has been commonly understood (Oakley, 1982). Acknowledging this is of some importance, for as in other aspects of psychosocial work with cancer patients, we need to be understanding of our own prejudices and perspectives in relation to patients and their families. Cultural and geographical influences modify the expectations and needs of families, patients and professionals alike. For example, in North America distance, geographical mobility, and very high divorce rates may all modify the patterns of response to 'bad news', life-threatening illness, palliative care and bereavement expectations. At the same time, good practice in the realms of communication, patient involvement in care and the growth of consumerism have all encouraged patients, families and the community into a more open dialogue with health care providers. Cancer is also more openly discussed.

In Europe, particularly in predominantly Catholic countries, divorce and family break-up have until recently been less common and this is still so in some areas. The traditional acceptance of the elderly or sick family member as the family's or community's natural responsibility is more common. Frequently the family is the only source of direct patient care in inpatient settings. Formal nursing is seen as too expensive or irrelevant to the day-to-day domestic needs of the patient and members are expected to participate actively in cooking, feeding and hygiene. The family, relative, or other key person is thus a crucial part of the patient's everyday care.

Where these cultural differences exist they must be recognized since they affect the provision of care that is appropriate to family's and patient's needs. In less sophisticated settings information or education which affect understanding of symptoms, progress, and treatment may be lacking and we must try to adapt the explanation and information given to the family accordingly. Although social factors are rapidly changing, people's expectations and behaviour, the apparently passive acceptance of the illness and death in some European countries may be difficult for us to understand. In fact although the Church and organized religious belief are supportive to families in the immediate mourning period, declining morbidity rates mean that there may be less understanding of the psychosocial factors involved in the transition from wife to widow and consequently poorer identification of those people with special needs.

A key person (who may be a neighbour, friend, homosexual partner or distant relative) may be much more significant to the patient than a biologically closer but uninvolved relative. The relationship of the key person to the patient may place them at the same degree of psychological risk following loss or death as a close partner in a conventional marriage or family. Despite increasing tolerance of 'unconventional' or homosexual relationships, these may not have been explicitly recognized by other biologically close family members, and fear of social disapproval may deny the partner or friend the support normally accorded to a spouse or close relative.

Even with a conventional family structure, whether apparently close and cohesive or detached and uninvolved, the individual members of a family may be functioning in unconventional ways. Thus an understanding of the role which each family member plays in the functioning of that family is important if adequate psychosocial care is to be provided. Individuals in families may adopt or be assigned positive or negative roles which are not at first apparent (such as the 'standard bearer', 'head of the clan', or the scapegoat) (Worden, 1983). Understanding these dimensions and their interrelationships helps to promote understanding of the effects of the illness or death of an individual. Their family will miss not only their physical presence but also the role fulfilled by that person and suffer from the resulting gap in the dynamic balance.

THE NEEDS OF THE FAMILY

Defining the family and identifying its immediate and long-term needs is an important part of early psychosocial assessment. It is important that this evaluation and care is not simply seen as treatment or palliation for pathology, traditionally a medical model approach. It is likely to be most effective if it seeks to identify and encourage coping skills, is constructive and affirms the individual's and family's strength and potential, and avoids fostering dependence and weakness which further serve to undermine confidence and the ability to cope.

Whilst hospitals can be extremely bewildering for many relatives unused to clinical settings, properly supported and encouraged the relative or family members can greatly assist the patient in carrying out simple domestic or personal tasks for them. They can learn to carry out more sophisticated procedures and techniques in hospital and at home, and provided that the patient has sufficient confidence, the ability to be of practical use to the patient confirms the relative in their previous function as a family carer, which is both comforting and reassuring for the patient, and greatly assists the family's feeling of competence and well-being. This in turn is likely to affirm their feeling of worth and self-esteem and, after a patient's death, family members often feel that they were able to make a sizeable contribution to the patient's comfort and well-being.

The professional helper however should be aware that delegating too many technical procedures to a family member, as sometimes happens when resources are scarce, may worry both the patient and the relatives. Encouraging relatives and friends to participate as much as possible in the care of the patient without provoking undue anxiety seems likely to improve bereavement outcome. Conversely, denying access or overprofessionalization of care can be isolating for patient and relative alike and may add to the understandable feelings of regret and guilt following the patient's eventual death. If we as professional care givers can be flexible and creative in our care for patients it is almost always possible to allow both patient and relative much greater autonomy than we imagine, and certainly more than has been the case in the past. Feelings of hopelessness and loss are exacerbated by loss of control (Seligman, 1975) and we should be striving to give back to the patient and relative the sense of mastery which they would have in their ordinary lives.

However much we encourage family members in their involvement with a patient, we must also continually monitor the situation. What is appropriate involvement at one stage of the disease may be quite different at another. Relatives who are supportive and energetic during the diagnostic phase of the illness may become completely exhausted by the necessity for hospital visits if single-handedly running a home, parenting, and working (Woods, 1989). The cost to the family in material, social and emotional terms may be considerable and should be regularly evaluated. One way of doing this (which is considered on page 163) is to encourage the patient's and family's free expression of their feelings. Some people are more able to express difficulties in shared group activities, supported by others in the same situation (Plant et al., 1987).

Family Needs at Different Phases

Treatment and care cannot be logically separated from preventative, health promotion approaches, but usually the needs of a particular patient and family will be quite different depending on the phase of the illness. Different phases and different forms of cancer may present different issues for patient and family care and support. The relapse/remission cycles of acute leukaemia are very different in nature from the slow but inexorable progression of some solid tumours. Similarly some types of therapy cause particular problems of loss of self-image and self-esteem for the patient, while primary or metastatic cerebral tumours may cause alterations of behaviour that family members find inexplicable, distressing or even unacceptable. Thus the individual situation has to be considered as unique, but some working framework is necessary.

Northouse (1984) suggested three major phases: initial, adaptive and terminal. Progress in the treatment of some cancers would suggest that long-term survival should be added as a fourth phase. Rait and Lederberg (1989) propose a more flexible and accurate terminology:

The acute phase around the time of diagnosis presents the whole family with a frightening crisis to which all members react in their characteristic ways. Some may be more acutely distressed than the patient. The crisis however allows for rallying and mobilization of help and support. Protective mechanisms may result in communication being resisted and creating a 'conspiracy of silence' which has negative effects on family relationships. This process may crystallize and become permanent if not recognized.

The mechanisms of the 'acute' period may also extend to treatment, relapse and unexpected complications.

The chronic phase involves different mechanisms when returning home, lengthy courses of treatment or hospitalization and periods of remission may be involved. At this time the family has to balance the needs of the patient with the needs of other family members and try to resume some normal life which may be difficult to achieve. Perceptions of different family members may be different. One member may become overprotective of the patient while other family members wish them to move on, psychologically speaking. Intrafamilial conflicts may arise with anger, jealousy, and the expression of different personal demands leading to a paradoxical increase in psychological symptoms during this phase. The support of extended family, friends and workmates may decline at this time when the family need most help.

Major decisions may be delayed by the family's preoccupation with long-term illness. The stress of this phase is indicated by a positive correlation between length and severity of illness and several measures of dysfunction in family members (Cancer Care Inc. and National Cancer Foundation, 1977; Koocher and O'Malley, 1981). Dysfunction however is not inevitable and some families may respond positively by adopting new roles and new goals.

The third or resolution phase covers the experience of bereavement and adaptation or recovery from the death of the patient. The adaptation of a particular family to this phase may be modified by the synchrony of 'timeliness' of fatal illness. A family may tolerate the cancer and eventual death of an elderly grandparent better than that of a child where future expectations are affected.

Talking to Patients and Families Together

The concept of the family as a unit in health and disease (Litman, 1974) is increasingly recognized in the field of psychosocial care and for professionals working in this field it is easy to forget that other professionals, perhaps more orientated to the medical model, or indeed family members themselves, may need gentle and tactful introduction to this approach. Practitioners who are at ease in individual work with a patient may find it difficult, unfamiliar or threatening to be asked or expected to work with several people whose competing and sometimes conflicting needs may require sensitive orchestration of the meeting. Many medical students admit that, unless family work has formed part of their child psychiatry or paediatrics instruction, they have never had the experience of interviewing a couple together, still less a large and extended family.

Many family members expect to have an individual consultation with the doctor, nurse, psychologist or social worker and, because of traditional medical practice, they often expect to be given the diagnostic 'bad news' with its accompanying burden of secrecy alone. It is therefore surprising to some patients and their relatives to have the opportunity to discuss the results of investigations and possible implications of a disease together. However, in the UK, at least, the move towards more open communication has been a direct response to the expressed wishes and needs of the families themselves.

Clear communication which is sensitive to the individual patient and their nonverbal behaviour, which includes use of open questions, entirely at the patient's and relative's own pace will, as Buckman (1988) has described, avoid the need for 'I never tell the patient' – 'I always tell the patient' conundrum. Manos and Christakis (1981, 1985) found that the solutions to this dilemma varied from country to country and culture to culture. According to their reviews of the literature in 1981, the practice varies widely from China, where truth appeared to be almost uniformly withheld, to the United States, where 97 per cent of physicians favoured giving honest information to the patient. The UK took up an intermediate position and inclined to more openness than France, Germany and Switzerland. In my experience, the past five years have shown an even greater swing in the UK towards reasonable honesty with the patient and relatives. It is wiser in any case to avoid overdogmatic, black-and-white 'prescriptions' and incline in the process of information sharing to the more reasonable course of 'how much, to whom and at what time'. The speed or pace of information sharing may similarly need to be tailored to the individual family.

While the figures quoted above in response to Manos and Christakis' enquiries of physicians' attitudes to 'truth telling' represent a trend, they should be interpreted with some caution. As Stedeford (1984) talking about diagnosis and prognosis, points out, in reality the situation is often much more complicated:

If he decides in an independent or arbitrary way how much it is good for the patient to know, he is not respecting the patient's right to knowledge about himself. The dilemma is that until the patient knows what the information is and feels its impact on him, he cannot be certain whether he would have wanted to be told or not. Therefore, the decision-making about the flow of information has to be carried out as a delicate negotiation between doctor and patient in which the doctor tries to ascertain how much the patient wants to know...

Clinical experience gives confidence but should not give complacency. Talking to patients and their families about diagnosis is not always a neat matter of consultation between an experienced consultant surgeon or physician and the patient. Often the relatively inexperienced or junior member of staff is confronted with important questions when the patient, feeling that they can trust this more approachable doctor or nurse, opens the dialogue. The inexperienced member of staff may feel unprepared for this opening. Conventional training does not always prepare staff for these issues and even 'trained' or more experienced staff are not always comfortable in this area. (Cassidy (this volume) gives guidance on how to break bad news.)

Learning how to promote a trusting and reasonably open relationship should improve the quality of communication and with it good quality care for the patient and family. Such learning experience should include the use of seminars, workshops and appropriate audiovisual resources with the help of which staff can explore and rehearse strategies (see Appendix for useful addresses). Written information helps to change attitudes but in this context there is no substitute for practical experience properly supervised, with the opportunity to try various appropriate communication techniques with guidance and encouragement. Direct and videotaped feedback from teacher to trainer has been shown to be effective (Maguire *et al.*, 1980).

Although much of this work is relevant to the initial diagnosis, it is also appropriate to the total care of the patient and family at all stages of the illness. Such an approach should make titrating the psychosocial care and support at all stages more appropriate.

Denial is a very strong psychological defence mechanism which often operates during the information-giving process. Some patients and families are very proud or very private and some individuals can only cope with the difficulties of life through the mechanism of denial. Well-meant attempts to test reality may not be productive or therapeutic in the long run; in fact it may be positively harmful. It is better to understand the mechanisms operating and to try to make the pproach appropriate to the current phase of illness or uncertainty rather than to make the individual fit the treatment. Examples of how to deal with strong or prolonged denial in such a way that the relatives can eventually find the information they require at their own pace are clearly described in Stedeford (1984). Patients and their families should always know what services and supports are available should their situation or needs change and be given the opportunity to participate later. Treatment, support or information which has the effect of rendering the individual uncomfortable or guilty is not appropriate. It is more helpful to assess family vunerability factors early and monitor progress in order to try to prevent or anticipate later difficulties.

THE STRESS OF TREATMENT

The burden of supporting a close family member with cancer is more than the sharing (of distressing knowledge) or 'the crisis of knowledge of death' (Mansell Pattison, 1977) or the reality of the 'living–dying interval' which the patient and their relatives may experience. With these complex and disturbing emotions go the practical, social, marital, domestic and often financial cost of chronic or life-threatening illness. Lansky *et al.*, (1979) and Bodkin *et al.*, (1982) have described the financial, non-medical costs of illness, the latter study in the UK, where 'socialized' medicine is thought to cover the cost of treatment. The fallacy that care at home is less costly than care in hospital was demonstrated by Murinen in a hospice study (1986) where the economic effect on primary care givers of voluntary resignation or job loss, particularly in lower income families who could least afford it, was documented in 25 per cent of primary care givers. Of the remainder, 60 per cent experienced a significant loss in income from absenteeism or less well-paid work. In this study the so-called financial savings associated with home care merely represented a shift from the 'formal' medical to the informal, that is, individual, family sources. Other authors (McCubbin, 1979; McCubbin and Figley, 1983; and McKeever, 1983) have discussed the longer-term implications of career disruption and loss of social mobility.

Relapse/Remission, 'Recovery' and Survival Phases

It is not commonly understood that a growing number of patients survive in a stable state for considerable periods of time. The adjustment involved in making the adaptation from the threat of death (Glaser and Strauss, 1966, 1968) only to discover that the fatal judgement has been revoked, proves difficult for some individuals. Teta *et al.*, (1986) in a large study drawn from the multi-centre National Cancer Institute study, investigated the psychosocial effects of long-term and adolescent cancer survival. While frequency of major depression in survivors did not appear to differ from that of their siblings and was similar to that of the general population, 80 per cent of the male survivors were rejected from the armed forces, 13 per cent from college and 32 per cent from employment. Other difficulties such as those of obtaining health and life insurance and in attaining major socioeconomic goals were described. Thus the family, having surmounted with the patient the threat of fatal illness, often discovers that quality of life and expectations are seriously curtailed.

The effects of life-threatening illness, overprotection of the sick family member, the guilt and resentment of some well siblings, together with the loss of expected attainments and independence for the young cancer survivor may perpetuate the parent–child relationship in a negative way. Family evaluation and support or intervention must obviously identify, monitor and try to modify the most negative of these effects.

Survival can involve other negative consequences. Problems relating to an unduly pessimistic prognosis are described by Stedeford (1984), in a case where a patient's wife prematurely developed a relationship with another man, needing his support and companionship for herself as well as for her children, in the expectation that her husband had only a few weeks to live. The relationship developed faster and further than she would have intended had she known that her husband would survive for longer. Psychological and material plans are often made in the expectation that death is not far off and an unexpected remission can cause problems for a family. In another case described by Bluglass (1986) everyone involved accepted that a patient's death was imminent, further efforts in active treatment were relinquished, 'acceptance' was accomplished and many of the psychological tasks in anticipating loss worked through. Meanwhile the patient actually lived on, and, as a consequence of both illness and treatment, was significantly changed in appearance and behaviour. Family members can be distressed by this sequence of events and may find it difficult to express their real feelings to the staff out of loyalty and concern for the patient. Staff members need to be aware and alert to these ambivalent feelings.

The nature of the tumour or cancer, its site and significance for the patient and the treatment involved may greatly modify the patient's and family's response during the remission/relapse or chronic phases. Since, for example, any changes to the breast have a highly significant effect on the patient's sense of attractiveness and self-esteem, partners and families need to be aware of this, and of the effect of their changed perception of the patient. Maguire *et al.* (1978,

1980) have drawn to the attention of the medical and nursing profession the psychosocial consequences, including undetected depression, of breast surgery. Broadwell (1987) found that adjustment was related to the level of social support experienced by both patients and their partners. Those who reported high levels of support had fewer postoperative adjustment difficulties. Patients and partners differed significantly in the levels of support they received over time, partners perceiving less support from friends, nurses and physicians (Northouse, 1988). Partners' assumptions about the most helpful attitude to develop towards the patient (protective, reassuring, minimizing) were perceived by their wives as rejecting and insensitive, and often led to relationship difficulties. This is commonly found in practice and often needs to be explored by the counsellor in discussion with the couple (Sabo *et al.*, 1986). Thus it seems that exploring families and patients' perceptions of each others' feelings and actions is likely to be most helpful and improve communication to lead to easier relationships and better adjustment.

The Chronic, Continuing and Terminal Phases

Stam *et al.* (1986) drew attention to cancer patients' concern about the effect of their illness on the family, which is often greater than their concern about the illness itself. This has to be managed sensitively and diplomatically, as both patient or relative may deny problems in order to protect one another.

A further factor in the adjustment of the family and patient in the chronic or continuing phase of cancer is the complex series of interacting factors between the frequent social ostracism of cancer patients and their sometimes self-imposed stigmatization. Verres (1985) discusses concepts of 'infectiousness', attribution of guilt and other fantasies as examples of lay perceptions of the disease. Neither are some doctors exempt from some of these attitudes, believing they can do nothing to overcome the social isolation of cancer patients. Improved public education may help to change attitudes. Teams who work with cancer patients and their families can help by preparing and distributing appropriate information; relatively informal work with groups (patients, families, and professionals) such as the Glasgow 'Tak Tent' organization (see Appendix) helps to break down these barriers.

In some communities there are of course facilities to cover night sitting, day sitting and other respite where appropriate, but these are not uniformly available and are usually hard pressed. In the UK, the Marie Curie Service and other organizations may help to provide specific additional care to lessen the load on relatives, for example at night, and in some areas good local voluntary care has developed. In others this has to be paid for. In some smaller communities informal support builds up through neighbours and concerned friends. It is as well however not to leave this to chance but for each team to try to develop such links as part of their help for patients and their families. Simonton (1984) described an interesting model in which offers of help from friends can be apportioned by drawing up a list of useful tasks. Friends then select one activity or task according to their preference or suitability, as from a list of presents.

Voluntary and informal self-help groups do invaluable work in supporting families. In a time of scarce resources however, befriending should not be confused with tasks which are the province of professionals. Very clear guidelines should be drawn up and distinctions made between befriending, support, counselling and other more complicated, sophisticated professional activities. The British Association of Counselling (see Appendix) is currently preparing guidelines for groups who use volunteers and befrienders to help them to clarify these distinctions.

In the continuing and chronic phases, or the beginning of the terminal or palliative phase of care, the family members, whose adjustment to the declining health of the patient may vary, will continue to modify their relationship to one another and to the patient. This is why continual monitoring of the family situation is important. If, for example, one family member has progressed psychologically while another is in a stage of fairly marked denial, there will be inevitable conflicts between themselves, the patient and the professionals involved. These situations are not irrevocable nor impossible to help, but do require careful attention to detail and an understanding of the family's composition and past history as well as its current functioning. Given these difficulties, it is encouraging and remarkable to see that many families do, with appropriate help, come through a most difficult period strengthened and more cohesive.

In a hospice setting, an example of good practice set by St Christopher's Hospice, London, in the 1960s, was to discourage visiting on one day a week. This gave a free day to family members or close relatives in which they could attend to their own business, domestic tasks or simply take some rest from what might be fairly intensive visiting and preoccupation with illness. It is an appropriate way in which to signal to the family that while their contribution to the care of the patient is important, they also need time to themselves and to recharge their batteries.

Ideally the care of the family will anticipate work in later bereavement, and begins (as in all other aspects of the illness) with establishing good contact, understanding, information and support at a very early phase of the disease, even if the longer-term difficulties are not in fact subsequently encountered or are long delayed. It is however not unusual for patients not to encounter a coherent plan for the care of their family until they and their relatives meet a team working in the terminal or palliative phase (for example a hospital support team, hospice staff or Macmillan nurses in the UK; in the United States this may be a hospice programme or a community out-reach programme rather than an inpatient unit). Saunders and McCorkle (1985) have thoughtfully described a variety of flexible models of care, which can be developed to support patients and other consumers in making informed decisions about treatment plans.

The last few years have shown an encouraging if qualitatively unequal increase in the number of studies on the quality of life in the final phase of an illness. It is also important to consider satisfaction with the actual quality of care. Kristjanson (1989) is engaged in a three-phase project designed to develop and test a tool to measure family satisfaction with terminal care. If this is successful it will be extremely important in the current debate since it is hard data (if truly measurable) about patient and family satisfaction and not soft, impressionistic hypotheses which will help us ultimately to determine the range of good practices which are most appropriate.

TREATMENT

Multidisciplinary Teamwork

The patient, individual family member and the constellation of individuals which go to make up the whole family will have different needs at different times. The ideal in any one unit or service is to ensure that a range of these facilities is available, including links with appropriate self-help groups and professionals from various psychosocial disciplines who can support, advise, lead if necessary, and provide consultation to such groups. Social workers and nurse therapists provide therapeutic skills, while clinical psychologists can assess needs and demonstrate behavioural management techniques for family members. An interested liaison psychiatrist with a practical, commonsense approach and ideally with an experience of the range of medical treatments encountered by cancer patients, can be aware of the likely effects of treatment on the patient's physical state, psychological functioning and likely psychosocial changes. An occupational therapist will help with hospital-to-home transitions and give advice about facilities and aids to daily living when activities are reduced or altered. An interested and experienced chaplain will provide appropriate explanation and spiritual support. Buckman (1988) describes an account of a fruitful co-operation between an effective chaplain and an oncologist.

Each of these professionals has a unique part to play in bringing their personal skills and talents to the continuing work with the patients' family, and has a responsibility for educating not only the family and the wider community, but other professionals on their team, in the range of skills which can be shared and acquired. A flexible approach and avoidance of demarcation disputes are more likely if the professionals in a unit or service are prepared to work together as a team.

Such a team is not an impossible ideal, and there are certainly many oncology units and services in existence, both in the UK, in Canada and the United States, where carefully thought-through co-ordination is working successfully. Although Europe has developed a little later than North America, it is rapidly catching up.

In psychiatric practice, particularly in large-scale mental health services, psychiatrists have had an opportunity during training to see the multidisciplinary team in practice and have come to accept their contribution to general care, and to understand the benefits of sharing tasks and expertise with others, nurses, psychologists, social workers. However in more traditionally orientated services, medical autonomy has been slower to change and until quite recently it was usually the hospice or support team which emphasized a team approach.

Teamwork has a supportive function for all the professionals concerned. As Stedeford (1984) has pointed out, it is all too easy in work of this kind for ideals to exceed capacity, for the single-handed or isolated staff member to feel that they cannot accomplish their targets or goals and to experience a sense of failure. Working together as a team helps avoid this, and fortunately the value of working together and sharing ideas, information and skills is now unchallenged.

Resources and Techniques

The work of the Lisa Sainsbury Foundation (see Appendix), a charitable organization set up in 1984 to support health care staff, has encouraged multidisciplinary ways of approaching the care of the cancer patient and their family, and has been enormously successful in changing attitudes and interprofessional rivalries. For the most part this has been achieved by an emphasis on experiential workshop seminars where staff from many disciplines learn how to work together as well as by teaching and lecturing. This concerted work provides a good model of cohesion for the family.

Many treatment approaches are available for families at all stages of the illness, ranging from cognitive and behavioural approaches, recreational and relaxational activities (Bailey, 1984; Johnson and Berendts, 1986), family-orientated multidisciplinary work or more sophisticated family therapy, normally carried out by professionals who have a special training and experience in this field, to the more formal psychotherapies, either group or individual.

Ideally, self-help or mutual aid groups work in very close collaboration rather than in competition with any of these approaches. They may be autonomous but will preferably have some professional input, supervision or leadership (Parkes, 1980). Berger (1984) described a drop-in support group for cancer patients and their families which is one variation of a relatively informal group. In the UK, patients and their families have increasingly voiced a need for facilities which encourage good communication between themselves and their professional care-givers, and the initiatives taken by groups such as 'Tak Tent' in Glasgow and the Bacup Organization have provided excellent models of ways in which information, feelings and help can be shared. (See Appendix for addresses.)

SPECIFIC TECHNIQUES

Improving Communication

As with more formal or traditional psychotherapies, interventions aimed at improving communication are available on an individual or group basis, and should be available for staff members too. The principles of preventative help for cancer patients and their families are described in detail in Moorey and Greer (1989). As they point out, there is evidence from at least two systematic studies (Lichtman and Taylor, 1986; Moynihan, 1987) concerning the general impression of those who work with cancer patients and their partners or families of a considerable undisclosed psychological morbidity. Moorey and Greer, in an approach which they call adjuvant psychological therapy (APT), explained the importance of evaluating, preventing or treating communication difficulties between partners (see also Moorey, this volume). This form of treatment, a cognitive-based therapy, is more properly considered as a form of psychotherapy. As with all therapies, the initial evaluation of need is paramount and a flexible approach is vital so that the patient, partner or family member may elect to have sessions together or separately.

Partners or family members may have even greater psychological needs than the patient with cancer. For example, one of my patients, faced with an equivocal but not life-threatening diagnosis wished to improve her psychological adjustment in order to minimize future stress, and maximize her 'fighting spirit' (Greer and Watson, 1987). She was helped on an individual basis using the principles of adjuvant psychological therapy. Her husband, a very anxious man, could not tolerate the explicit discussion of her symptoms, regularly saw her future and prognosis in excessively negative terms, and although from time to time we undertook joint sessions, it proved necessary for him to have some cognitive intervention on his own account before he could tolerate these. Far from adopting the typical denying, cheerful stance often described in such situations (Sabo *et al.*, 1986) the husband's overpessimistic reaction led to excessive strain on the patient who was herself determinedly and realistically optimistic.

Group Treatment

Couples treated together (Heinrich and Schag, 1985) derive equal benefit and improvement in knowledge about cancer in group therapy. The experimental group received cancer education, relaxation and a cognitive approach to problem-solving and activity management while a control group received conventional, routine care with group discussion.

Group and Individual Psychotherapy

Some recent studies (Baider, 1989; Maguire *et al.*, 1980) have questioned the universal assumption that all insight-giving psychodynamic orientated psychotherapies are necessarily helpful. Others (Saravay *et al.*, 1988) have proposed a simple framework with an emphasis particularly directed to providing a limited and practically-based form of psychotherapeutic intervention which will overwhelm neither patient nor therapist. One approach which has the value of clarifying the patient's and family's needs in relation to available services is described by Vess *et al.* (1988). By clarifying the subjects' concerns about family functioning (obtained from taped interviews with patients and spouses) and the interaction between themselves and the health care systems, health care providers can respond more effectively to their psychosocial needs.

A positive, non-pathology based approach is proposed by Pedersen and Valanis (1988) which steers emphasis away from the problems of the individual patient and towards identifying high-risk families who cannot adapt successfully. They suggest that further research should usefully compare families who enhance their lives positively and cope well with those who cope dysfunctionally or with difficulty.

In this family-orientated work we will sometimes meet an individual with previous psychological morbidity, or who is at increased risk of developing this, or who is currently displaying problems which may be only tangentially, if at all, related to the cancer of their close family member. Detecting such morbidity of course calls for imperative intervention if the symptoms or problems disclosed are likely to cause real difficulty either to the individual concerned, to the family as a whole, or are likely to have some negative impact on the patient. In this situation, as elsewhere, the skills available in a particular team may not be sufficient to deal effectively with psychological difficulties and the liaison psychiatrist or psychotherapist, if part of the team, may need to refer outside. Good liaison with a range of therapists working in different modalities is desirable, both for direct treatment from time to time, and to provide advice for the team.

Klagsbrun (1983) discusses the attributes and qualities of such a psychotherapist. He himself works with individuals and with small groups of cancer patients and their relatives. His clinical orientation, born of years of experience, is one of extreme flexibility of application of the psychotherapeutic skills involved in psychodynamic psychotherapy to the particular nature and set of difficulties encountered by the cancer patient and their family. Most psychiatrists in the UK who have had some experience of working over a period of time with cancer patients and their families (particularly chronically or terminally ill patients) and who have had contact with hospices (Parkes *et al.*, 1981) adopt this model.

For those who have not had this experience or who are diffident about putting their psychotherapeutic skills into practice for a group of people with such particular problems and crises to overcome, Whitman and Gustafson (1989) describe how to initiate, lead and analyse supportive group therapy meetings for families of individuals with cancer based on their experience of conducting more than 600 group sessions over 12 years. They suggest that most families will benefit from multiple therapy sessions and that even highly stressed families can benefit significantly from both multiple- and single-family therapy meetings. They emphasize the need for therapists to attend to nonverbal as well as verbal communications in families and to be flexible in adapting different interacting techniques for each type of therapy group. The meetings aim to overcome family members' resistance to discussing the real distress caused by the disease and to work through difficulties from the past, anxieties about the present, and fantasies about the future. Cain *et al.* (1986), Kreech (1975), Cunningham *et al.* (1978), Ferlic *et al.* (1979), Holland and Rowland (1989), Maguire *et al.* (1980), and many other authors have discussed the use of various psychotherapies with patients, ranging from short-term supportive and counselling approaches to more analytical therapies, for example, Bard (1959). Relatively few, have formally described work with heterogeneous groups including patients and their family members (Goldberg and Wool, 1985; Vess *et al.*, 1988; Whitman and Gustafson, 1989).

Educational Interventions

Educational interventions are useful because of the fear of patients and families with 'bothering' staff members. Many self-help groups, both locally and nationally, use a modified form of educational approach, bringing in 'experts', that is professionals, to explain and discuss some of the available treatments or deal with myths and fantasies which may exist about responses to treatment. Educational interventions may be required in the patient's social environment, family, the primary care physician or their staff, and in the patient's work place or school. Cassileth *et al.* (1982) demonstrated lowering anxiety levels in families who had access to audiovisual teaching materials prepared to enhance their understanding of the treatment programme. Similarly Rudolph *et al.* (1981) reported positive results of an extensive 'teaching' programme in a paediatric context. There is no reason of course why this should not be extended to the families and support systems of adult patients. Many other support groups, for example Berger (1984), have incorporated a teaching or educational component into their support system.

TABLE 1 *Educational interventions*

Recipient	Interventions
Patient	Classifying information about the medical condition (tests, diagnosis); treatment side-effects (and control of side-effects); medical system (costs, access)
	Reinforcing information from staff
	Identifying community resources
	Explaining expected emotional reactions
Family	Encouraging asking questions as needed (ways to cope)
	Preparing for common problems encountered at home and at work
	Facilitating their communication

The provision of educational information for patients and relatives, developing written materials, videotapes and written instruction, as well as 'live' presentation by staff, should all help to make the patient and family feel more involved, more active than passive in treatment. This leads naturally on to consideration of the place in psychosocial intervention of the 'fellow sufferer', befriender or self-help group. Self-help or mutual support groups, often involving patients and families with similar diagnosis and treatment, focus on education, practical advice and modelling of good coping styles (Cordoba *et al.*, 1984).

Unfortunately until quite recently many professionals have been oversensitive to the 'consumerist' and antiprofessional issues (such as may arise from misunderstandings over treatments or cause of death) with which they identify these groups. My own experience of working closely with such groups, drawn from patients and clients with quite widely differing psychosocial difficulties, has been nothing but educational and rewarding. The indications are that when the client/patient and family member feels that their needs are being understood and heard, particularly where other fellow suffers can validate their own experience and make them feel less strange or different, this is of undeniable reassurance to them.

Creativity as a Therapeutic Technique

Such studies as exist of the power of creative activity to improve the quality of life for patients using music and art therapy (Bailey, 1984; Johnson and Berendts, 1986) usually involved mixed patients and family groups. The value of the creative experience should not be underestimated as it can give patients and their families an opportunity for expression which does not necessarily depend on a high degree of skill and talent. Opportunities for music, art and drama therapy promote relaxation and distraction from current problems, as well as the opportunity to express emotion which they cannot articulate in words. A collection of poetry recently published (Stedeford, 1990) shows the value of poetry as a means of expression, by no means sad or morbid but very moving, in conveying the thoughts and feelings of patients and family members. Not all are as talented as she, but even a very busy team or unit might try a creative seminar or workshop with an invited experienced leader from the world of poetry or the arts, to stimulate experiments in this way. Existing anthologies of poetry (Whittaker, 1983), which largely deal with bereavement, or individual collections (Stedeford, 1990) can be used in informal discussion groups if participants lack the confidence to create their own works.

Family Therapy

Family therapy has become a highly sophisticated technique, although it is important for the team which has only limited access to a professional in the psychosocial field with suitable training and experience to take a family-centred approach. Rait and Lederberg (1989) urge all teams to look for problems in family members and to refer promptly before the situation becomes chaotic, but further urge that all professionals working in this field should learn to 'think family' even although they may not be trained family therapists. They provide an excellent review of the problems and approaches to family difficulties caused by the stress of cancer in one of their members. They quote Eisenberg *et al.* (1984) in an extensive survey and discussion of the effect of chronic illness on the family by developmental stage. Key sources for an understanding of the classical family therapy approach are Minuchin (1974), Cleese and Skynner (1983) and Minuchin and Minuchin (1987). These authors emphasize the need for flexibility and capacity to adapt and change under stress.

The family has a rich past experience, family myths and traditions, as well as recognized and unrecognized past events or personalities which have contributed to its present make-up. In the areas of past illness and loss much of the response to the present crisis can be understood, and even in the least sophisticated team, valuable information is obtained by helping the family to draw a genogram (a diagrammatic representation of the family tree). In this way gaps, deaths, significant events in the past, may guide our understanding of the present, and in particular may help to define and explain the interaction between family members and their past, present and future roles.

By taking this perspective on the family we can help to demonstrate the relationship between the family members and the health care team with its important implications for compliance, management and relationships. Cassileth (1979) reviews the 'socialization' of the family to the medical system. If oversocialization occurs the family may become too passive or unassertive. If there is too much conflict between the team and the family – a 'bad fit' – then the course of treatment becomes fraught with problems and complications, and the family may be scapegoated by the professions.

Imber-Coppersmith (1985) develops this theme further. This review should be read by any team which seriously wishes to achieve the right level of communication with families. The risks of overcompliance on the patient's/family's part and overcontrolling on the part of the professional are ever-present. Overcompliant families are passive and identify deeply with the treatment team ('good' families from the staff's point of view). Other reactions include surface compliance but hidden ambivalence, which may be expressed in disappointment, anger and blame, and may seriously disrupt the relationship between the family and the team. It is suggested (Rait and Lederberg, 1989) that this is less likely to occur when good open communication and trust have previously been established, but this is by no means always the case. Concerned staff on the team, working in often tiring and stressful conditions, naturally find, unless well-supported and with great psychological insights themselves, protesting and arguing families are extremely difficult and exhausting. It is important that someone on the team, or preferably an outside consultant providing staff support (who can be a professional in the psychosocial area with the appropriate skills, and need not be restricted to one particular discipline) can interpret the difficult behaviours for the staff so that they become more understandable.

Where these skills are not readily available, the team or unit which is planning good psychosocial care should try to achieve some instruction and training by sending a staff member to appropriate educational activities such as a short course on family therapy, or by inviting a suitable speaker to visit the unit to augment appropriate reading.

Treatment of Sexual Problems

It is increasingly being recognized that the problem of impaired sexual functioning in patient or partner must be addressed (Moorey and Greer, 1989; Maguire *et al.*, 1978; Moynihan, 1987 and this volume). Many professionals have previously failed to recognize, or ignored through inexperience or lack of ability, to take a sexual history of the various sexual disfunctions which are common. Severe illness, pain, depression or anxiety may indeed diminish sexual interest. This area is now recognized as an important area of stress for patients and their families, as reflected in the demand for seminars and workshops led by experienced facilitators from the Lisa Sainsbury Foundation. It is very important to assess what is appropriate and what does or does not represent a problem to the patient or partner. Buckman (1988) is particularly readable and practical on this point.

Moorey and Greer set out helpful models for assessment and treatment of sexual difficulties. The value of cognitive behavioural training with an emphasis on the processes of psychosocial problem solving when a complementary therapy such as relaxation is also used (Weissman *et al.*, 1980). Watson (1983) has carried out an extensive review of psychosocial interventions with patients covering the range of techniques available and their efficacy. There are often difficulties in interpreting or generalizing results to families, and researchers should study this review to appreciate the minefield of methodological problems. Vachon *et al.* (1982), Forester (1982) and Gordon *et al.* (1980) describe various approaches. If the whole family is the unit of care, then it is reasonable to suppose that a more general approach which can include any of the following: education, counselling, communication, psychodynamic exploration and environmental manipulation which have been used to benefit patients apply to the family as a whole. Practically orientated, non-invasive, supportive behavioural treatments are unlikely to do harm and may confer great benefit to families, spouses and partners.

BEREAVEMENT

Unlike sudden death from cardiovascular causes, road traffic accidents and other violent deaths, the death of the cancer patient is almost always anticipated, even though the exact prognosis and length of life span is, in many cases, difficult to calculate. So, in theory, there may well have been the opportunity for the family to be helped to prepare to some extent for the death and, given the right psychological circumstances, there may have been a period of anticipatory grieving. Even here, however, many families will say that when it happened, the death came as a shock and was too sudden, that they were still relatively unprepared.

The team caring for the family from the point of first contact throughout the illness should understand that the foundation of preparing the family for an eventual death is really laid at their first encounter. To do this they must have a thorough grounding in the theory and practice of bereavement care. Bereavement or loss is not in itself an illness or disease but the process whereby we separate from someone or something we have lost and this implies a previous attachment. Grief and mourning are the emotions felt during this state and different individuals encounter and experience this in different ways. Not all will require intensive intervention, but studies by Parkes (1980) have confirmed the increased risk of psychiatric and psychosomatic disorders associated with disruption by death of a close relationship. Personal counselling early in bereavement to prevent later problems may be required by up to a third of widows and widowers to reduce the likelihood of psychosomatic symptoms. It is important to distinguish the principles of bereavement counselling to facilitate the expression of normal grief (see Table 2) and the tasks of grief therapy, which is a more sophisticated professional task usually requiring a professional, as opposed to a lay or befriending, background. Some knowledge of behavioural modification principles and

---

TABLE 2   *Principles of bereavement counselling (from Worden, 1984)*

- Recognize the loss
- Identify and ventilate feelings
- Explore life without the deceased
- Discourage emotional withdrawal
- Allow time for grief
- Allow for individual differences
- Provide continued support
- Examine coping styles (defences)
- Identify pathology (may require specialist referral)

---

some knowledge of psychodynamic processes and psychopathology are also helpful. The most useful small text in this context is by Worden (1984). Members of the team should understand the advantages and disadvantages of preparation or anticipatory grief, 'worry work', and how these processes affect different people and may be modified by special circumstances (Worden, 1983; Raphael, 1985; Stroebe and Stroebe, 1987).

Good practice includes an attempt to identify for special monitoring and follow-up those at particular risk of difficulties following bereavement (see p. 183). Whilst encouraging and developing the potential for growth and change in all family members the team should not undermine the coping capacity of the great majority. It has been suggested that there is both an opportunity and an obligation for oncology specialists and their teams to provide care and comfort of the patient, with guidance of the family through the phases of terminal illness and death, Koocher (1986). It is certainly true that, as outlined earlier in this chapter, careful and sensitive handling of the family, clear communication and understanding of the group and individual sensitivities of families members, can greatly improve the prospects of a good outcome from the bereavement phase. Families recall vividly how the initial diagnosis was handled, how accessible the team was throughout all phases of the illness and how the last phase of illness was managed.

Chochinov and Holland (1986) remind us that survivors may have intense but ambivalent feelings about the oncologist and support staff because of this special relationship and because of the memories which they evoke. The family and their sick relative were dependent on them for care and are usually grateful to them, yet they may be the focus for nagging questions of doubt or 'bargaining' which follows any loss: 'Was everything done correctly? Could it have been prevented? Did anything go wrong?' Individuals who have not resolved past losses, separations or bereavements may have difficulty in facing the prospect of loss by death.

Chochinov and Holland further suggest that the oncologist is uniquely placed to assist the relatives through anticipated bereavement. This, too, perhaps reflects a North American experience based on extensive work at the Memorial Sloan Kettering Institute and the highly sophisticated application of a wide range of skills in the oncology team. In the UK, the oncologist in person may not necessarily have access to appropriate psychosocial skills but, ideally, working within a multi-disciplinary team they will be able to make contributions towards the care of the patient and family and will both learn from other team members, with psychosocial backgrounds, as well as contributing to their colleagues' understanding of the disease.

Earlier estimates of substantial mortality from cardiovascular causes, 'dying of grief' and 'a broken heart' have been modified by better controlled studies and appear to be rather less. However bereavement morbidity is still substantial. Increases in smoking, alcohol and frequent visits to the general practitioner have all been documented. More recently, Schleifer (1983) and others have prescribed alterations of immune function following bereavement. Apart from physical risks, the psychological risks and morbidity still appear to be significant. Stroebe and Stroebe (1987) have carefully re-examined the evidence for some of the above assumptions and for a detailed discussion of this area the reader is advised to consult their excellent work.

Definitions of Grief and Bereavement

The team should at least be able to understand the processes of preparation for bereavement, the features of normal grieving and be able to identify abnormal patterns of grief reaction, for which specialist help or referral is necessary. Osterweiss *et al.*'s 1984 definitions are given below:

Bereavement refers to the loss of someone through death. Bereavement reactions are the psychological, or behavioural responses to bereavement.

Grief is the feeling (affect) resulting from the loss and associated behaviour, such as crying; the grieving process is the changing affect over time.

Mourning is used to refer to the social expressions in response to loss and grief, including mourning rituals and behaviours specific to each culture and religion. Bowlby (1961, 1980) and Parkes (1986), have helped us to understand the psychological process involved in loss based on attachment theory. Understanding separation and loss involves understanding the processes involved in the rupture of affectional and attachment bonds. Parkes (ibid) whose description of the initial phases of numbness, yearning, searching, motor restlessness, leading to disorganization, disinterest, depression and despair, finally achieving, if possible, some degree of acceptance, helps us to understand the emotions of the newly bereaved. Education of the public and the individual in these areas, once death has occurred, helps the bereaved to understand their experience and to reassure them that they are not 'going mad' as some fear.

Bereavement can also be understood in the light of *crisis theory*, for loss of spouse has been regarded as the event resulting in most change in adult life (Holmes and Rahe, 1967). Failure of adaptation can result in profound disorganization, whereas effective coping may lead to adaptations, emotional growth and change.

Vachon, in 1987, drew attention to the effect of unresolved losses on the resolution or adaptation to a current bereavement. It is simple and important to take a history of previous losses, particularly identifying those that seem not to have been adequately worked through. A similar technique which frequently produces extremely helpful information in working with bereaved relatives is to take a separation history. A past history of difficult separations, clinging and dependent behaviour, whether or not accompanied by overprotection on the part of parents or other relatives, can often indicate a likely difficulty in separating effectively from the deceased. Certainly in clinical practice with bereaved people referred for bereavement difficulties, especially chronic grief reactions, I find that this is often useful in clarifying particular forms of response which have developed following a major loss.

Fortunately the team is not alone in its efforts to counsel or treat bereaved people. In the UK, particularly in the last ten years, the level of professional and public re-education about bereavement has undergone an enormous change, largely thanks to the initial efforts of psychiatrists such as Colin Murray-Parkes, the organization Cruse (see Appendix) for the bereaved, and many smaller organizations which have evolved to help the bereaved in particular forms of loss. In many areas, whether or not there is a Cruse group, health authorities and others are now recognizing the value of this work and setting up bereavement services of their own. The principles are to establish that the need for appropriate grieving and expression of feeling is natural, normal, to be encouraged, and that suppression of feelings may lead to later difficulties; to help to identify those people whose bereavement reaction is not proceeding at an appropriate rate or in an appropriate manner, and to provide special help for those in this category.

Unfortunately there are still many people who fall through the net of these various services. The resulting economic and health costs to the individual, the family and the state are, of course, enormous.

The loss effect.   Stroebe and Stroebe (1987) re-evaluated the relationship between bereavement and physical health and this now appears to be a weaker association than that between bereavement and mental health. The most convincing evidence of a relationship between bereavement and general health comes from the association with mortality. Overall, although available studies are not without inconsistencies and problems, there is convincing support for the loss effect. Whether one looks at the rate of psychiatric disorder, physical illness or mortality, comparisons of married and widowed people support the conclusion that the experience of partner loss is associated with health deterioration.

Risk factors. If the main effects of gender on health are controlled, widowers are found to suffer greater detriments compared with married men than are widows compared with married women. In fact, it has sometimes been found that depression in samples of widowers is greater than in widows even when non-bereaved controls are not included.

This leads us to a consideration of the effect of social support. Personality traits are also relevant to the impact of bereavement or loss on individuals. However, many of the reported studies lack non-bereaved control groups and it is often difficult to draw other than anecdotal conclusions about the importance of personality factors as moderators of bereavement reactions. Of all the factors suggested as predicting poor outcome after bereavement (age, gender, social support, socioeconomic status, previous bereavement, health before bereavement, antecedent and current stresses, religion and personality, the mode of death and duration of terminal illness) conclusions from many studies seem to implicate gender, age, anticipation of the loss and dependency or ambivalence in the relationship, particularly in work relating to spouse bereavement – for example, Parkes (1975), and the study of Chicago widows by Lopata (1979).

While it may seem strange that partners who have happy marriages and loving relationships may have better health outcomes in bereavement than those who are intensely involved and dependent or whose marriages are full of conflict, this may not be so paradoxical as it appears. Children securely attached to their mothers do not need to cling to them, whereas in insecure relationships overdependent or ambivalent feelings may produce the same reaction as the clinging attachments of small children and an intolerance of separation.

Finally most of this work confirms the generally positive effect of good social support, and conversely, the risk of poor outcome if social support is generally lacking. In the clinical situation, although it may be easy to identify an individual who has a large number of risk factors, the exact prediction of risk is difficult and has to be made on the best available evidence in each case, taking into account the potential interactions between positive and negative risk factors.

SERVICE ORGANIZATION SUMMARY

Good care of the cancer patient's family depends on the individual contributions of patients, families and the team. It is therefore important to:

(1) Recognize the individual worth and contribution of each profession in the team; skills are complementary, not competitive.

(2)   Try to ensure representation of at least one of each 'contributor' to psychosocial care of the family (liaison psychiatrist, clinical psychologist, general practice liaison nurse, social worker). Remember the need for holidays and sick leave; duplicate if possible or arrange for back-up. Balance continuity with need to allow staff to move on, seek promotion or leave unit gracefully.

(3)   Discourage exclusivity of involvement (which leads to dependence of families and patients and 'battle fatigue' of professionals). Rather, allow sharing of tasks and information with team and family.

(4)   Enlist if possible outside 'informal' and if necessary voluntary support in order that staff members have access to personal support/supervision to preserve objectivity and reduce stress.

(5)   Consider whether team 'staff support' person should not be member of team but rather from outside the unit.

(6)   Plan regular clinical meetings but take time for social/sports activity as a group, too. Continuing education is also stress reducing; family therapy workshops, Cruse courses and workshops from outside agencies help staff to learn other techniques and improve confidence.

(7)   Try to allow families *flexible time* and *space* on the unit, but also consider organized group meetings. These allow sharing of feelings and ideas between families and team, and also help them to relax and to feel less threatened and more supported. Sometimes such meetings can be used for general information and education (for example, procedures on unit, patient care on discharge home, likely later symptoms, prognosis, etc.). Contributors can include oncologist, specialist nurse, indeed any member of the team with information to share.

(8)   Monitor emotional as well as social needs of family members (through the team's social worker, clinical psychologist, for example).

(9)   Refer for consultation (e.g. to liaison or local psychiatrist) vulnerable people or those with persistent or inappropriate response or behaviour early rather than late, making or maintaining good links for them with community resources, voluntary and 'befriending' agencies.

(10)   Co-ordinate and plan bereavement care. Follow-up support meetings are helpful and staff such as psychiatric social workers and clinical psychologists allow further monitoring of family bereavement response. Be sure to establish referral consultation

links first to general practitioner, Cruse counsellors and psychiatrists where necessary.

APPENDIX   *Useful addresses*

The Lisa Sainsbury Foundation
8–10 Crown Hill
Croydon
Surrey CRO 1RY
Tel: (081) 686 8808

(An invaluable source of workshops, with a comprehensive reading and audiovisual list; videotapes are also available.)

Tak Tent/Cancer Support
Organization
G Block
Western Infirmary
Glasgow G11 6NT
Tel: (041) 332 3639

The Bacup Organization
The British Association of Cancer
Patients
121–123 Charterhouse Street
London EC1M 6AA
Tel: (071) 608 1661

The British Association of
Counselling
37a Sheep Street
Rugby
Tel: (0788) 78328/9

Cancer Link
46 Pentonville Road
London N1 9HF
Tel: (071) 833 2451

Cruse
Cruse House
126 Sheen Road
Richmond
Surrey TW9 1UR
Tel: (081) 940 4818

(Provide an extensive professional reading list as well as suitable books for bereaved people.)

References

BAIDER, L. and DE NOUR, A.K. (1989) Group therapy for adolescent patients. *Journal of Adolescent Health Care, 10*, 35–38.

BAILEY, L.M. (1984) The use of songs in music therapy with cancer patients and their families. *Music Therapy, 4*(1), 5–17.

BERGER, J.M. (1984) Crisis intervention: A drop-in support group for cancer patients and their families. *Social Work Health Care, 10*(2), 81–92.

BLACK, D. and URBANOWITZ, M. (1987) Family intervention with bereaved children. *Journal of Child Psychology and Child Psychiatry, 28*, 467–476.

BLUGLASS, K. (1986) Caring for the family. In B.A. Stoll (Ed.), *Coping With Cancer Stress*. Lancaster: Nijhoff.

BODKIN, C.M., PISOTT, T.J. and MANN, J.R. (1982) Financial burden of childhood cancer. *British Medical Journal, 284*, 1542–1544.

186 *Kerry Bluglass*

BOWLBY, J. (1961) Process of mourning. *International Journal of Psychoanalysis*, 42, 317–340.
BOWLBY, J. (1980) Loss, Sadness and Depression. London: Hogarth Press.
BROADWELL, D.C. (1987) Rehabilitation needs of the patient with cancer. *Journal of Cancer*, 60, 563–568.
BUCKMAN, R. (1988) I don't know what to say: How to help and support someone who is dying. London: Macmillan.
CAIN, E.N., KOHORN, E.I., LATIMER, K. and SCHWARTZ, P.E. (1986) Psychosocial benefits of a cancer support group. *Cancer*, 57, 183–189.
CANCER CARE, INC and NATIONAL CANCER FOUNDATION (1977) *Listen to the Children: A study of the impact on the mental health of children of a parent's catastrophic illness.* New York: Cancercare Inc. and National Cancer Foundation.
CASSILETH, B.R. (Ed.) (1979) The Cancer Patient: Social and medical aspects of care. Philadelphia: Lea Febiger.
CASSILETH, B.R., HEIBERGER, R.M., MARCH V. and SUTTON-SMITH, K. (1982) Effect of audiovisual cancer program on patients and families. *Journal of Medical Education*, 57, 54–59.
CHOCHINOV, H. and HOLLAND, J.C. (1986) Bereavement: A special study in oncology. In J.C. Holland and J.H. Rowland (Eds), *Handbook of Psychosocial Oncology: Psychological care of the patient with cancer.* New York: Oxford University Press.
CLEESE, J. and SKYNNER R. (1983) *Families and How to Survive Them.* London: Tavistock.
CORDOBA, C., SHEAR, M.B., FOBAIR, P. and HALL, J. (1984) *Cancer Support Groups' Practice Handbook.* Oakland, California: American Cancer Society.
CREECH, R.H. (1975) The psychologic support of the cancer patient: A medical oncologist's viewpoint. *Seminars in Oncology*, 2, 285–292.
CUNNINGHAM, J., STRASSBERG, D. and ROBACK H. (1978) Group psychotherapy for medical patients. *Comprehensive Psychiatry*, 19, 135–40.
EISENBERG, M.G., SUTKIN, L.C. and JANSEN, M.A. (Eds) (1984) *Chronic Illness and Disability Through the Life Span: Effects on self and family.* New York: Springer.
FERLIC M., GOLDMAN A. and KENNEDY B.J. (1979) Group counselling in adult patients with advanced cancer. *Cancer*, 43, 760–766.
FERRARO, K.F. (1985) The effect of widowhood on the health status of older persons. *International Journal of Ageing and Human Development*, 21, 9–25.
FORRESTER, B., KORNFIELD, D.S. and FLEISS, J. (1982) Effects of psychotherapy on patients' distress during radiotherapy for cancer. *Psychosomatic Medicine*, 44, 118.
GLASER, B.G. and STRAUSS, A.L. (1966) *Awareness of Dying.* Chicago: Aldine.
GLASER, B.G. and STRAUSS, A.L. (1968) *Time For Dying.* Chicago: Aldine.
GOLDBERG, R.J. and WOOL, M.S. (1985) Psychotherapy for spouses of lung cancer patients: Assessment of an intervention. *Psychotherapeutic Psychosomatics*, 43(3), 141–150.
GORDON, W.A., FREIDENBERGS, I., DILLER, L., HIBBARD, M., WOLFE, C., LEVINE, L., LIPKINS, R., EZRACHI, O. and LUCIDO, D. (1980) Efficacy of psychosocial intervention with cancer patients. *Journal of Consulting and Clinical Psychology*, 48, 743–759.
GREER, S. and WATSON, M. (1987) Mental adjustment to cancer: Its measurement and prognostic importance. *Cancer Survey*, 6, 1439–1453.
HEINRICH, R.L. and SCHAG, C.C. (1985) Stress and activity management: Group

treatment for cancer patients and spouses: *Journal of Counselling and Clinical Psychology*, 53, 439–446.

HOLLAND, J.C. and ROWLAND, J.H. (1989) *Handbook of Psychosocial Oncology: Psychological care of the patient with cancer*. New York: Oxford University Press.

HOLMES, T. and RAHE, R.H. (1967) The social readjustment rating scale. *Journal of Psychosomatic Research*, 11, 213–218.

IMBER-COPPERSMITH E. (1985) Families and Multiple Helpers. In D. Campbell and R. Draper (Eds) *Application of Systemic Family Therapy: The Milan approach*. London: Grune and Stratton.

JOHNSON, J.L. and BERENDTS, C.A. (1986) Arts and Flowers: Drawing out the patient's best: The 'we can' weekend. *American Journal of Nursing, Feb*, 86(2), 164–166.

KLAGSBRUN, S. (1983) The making of a cancer psychotherapist. *Journal of Psychosocial Oncology*, 1, 55–60.

KOOCHER, G.P. (1986) Coping with a death from cancer. *Journal of Consulting and Clinical Psychology, Oct*, 54(5), 623–631.

KOOCHER, G. and O'MALLEY, J. (1981) The Damocles Syndrome: Psychological consequences of surviving childhood cancer. New York: McGraw-Hill.

KRISTJANSON, L.J. (1989) Quality of terminal care: Salient indicators identified by families. *Journal of Palliative Care, Mar*, 5(1), 21–30.

LANSKY, S.B., CAIRNS, N., CLARKE, G., LOWMAN, J.T., MILLER, L. and TRUEWORTHY, R.C. (1979) Childhood Cancer: Non-medical costs of the illness. *Cancer*, 43, 403–408.

LICHTMAN, P.R. and TAYLOR, S.E. (1986) Close relationships and the female cancer patient. In B.L. Anderson (Ed.) *Women with Cancer*. New York: Springer.

LITMAN, T.J. (1974) The family as the basic unit in health and medical care. *Social Science and Medicine*, 8, 495–519.

LOPATA, H.Z. (1979) *Women as widows: Support systems*. New York: Elsevier.

MAGUIRE, G.P., LEE, E.G. and BEVINGTON, D.J. (1978) Psychiatric problems in the first year after mastectomy. *British Medical Journal*, 1, 963-969.

MAGUIRE, G.P., TAIT, A., BROOKE, M., THOMAS, C. and SELWOOD, R. (1980) Effect of counselling on the psychiatric morbidity associated with mastectomy. *British Medical Journal*, 281, 1454–1456.

MANOS, N. and CHRISTAKIS, K. (1981) Attitudes of cancer specialists toward their patients in Greece. *International Journal of Psychiatry in Medicine*, 10, 305–313.

MANOS, N. and CHRISTAKIS, J. (1985) Coping with cancer: Psychological dimensions. *Acta Psychiatrica Scandinavica*, 72, 1–5.

MANSELL PATTISON, E.M. (1977) *The Experience Of Dying*. London: Prentice-Hall.

MCCUBBIN, H.I. (1979) Integrating coping behaviour in family stress theory. *Journal of Marriage and Family*, 41, 237–244.

MCCUBBIN, H.I. and FIGLEY, C. (Eds) (1983) *Stress and the Family*. New York: Brunner-Mazel.

MCKEEVER, P. (1983) Siblings of chronically ill children: A literature review with implications for treatment and practice. *American Journal of Orthopsychiatry*, 53, 209–217.

MINUCHIN, S. (1974) *Families and Family Therapy*. Cambridge, Mass: Harvard University Press.

MINUCHIN, P. and MINUCHIN, S. (1987) Family as the context for patient care. In

L.H. Bernstein, A.J. Grieco and M. Dete (Eds). *Primary Care in the Home*. Philadelphia: Lippincott.

MOOREY, S. and GREER, S. (1989) *Psychological Therapy for Patients with Cancer: A new approach*. Oxford: Heinemann.

MOYNIHAN, C. (1987) Testicular cancer: The psychosocial problems of patients and their relatives. *Cancer Surveys, 6*, 477–510.

MURINEN, J.M. (1986) The economics of informal care. Labor market effects in the National Hospice Study. *Medical Care, 24*, 1007–1017.

NORTHOUSE, L. (1984) The impact of cancer on the family: An overview. *International Journal of Psychiatry and Medicine, 14*, 215–242.

NORTHOUSE, L.L. (1988) Social support in patients' and husbands' adjustment to breast cancer. *Nursing Research, 37(2)*, 91–95.

OAKLEY, A. (1982) Conventional families. In R.N. Rapoport, M.P. Fogarty and R. Rapoport (Eds). *Families in Britain*. London: Routledge & Kegan Paul.

OSTERWEIS, M., SOLOMON, F. and GREEN, M. (1984) *Bereavement: Reactions, consequences and care*. Washington: National Academy Press.

PARKES, C.M. (1975) Determinants of outcome following bereavement. *Omega, 6*, 303–323.

PARKES, C.M. (1980) Bereavement counselling: Does it work? *British Medical Journal, 281*, 3–6.

PARKES, C.M. (1986) *Bereavement: Studies of grief in adult life*. London: Penguin. (Originally published in 1972.)

PARKES, C.M. and STEVENSON-HINDE, T. (1982) The Place of Attachment in Human Behaviour. London: Tavistock.

PARKES, C.M., FRYER, J. and KLAGSBRUN, S. (1981) The role of the psychiatrist in the care of the dying. *Bulletin of the Royal College of Psychiatrists, October, 5*, No 10.

PEDERSON, L.M. and VALANIS, B.G. (1988) The effects of breast cancer on the family: A review of the literature. *Journal of Psychosocial Oncology, 6(1/2)*, 95–118.

PLANT, H., RICHARDSON, J., STUBBS, L., LYNCH, D., ELLWOOD, J., SLEVIN, M. and DE-HAES, H. (1987) Evaluation of a support group for cancer patients and their families and friends. *British Journal of Hospital Medicine, Oct. 38(4)*, 317–322.

RAIT, D. and LEDERBERG, M. (1989) The family of the cancer patient. In J.C. Holland and J. Rowland (Eds) *Psychosocial Oncology*. Oxford University Press.

RUDOLPH, L.A., PENDERGRASS, T.W., CLARKE, J., KJOSNESS, M. and HARTMANN, J.R. (1981) Development of an education programme for parents of children with cancer. *Social Work Health Care, 6*, 43–54.

SABO, D., BROWN, J. and SMITH, C. (1986) The male role and mastectomy: Support groups and men's adjustment. *Journal of Psychosocial Oncology, 4*, 19–31.

SARAVAY, S.M., LOVETTE, E., TANENBAUM, C. and MCCARTNEY, L. (1988) Psychotherapeutic approaches to the cancer patient. *Clinical Social Work Journal, 16(1)*, 43–51.

SAUNDERS, J.M. and MCCORKLE, R. (1985) Models of care for persons with progressive cancer. *Nursing Clinics of North America, 20(2)*, 365–377.

SCHLEIFER, S.J., KELLER, S.E., CAMERINO, M., THORNTON, J.C. and STEIN, M. (1983) Suppression of lymphocyte stimulation following bereavement. *JAMA, July 15, 250, 3*, 374–377.

SELIGMAN, M.E.P. (1975) *Helplessness*. San Francisco: Freeman.

SIMONTON, S.M. (1984) *The Healing Family*. London: Bantam.

STAM, H.J., BULTZ, B.D. AND PITTMAN, C.A. (1986) Psychosocial problems and interventions in a referred sample of cancer patients. *Psychosomatic Medicine*, 48, 539–548.

STEDEFORD, A. (1984) *Facing Death: Patients, families and professionals*. Oxford: Heineman Medical Books.

STEDEFORD, A. (1990) *Elipse*. Oxford: Amate Press.

STROEBE, W. and STROEBE, M.S. (1987) *Bereavement and health. The psychological and physical consequences of partner loss*. Cambridge: Cambridge University Press.

TEETER, M.A., HOLMES, G.E., HOLMES, F.F. and BAKER, A.B. (1987) Decisions about marriage and family among survivors of childhood cancer. *Journal of Psychosocial Oncology*, 5(4), 59–68.

VACHON, M.L.S. (1987) Unresolved grief in persons with cancer referred for psychotherapy. *Psychiatric Clinics of North America*, 10(3), 467–480.

VACHON, M.L.S., LYALL, W.A.L. and ROGERS, J. (1982) The effectiveness of psychosocial support during post-surgical treatment of breast cancer. *International Journal of Psychiatry and Medicine*, 11, 365–372.

VERRES, R. (1985) The cancer patient and his environment. *Geburtshilfe: Frauenheilkund*, 45(9), 583–591.

VESS, J.D., MORELAND, J.R., SCHWEBEL, A.I. and KRAUT, E. (1988) Psychosocial needs of cancer patients: Learning from patients and their spouses. *Journal of Psychosocial Oncology*, 6(1/2), 31–51.

WATSON, M. (1983) Psychosocial intervention with cancer patients: A review. *Psychological Medicine*, 13, 839–846.

WHITMAN, H.H. and GUSTAFSON, J.P. (1989) Group therapy for families facing a cancer crisis. *Oncology Nursing Forum*, 16(4), 539–543.

WHITTAKER, A. (1983) *All in the End is Harvest*. London: Dartman, Longman Todd in association with CRUSE.

WOODS, N.F., LEWIS, F.M. and ELLISON, E. (1989) Living with cancer: Family experiences. *Cancer Nursing, Feb*, 12(1), 28–33.

WORDEN, J.W. (1983) *Grief Counselling and Grief Therapy*. London: Tavistock.

Part II

Treatment methods for specific diagnostic groups

LUNG CANCER

Ann Cull

There are over three quarters of a million cancer deaths in the twelve member countries of the European Community each year. Lung cancer is the leading cause of cancer deaths in males, responsible for 28 per cent of all male cancer deaths (CRC, 1988). Lung cancer is the commonest cancer in the UK causing a quarter of all cancer deaths (CRC, 1989). The incidence rates in Scotland are among the highest in the world – 113 per 100,000 men and 52 per 100,000 women (Registrar General Scotland, 1988).

The Edinburgh Lung Cancer Group reviewing a series of patients newly diagnosed with lung cancer between 1981 and 1984 reported a median age at diagnosis of 66.8 years. The age distribution of this sample of 2586 patients, which is not atypical, is shown in Table 1 (Capewell, 1985).

TABLE 1 *Age distribution of newly diagnosed lung cancer patients*

Age in years	50 years	50–59	60–69	70 yrs	
Percentage distribution	4%	20%	39%	36%	n = 2586

Thus group data refer predominantly to middle-aged and elderly men and acknowledgement of their life stage and consequent personal concerns is an important consideration in psychological care. The pattern is however changing.

The proportion of women among lung cancer patients has doubled in the last 25 years and the absolute incidence rate has more than trebled since 1960 (Registrar General Scotland, 1988). Lung cancer has overtaken breast cancer as the commonest cause of death from cancer among Scottish women (Scottish Home and Health Department, 1985).

Incidence rates, which rise steeply with increasing age, are closely related to trends in cigarette smoking, with a lag period of 20-30 years (Geddes, 1979). Between 1976 and 1984 the per capita consumption of cigarettes has increased in Spain, Portugal, Italy and Greece, which will lead to higher death rates from lung cancer in the future. Other EC nations (except France) show promising decreases in per capita cigarette consumption (CRC, 1988). As the prevalence of smoking is slowly falling so lung cancer mortality rates are beginning to fall in younger age groups in Britain though for women mortality rates are still rising in the older age groups (see Figure 1).

In 1958 there were no major social class differences in smoking behaviour. Now unskilled working men are twice as likely to smoke as professionally employed men. Smoking behaviour among women shows similar but less marked social class differences. These trends may be expected to influence future demographic patterns of incidence of lung cancer.

There are also worrying data about the smoking behaviour of contemporary young people. By the age of 15–16 24 per cent of boys and 26 per cent of girls in Scotland will have become regular smokers. In England the figures are 18 per cent and 27 per cent respectively (Goddard and Ikin, 1987).

There are three strategies for the control of cancer: prevention, screening for earlier detection and treatment. The impact of screening on mortality from lung cancer has been disappointing. There have been no major developments in treatment which have significantly improved survival. A small number of patients may be cured by surgery but the overall five-year survival rate for lung cancer remains less than 10 per cent. Generally then it is the need for prevention which must be emphasized if lives are to be saved and it can be argued that the main thrust of psychological intervention should be to this end.

Given public awareness of the link between cigarette smoking and lung cancer and the fact that the proportion of non-smokers developing the disease is about 3 per cent (Capewell, 1985), the majority of patients presenting with lung cancer have to deal with the uncomfortable knowledge of having contributed to their own life-threatening disease. Sensitivity to the issues which this raises for patients is an important aspect of their psychological care.

LUNG CANCER AND SMOKING

The Royal College of Physicians first drew public attention to the health risks of cigarette smoking in 1962. Since then a huge research literature has grown up reinforcing the conclusion that cigarette smoking causes lung cancer and extensive health education campaigns have sought to publicize this information. The vast majority of the population now knows of the risks of smoking and most smokers say they want to stop smoking. Progress has however been slow. Smoking behaviour has proved notoriously resistant to intervention. The typical success rate of specialized smoking clinics at one year

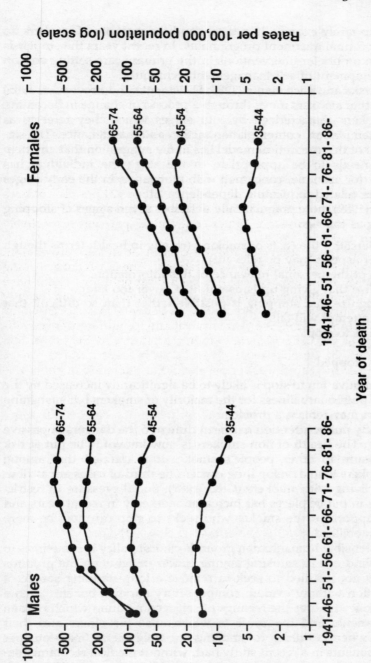

FIGURE 1 Mortality time trends in England and Wales 1941–1985

follow-up rarely exceeds 15 per cent and the majority of smokers do not seek formal treatment programmes. In recent years the emphasis has been on briefer interventions in the primary care setting and on the development of self-management techniques.

Prochaska and Diclemente (1983; Diclemente and Prochaska, 1985) suggest that smokers move through a process of change in becoming non-smokers characterized by four stages which they refer to as pre-contemplation, contemplation, action and maintenance. The significance of this theoretical model lies in the suggestion that any help offered needs to be appropriate to the stage the individual has reached (for example, concerned with motivation in the early stages and more related to nicotine dependence later).

Jarvis (1989) more pragmatically describes seven stages of stopping smoking as follows:

(1) Understand the costs of smoking (chiefly in health terms though other aspects may be relevant).
(2) Accept the personal relevance of this information.
(3) Realize that giving up is useful (it is never too late).
(4) Recognize that stopping is possible rather than so difficult that any attempt will fail.
(5) Decide to stop.
(6) Stop.
(7) Stay stopped.

Clearly motivation to stop is likely to be significantly increased by the onset of pulmonary illness for the majority of smokers but sustaining the effort may remain a problem.

Recently public attention has been drawn to the dangers of passive smoking. The health of non-smokers is now known to be put at risk by exposure to other people's smoke. It is claimed that among non-smokers who develop lung cancer one third of cases are attributable to living with smokers (CRC, 1989). Social pressure to restrict smoking in public places has increased markedly in recent years and social support for the smoker who seeks to stop can now be more readily mobilized.

On ostensibly humanitarian grounds clinical policy is sometimes to turn a blind eye to smoking among cancer patients on the grounds that it is not justified to seek to remove a long-standing source of gratification without evident compensatory survival benefit. Such a global policy ignores the feelings of self-recrimination which burden some patients and the conflicts which arise for others and their families where attitudes to smoking are ambivalent. Sixty-four per cent of patients in a recent study had, without medical recommendation, stopped smoking on becoming ill. However it is difficult for them to 'stay stopped' without appropriate support. Furthermore in avoiding this issue an important opportunity to influence the smoking behaviour of other family members is missed.

This is not to advocate an evangelical crusade toward lung cancer patients and their families. Jarvis (1989) outlined a brief procedure for raising the issue of smoking in a primary care setting. This simple approach could be incorporated by any health professional into everyday clinical routines and would allow patients who so wish the opportunity to talk about and/or modify their smoking behaviour without coercing those who do not. Against this background it is also legitimate to enquire about the smoking behaviour of those who share the patient's home environment.

(1) Ask all patients about their smoking and record it in the notes.
(2) Advise all smokers to stop. Do not press the reluctant but use the record in the notes as a prompt to raise the issue again.
(3) For those who want to stop offer advice about how to go about it and set a target day for stopping.
(4) Jarvis recommends nicotine chewing gum for those who have tried unsuccessfully to stop smoking in the past. He emphasizes the importance of giving these patients a clear rationale and specific instructions for the use of the gum.
(5) Offer supportive follow-up within a few days of the chosen quit date.

Realistically the response rate may be quite low but current opinion is now in favour of persuading health professionals that such simple efforts sustained over time can make a useful contribution to reducing smoking.

What Help Can Be Offered?

Coping with feelings. An important element of counselling is often helping people to let go of unsatisfactory aspects of the past which cannot be changed in favour of focusing on the present where positive change is still possible. Some lung cancer patients need to deal with self-recrimination about their smoking behaviour, particularly intentions to quit that were never actualized or previously failed attempts. It may be necessary for them to reflect on their smoking behaviour in the light of social trends as a means of relieving some personal guilt; for example, many current patients formed the habit during the war years when smoking was actively encouraged. For those patients the motivation to stop smoking is often high but help may be needed in overcoming dependency. Others who have successfully defended themselves against health education propaganda in order to continue smoking may experience more conflict on diagnosis as to whether it is now worth stopping. Tension results when the patient and their family resolve this conflict differently. Some families need a safe outlet for anger and blame of the patient for having brought on his or her own illness, particularly if smoking has been a contentious issue in the family and continues after the diagnosis.

Stopping smoking.   There are a number of publications available to help people stop smoking (Glasgow and Rosen, 1978; 1979) and some written information can usefully be offered when the recommendation to stop is made. Usually it is suggested that patients stop completely on a target date but if this is impossible some goal of limiting consumption (for example, number of cigarettes smoked, lower tar content) may be agreed.

The evidence suggests simple self-help strategies tailored to individual needs are most effective in helping patients to stop and avoid resuming smoking. Cognitive, behavioural and social techniques may be employed:

Cognitive – to sustain motivation patients will need to maintain a positive attitude to themselves and the value of stopping smoking. Being able to identify and challenge self-defeating thinking using the methods of cognitive therapy (described by Moorey in this volume) can be helpful.

Behavioural – appetitive habits are often under stimulus control; that is, the patient learns an association between certain situations (for example having a cup of tea or feeling upset) and having a cigarette. These situations then become powerful cues to lighting up. Smokers can be helped by identifying such situations in their own lives which trigger smoking and then working out how to avoid or deal differently with them. Hospital attendance could provide not only a useful interruption to the smoking habit but an opportunity to learn other coping strategies (such as relaxation techniques for managing tension). Giving up something pleasurable requires compensatory reward and patients may need encouragement to find positive reinforcement for their efforts particularly at a time when potential rewards may be curtailed by illness and treatment.

Social – social support from family members and fellow patients can be an important aid to stopping smoking. Involving others offers the opportunity to influence the health of a wider group as well as providing a source of reinforcement for the patient.

Not stopping smoking.   Realistically, a significant proportion of patients will be unwilling or unable to stop smoking even following the diagnosis of lung cancer. Effective defences such as denial probably need to be left intact at this stage. Patients may none the less benefit from some monitoring of their smoking which may in some cases be liable to increase with the stress of illness and treatment. It can still be helpful to offer alternative coping strategies to help the patient avoid developing the classic vicious circle of feeling bad – increasing substance abuse – feeling worse.

For a fuller review of self management techniques see Glasgow (1986).

Clinical Presentation

Most patients with lung cancer present with symptomatic disease. Symptoms may be attributable to the primary tumour, to metastatic spread or systemic indicators of the malignant process. The most common presenting symptoms overall are listed in Table 2 (from Doyle and Aisner, 1989).

TABLE 2 *Common presenting symptoms of patients with lung cancer*

Finding	Percentage
Cough	74
Weight loss	68
Dyspnoea	58
Chest pain	49
Sputum production	45

It is common for lung cancer patients to delay seeking medical attention for several months, attributing symptoms to a smoker's cough or the common cold. Several additional months may be spent in symptomatic treatment (for example, antibiotics from the GP) before the diagnosis is made. Dealing with feelings about the individual circumstances of any such delay can be an important issue for some patients in coming to terms with the diagnosis.

The site of metastatic spread is important to the patient's experience of symptoms. Lung cancer frequently metastasizes to bone causing pain, to the liver causing fatigue, nausea, malaise and jaundice and to the brain disturbing a range of higher mental functions. The neuropsychiatric sequelae of central nervous system (CNS) involvement have particular implications for psychological assessment and care which will be reviewed in the discussion of cranial irradiation.

PSYCHOLOGICAL IMPACT OF SYMPTOMS

More systematic recording of patients' subjective experience of lung cancer symptoms has been promoted by the Medical Research Council in Britain and the European Organization for Research in the Treatment of Cancer, both of which encourage quality of life assessment in clinical trials. This has allowed some documentation of the psychological distress of both patients and their care givers which can be associated with some symptoms. Bakker (1986) particularly identifies pain, insomnia, respiratory distress and cachexia in this regard. Clinically it is clear that such physical problems can be compounded by emotional distress and that on occasion psychological principles and techniques can provide a useful adjunct to standard medical care.

Pain

The psychological contribution to the management of pain has been fully discussed by Turk and Fernandez in this volume and the general principles described can usefully be applied to lung cancer patients.

Insomnia

Insomnia or expressed dissatisfaction with the duration or quality of sleep can be a significant problem for lung cancer patients, rendering them more emotionally distressed and less able to cope with other aspects of the disease or treatment. Sleep may be disturbed by physical factors such as coughing, the action of some medication (for example corticosteroids) or psychological factors such as depression. Clearly the primary cause needs first to be assessed and treated where possible.

An extensive study involving a mixed group of 1579 cancer patients in the United States found hypnotics were the most frequently prescribed psychotropic medication accounting for 48 per cent of the total prescribed for these patients and consumed by 24 per cent of the sample (Derogatis et al., 1979). At that time approximately 4 per cent of the general adult population of the United States was prescribed hypnotics (Solomon et al., 1979).

Among patients aged 45 to 60 years treated with chemotherapy Coates et al. (1983) found disturbed sleep ranked next in severity after nausea, vomiting and hair loss on the list of complaints.

Lung cancer patients have been investigated in the sleep laboratory at Dartmouth Medical School (Silberfarb, 1986). Relative to normal controls they spent more time in bed but less time asleep, showed more sleep latency, lower sleep efficiency, more body movements in sleep and were awake after falling asleep three times more often.

Silberfarb *et al*. (1985) also reported lung cancer patients spend more time in REM and Stage I sleep and less time in Stage II and non-REM (delta) sleep than normal controls. Cancer patients' satisfaction with their sleep related solely and significantly to the amount of non-REM sleep. These are preliminary findings from a small sample but they may be important for the future management of insomnia in cancer patients since there is some evidence that delta sleep is a restorative stage of sleep related to biological recovery. All body processes tilt towards anabolic activity from catabolic activity and this may be critical for cancer patients (Adam and Oswald, 1977). Benzodiazepines which are frequently prescribed in this situation suppress delta sleep and may thus be contraindicated (Williams and Karacan, 1976). Further work is needed in this area.

Patients can however develop maladaptive habits with respect to sleep, for example, reversing night and day arousal patterns. Since fear, distress and confusion are generally worse at night, some intervention may be indicated and psychological principles may be helpful in combating this aspect of insomnia.

Fearful of the consequences of overexertion, patients, sometimes at the insistence of their partners, may settle for a more restricted lifestyle than is warranted by day with a consequently reduced sleep requirement at night. Enforced inactivity resulting from breathlessness or fatigue can also be a problem resulting in boredom from which the patient withdraws into sleep during the day. In either case providing appropriate stimulation to keep the patient alert and engaged for a greater proportion of the day may require some ingenuity but efforts are rewarded by an increased sense of mastery and pleasure for the patient by day and a greater need for rest thereafter.

The development of behavioural routines which signal the transition from daytime activity to night-time rest (for example, warm bath, milky drink) can be helpful although there is controversy over whether the bedroom itself should be regarded as a cue for sleep (Turner and Ascher, 1979) or whether it is merely a cue for relaxation (Zwart and Lisman, 1979). In the latter case activities such as reading or watching TV which are incompatible with sleep can be encouraged since they do at least allow the patient to be relaxed. Where sleep is the sole goal such distracting activities may be better associated with another place so that bed becomes the cue for sleep.

Relaxation training is the most commonly used psychological intervention for sleep problems (Griffiths, 1981). Although there are several approaches to relaxation (for example progressive muscular relaxation) (Jacobson, 1938; 1964), autogenic methods requiring less movement may be preferred, particularly by patients with difficulty in finding a comfortable posture and those concerned about disturbing their partner (Schultz and Luthe, 1959).

TABLE 3 *Challenging negative thinking*

Challenge	Specific questions
What is the evidence	– to support these thoughts? – against them?
What alternative views are there?	– How would someone else view this situation? – If this were happening to someone else how would I view it?
Is the thinking distorted?	– Am I attending only to the black side of things? – Am I predicting the future instead of experimenting with it? – Am I assuming I can do nothing to change things?
What action can I take?	– Where does thinking like this get me? – What can I do to change my situation?

Cognitive strategies for dealing with self-defeating or alarming thoughts may be helpful to the patient beset with fears at night. Sometimes recurrent themes are troublesome until a satisfactory riposte is found and patients can be helped to generate questions such as those listed in Table 3 to challenge negative thinking whenever it occurs (Beck, 1979). For a fuller discussion of this approach see Moorey, this volume.

Sometimes writing the worry down as a means of discharging it till morning is helpful; at other times distraction works more satisfactorily. Finally it sometimes helps to de-emphasize sleep as the goal. Aiming only for peaceful rest may allow the insomniac to approach night with equanimity.

Respiratory Distress

Respiratory distress can be alarming for patients and fear of suffocating to death may exacerbate the existing problem. As in the management of other respiratory crises such as asthma or chronic obstructive airways disease, a cognitive-behavioural approach can be helpful in breaking the vicious circle of symptoms that increases anxiety and worsens symptoms. A simple physiological explanation of the effect of mounting panic on breathing is a helpful basis for demonstrating to patients that some control can be regained over the respiratory problem and for making sense of their somatic experience. Again relaxation techniques and means of dealing with frightening thoughts are a valuable adjunct to physical management. Since panic disorganizes thinking and behaviour it is helpful to give such patients tangible prompts to have by them in case of panic. We have found a written list of instructions for coping with panic (see Table 4) and an audiotape of relaxation exercises useful under these circumstances.

TABLE 4   *Rules for coping with panic*

---

(1) Remember the feelings are an exaggeration of your body's normal reaction to stress.

(2) They are not harmful or dangerous, only unpleasant. Nothing worse will happen.

(3) Stop adding to the panic with frightening thoughts, especially 'what if . . .'.

(4) Notice what is happening in your body *now*, not what you fear might happen.

(5) Notice that when you stop adding to it with frightening thoughts the panic stops rising.

(6) Now you can help the fear to subside by using your relaxation exercises.

(7) Remember the reason for practising these things is to learn how to cope with fear. An episode of panic does not mean you cannot cope. What can you learn from this episode to help you for the future?

Appetite and Weight Loss

Appetite and weight loss associated with cancer can become highly emotionally charged for patients and their care givers. The concept of small amounts of a variety of preferred foods, attractively and frequently offered is a counsel of perfection which may be unattainable in institutional catering or for the patient living alone or with limited means. Although dietary supplements are widely available they are not always palatable. The contribution of 'alternative' therapies in recommending restrictive diets of unproven value has not been helpful in this regard.

The pathogenesis of weight loss in patients with cancer is not completely understood. Lung cancer cachexia may reflect a reduced appetite due to metabolic disturbances induced by the tumour, but it may occur despite an adequate calorie intake (Chlebowski *et al.*, 1983). The problem may be compounded by disturbance of taste and/or smell caused by the action of some cytotoxic agents or by conditioned association of certain foodstuffs with emetogenic therapy resulting in specific aversions.

Patients often feel very self-conscious about weight loss. Lung cancer patients tend to question whether it is worth replacing clothes which no longer fit while others are deterred by the reactions of others to their changed appearance. Some patients respond by social withdrawal, distressing in itself but increasing vulnerability to depression. Starting with some brief and relatively easy social contact, patients' self-confidence may be increased and social anxiety desensitized by encouraging gradual progress through more demanding encounters towards the patients' preferred level of social activity.

Coping with appetite and weight loss can become a focus for strong feelings about fighting the disease for both patients and care givers. Patients are often worried and depressed by their appetite loss, not only for the loss of a former source of pleasure but with concern for increasing weakness and debility. A commonly expressed fear is of facing a lingering and wasting death. Carers feel rejected and impotent when in spite of their best efforts the patient is unable to eat. Relatives may feel anger as well as distress that the patient is 'turning their face to the wall' in refusing food and access to supportive services is likely to be helpful to those caring for cachetic patients.

Predicting Psychological Distress

Knowing the extent to which medical variables can account for psychological distress is important in predicting 'at risk' patients for whom early intervention may be indicated. Cella *et al.* (1987) reported a useful study of a large sample of 455 small cell lung cancer patients (SCLC) which confirmed a statistically significant connection between extent of physical impairment and mood disturbance. The increased mood disturbance with poorer performance status was more marked in patients with extensive disease. Women exhibited more mood disturbance on the measure used, but this is not a cancer specific finding (McNair *et al.*, 1971). Knowledge of these factors alone is insufficient to predict clinically significant distress but they can contribute to a larger model of risk assessment.

Depressive illness secondary to organic brain syndromes or reactive to the physical and psychological impact of symptoms is not uncommon in cancer generally and depression has been described as a presenting feature of lung cancer. Hughes (1985a) found an excess of depressive illness among patients attending a chest hospital prior to the diagnosis of lung cancer when compared to the general population or to patients in hospital for elective surgery. The prevalence of 16 per cent was also higher than among patients with nonmalignant chest conditions. A past history of psychiatric and/or recent social stress were the most significant factors, although patients with more extensive disease were also more likely to be depressed. In three out of four cases the depression was unrecognized and untreated. Thus a subset of patients may be identified as being at greater risk following the diagnosis of lung cancer of becoming significantly psychologically distressed to a degree warranting at least closer assessment and possible intervention. Table 5 shows the risk factors for psychological distress.

TABLE 5   *Risk factors for psychological distress*

Poor performance status
Extensive disease
Past psychiatric history
Lack of family support
History of recent life stress
Female sex

A multicentre cross-cultural clinical trial which included quality of life assessment reported baseline (i.e. pre-treatment) measures from 80 small cell lung cancer patients (Aaronson *et al.*, 1986). The clinical significance of the degree of distress reported was not assessed but the authors found 45 per cent of the sample tense, 44 per cent worried, 34 per cent depressed and 21 per cent irritable to degrees that were rated 'quite a bit' or 'very much' on their self-report measure.

TREATMENT OPTIONS

It is necessary to discriminate between tumour types to appreciate current issues in medical management which are central to the patient's experience of treatment. The term 'lung cancer' refers to a heterogeneous group of neoplasms but for the purpose of this chapter it is sufficient to distinguish two broad groups: small cell lung cancer (SCLC) and non small cell lung cancer (NSCLC) reflecting different treatment strategies. Unfortunately the prognosis for all groups remains generally poor and quality of life issues are increasingly being recognized as important in clinical decision making and in the evaluation of new treatment efforts.

Non Small Cell Lung Cancer

Complete surgical resection offers the best hope of cure, but most tumours are inoperable. In the Edinburgh series described by

Capewell (1985) 19 per cent of lung cancer patients were referred for surgery. Even in this highly selected group five-year survival was of the order of 30 to 40 per cent. The majority of surgically treated patients develop local recurrence or distant metastatic spread within two years (Weisenburger, 1989). There has therefore been interest in combining surgery with radiotherapy and/or chemotherapy in an attempt to improve the outcome of primary treatment. Any gains achieved have to be balanced against increased treatment time and morbidity. Although improvement in response has been reported for multimodal therapy, over surgery alone no major impact on survival has been achieved, and there is a dearth of published data to document the patient's subjective experience.

Although lung cancer patients have been treated with radiotherapy since the late 1940s, the exact role of this modality remains controversial. Patients with inoperable but localized small volume disease and no evidence of distal metastases may be offered radical radiotherapy with curative intent but there are unresolved controversies about the optimal schedule for delivery of treatment and increasing the dose to improve local control increases the potential for damage of normal tissue. Without doubt local radiotherapy can offer significant palliation of symptoms, for example, effectively relieving haemoptysis for 84 per cent of patients and pain or dyspnoea in about 60 per cent of cases (Slawson and Scott, 1979). For the patient without troublesome symptoms optimal timing of radiotherapy remains controversial and a wait-and-see policy may be advocated, although Hughes' (1985) study of lung cancer patients showed that those who did not receive active treatment were more likely to be depressed and dissatisfied.

Since approximately 50 per cent of NSCLC patients have distant metastases at the time of diagnosis and a further 40 per cent will develop metastases after treatment by surgery or radiotherapy, the majority of patients could logically be candidates for systemic therapy. Unfortunately NSCLC has shown greater resistance to known cytotoxic agents than SCLC. Response rates to standard chemotherapy regimens have remained poor, producing 20 to 40 per cent predominantly partial regressions of short duration. The most effective agents (for example platinum-based combinations) are highly toxic. It is of interest then that in a randomized trial of chemotherapy versus radiotherapy for patients with inoperable NSCLC. Kaasa *et al.* (1988b) found no significant difference in measures of physical function and everyday activity between the two groups although in this study the complete response rate was low for both. Both groups of patients reported an increase in psychosocial well-being following treatment. In the radiotherapy group this improvement in the quality of life began from the start of treatment and was maintained over the first three months of the study for which reliable data were available. The chemotherapy patients displayed a significant drop in their quality of life after two weeks but thereafter an improvement was observed (Kaasa *et al.*, 1988c). Although the authors attributed this difference to organizational differences which may have meant that radiotherapy patients received more support, they concluded from taking patients' subjective experience and the need for secondary treatment into consideration that radiotherapy was the treatment of choice (Kaasa *et al.*, 1989).

Thus the role of chemotherapy in the management of NSCL remains controversial. It is argued it should be explored only through clinical trials which take account of quality of life assessments rather than routinely without protocol (Greco, 1988). The case for palliative chemotherapy rests on the selection of patients of good performance status and emphasizes that the duration of treatment need not be protracted since response can be determined early to indicate whether there is any value in continuing the medication. There is considerable morbidity to the patient associated with untreated disease and many patients prefer active intervention, though in some centres supportive care will be the preferred strategy.

There is no standard therapy for this group of tumours. Among doctors, attitudes to the disease are gloomy and attitudes to treatment may vary across medical specialties. Patients with comparable disease are likely to be managed differently in different centres.

Small Cell Lung Cancer

Small cell lung cancer represents 20 to 25 per cent of all lung cancers and is characterized by a more rapid growth and earlier metastasis than other tumour types. Depending on the extent of the disease at diagnosis the median survival of untreated patients is 5 to 12 weeks. A recent study reported a five-year survival rate of 35 per cent for patients with Stage I disease and 23 per cent for those with Stage II disease following surgical resection (Prasad *et al.*, 1989) but reviewing this study Crompton (1990) emphasizes that most patients have inoperable disease.

Combination chemotherapy has been the treatment of choice for the majority (Smyth *et al.*, 1986). A variety of combinations of cytotoxic agents appear equally effective in achieving response rates of 70 to 90 per cent, with 25 to 50 per cent complete responses, depending on the extent of the disease initially. This has led to greater attention being given to determine how maximal effectiveness of treatment could be maintained for least toxicity. However the emergence of a few patients as long-term survivors has maintained the intriguing possibility of cure as a goal and has encouraged a continuing search for more prognostic indicators to help identify this group of patients for whom more aggressive therapy may be justified.

Efforts to increase the rate of treatment response by late intensification of therapy have been disappointing and prolonging chemotherapy does not appear to improve the quality or duration of patients' survival (Leonard, 1989).

Although the specific agents used may vary patients are now likely to be offered a relatively short induction course of chemotherapy, the effectiveness of which will probably be apparent after six weeks. Some time off treatment, perhaps with chemotherapy on relapse, is now preferred to continuous therapy and there is renewed interest in including quality of life measures in clinical trials involving these patients.

For elderly patients and those with a poorer prognosis (through more extensive disease or poorer general health), considerable effort has gone into the selection of a chemotherapy regime which achieves effective palliation without the toxicity associated with more aggressive therapy (Allan et al., 1984).

The question of combining therapies for patients with SCLC remains controversial. For patients with limited disease efforts to improve local control of the disease have led to the combined use of chemotherapy and radiotherapy to the chest (Arriagada, 1985). There are significant problems of morbidity and it remains unclear whether these modalities should be delivered concurrently or sequentially. Clinical trials to address this question are underway.

A further problem for this group of patients is the high risk of developing intracranial metastases, a risk which increases with increasing survival time: 50 per cent at 1 year and 80 per cent for patients alive at two years after diagnosis (Nugent et al., 1979). Cerebral metastases cause greater deterioration in performance status and require more hospitalization for patients than relapse at other sites (Felleti et al., 1985). Silberfarb (1986) points out that many types of abnormal behaviour can result, causing great distress to the patient and their family. Cognitive functions such as orientation, attention and memory may be impaired and aspects of the patient's personality, emotional and/or behavioural control may be disturbed. A mental state examination, including neuropsychological assessment, may be useful in discriminating and monitoring organic impairment which is often missed particularly when deficits are subtle.

Palliative radiotherapy for cerebral metastases is relatively unsuccessful with complete response rates of around 20 per cent; thus a case has been made for prophylactic use of cranial irradiation. This does significantly lower the incidence of cerebral metastases, thereby reducing the physical morbidity and social consequences of cranial relapse (Hansen et al., 1980). However prophylactic cranial irradiation does not improve overall survival (Rosen *et al.*, 1983) and it is only potentially curative when non-CNS disease has been eradicated. The policy tends to be for prophylactic cranial irradiation to be offered only to those patients who have achieved a complete response to induction chemotherapy (Aroney *et al.*, 1983, Lucas *et al.*, 1986).

Thus the situation for patients with SCLC is that chemotherapy with or without radiotherapy can improve symptoms and extend survival for most patients but with considerable risk of toxicity and only a small chance of long-term survival.

EVALUATING TREATMENT OPTIONS

All treatment modalities involve risk to normal structures and the possibility of toxicity which may impair the patient's quality of life. When, as for the majority of lung cancer patients, treatment is given with palliative intent and the prognosis is poor, costs and benefits have to be carefully weighed. More information is required about subjective experience of toxicity for all modalities of lung cancer treatment. Patients' attitudes to these therapies and the risks involved are incompletely understood. The requirements of informed consent procedures may place considerable strain on patients in confronting them with current treatment dilemmas.

Surgery

As with all surgical procedures, postoperative pain is to be expected at the site of the wound. Postoperative complications may include respiratory failure, infection and cardiac arrythmias. The operative mortality rate is small but significant: 2.9 per cent for lobectomy and 6.2 per cent for pneumonectomy (Ginsberg *et al.*, 1983). The quality of survival of patients cured by pulmonary resection has been described as excellent (Nou and Aberg, 1980) though the Carlens Vitagram method used assesses only working capability, symptoms and time in hospital. In the same study, patients who were not cured scored poorly in this measure for the rest of their lives, and slightly worse than matched controls who were not operated on. There are no published data on the psychological outcome of lung cancer surgery beyond an affirmation of the role of personality factors in reported post-thoracotomy pain (Bachiocco *et al.*, 1988) and more systematic assessment of the subjective intensity and duration of postoperative pain, fatigue and dyspnoea is called for.

In a hypothetical model lung cancer patients asked to choose between a fixed period of assured survival with radiotherapy and a gamble on longer survival with surgery preferred not to take surgical risks (McNeil *et al.*, 1978). Although this study has been criticized for the specific options presented (Bakker, 1986), the general finding is supported by clinical experience that, in general, younger patients more readily accept higher risks for the potential cure than older patients whose priorities may be to secure short-term personal goals.

Radiotherapy

The general view is that radiotherapy effectively palliates symptoms in most lung cancer patients (Cox *et al.*, 1985), although the response criteria are rarely based on systematic self-report data from patients and the duration of the response and time in treatment as a proportion of survival time are rarely cited. Common early side-effects of thoracic radiotherapy include oesophagitis and pneumonitis. Late morbidity involving the heart or spinal cord is a serious risk for longer-term survivors which clinicians try to reduce in their treatment planning.

The psychological impact of radiotherapy is mediated by management as well as by physical side-effects of the procedure. Fears about the machinery and practicalities of the administration of treatment (for example, being alone) are not uncommon and misconceptions about the nature of radiotherapy still abound (for example, fear of being burned, confusion between the therapeutic and carcinogenic properties of radiation). These can be reduced with more attention to early information giving when preparing the patient for treatment.

Patients commonly experience generalized malaise and fatigue after radiotherapy. The interpretation placed on these side-effects can significantly influence their emotional impact. Lethargy interpreted as a side-effect of effective treatment is better tolerated than when it is interpreted as evidence of progressive disease. The importance of information for patients about what to expect of treatment cannot be overstated. Such information often needs to be repeated and should include some practical advice about coping. Written or taped information can be particularly helpful (Hogbin and Fallowfield, 1989).

Peck and Boland (1977) found a mixed group of cancer patients more depressed and anxious on completing radiotherapy than at the outset. Forester *et al.*, (1978) described apprehension, anxiety, depression and social withdrawal among lung cancer patients treated with radiotherapy. Distress diminished over the course of therapy only to increase again at the end of treatment. The same authors have shown a reduction in both emotional and physical symptoms (for example, anorexia and fatigue) in response to psychotherapy in this situation relative to randomized controls who had routine care (Forester *et al.*, 1985).

The psychotherapeutic intervention offered was unstructured and tailored to individual needs. Three aspects of supportive intervention were identified:

education   – listening, answering questions
interpretive – pointing out psychological mechanisms for dealing with
                distress
cathartic   – encouraging expressing of emotion

These were broadly concerned with helping patients make sense of their physical and emotional experience.

Janis (1958) first described the importance of preoperative anxiety as a factor in postoperative recovery. Andersen and Tewfik (1985) point out that using this theoretical model in the context of coping with repeated treatments and adjustment to the treatment for a chronic illness, the maintenance or attainment of a moderate manageable level of anxiety might be expected and facilitates coping responses. The goal of intervention realistically then would not be to eliminate anxiety, but to help the patient keep worry within manageable proportions. The 'work of worrying' (Marmor, 1958) facilitates attending to information and treatment, seeking reassurance from others and warding off feelings of helplessness. This active coping style has been suggested by some authors to convey a survival advantage.

There are particular concerns about the neuropsychiatric sequelae of cranial irradiation. The problems described range from mild impairment of intellectual function to severe dementia (Looper *et al.*, 1984; Johnson *et al.*, 1985). It remains unclear to what extent these abnormalities reflect the influence of previous cytotoxic therapy, the scheduling of drugs in relation to prophylactic cranial irradiation and radiation-dose time factors. A number of trials are underway to evaluate the effectiveness of prophylactic cranial irradiation in the management of SCLC patients but in the meantime this issue raises worrying uncertainties for patients and their families.

Chemotherapy

A range of chemotherapeutic agents may be used with toxicities which can adversely affect patients' quality of life. The commonest side-effects are nausea, vomiting and alopecia, and their implications for psychological care are obviously not unique to the experience of lung cancer patients. As well as being distressing in their own right the more emetogenic regimes place patients at increased risk of developing conditioned responses which compound distress and threaten compliance. Intervention strategies are reviewed in Black and Morrow, this volume.

Although women may be more likely to voice their distress about hair loss, the impact on the personal and social functioning of male patients should not be overlooked. Attitudes to hair loss have not been adequately explored among men of this age for whom wigs are often less satisfactory than for women. Embarrassment about alopecia may cause considerable personal distress and social withdrawal. Patients seldom volunteer this information, feeling admissions of vanity or concerns about social activity to be inappropriate concerns on the face of life-threatening illness. More sympathetic enquiry may be called for since cognitive-behavioural approaches can be effective in encouraging the recovery of self-confidence and social interaction.

In lung cancer when the survival gain may be small the impact of side-effects comes under close scrutiny; for example Bakker et al., (1986) confirmed the antitumour effect of a combination of vindesine, cisplatin and bleomycin in patients with advanced NSCLC but concluded that treatment-associated toxicity, particularly nausea and vomiting, and deterioration of patients' well-being offset any potential survival advantage.

The range of side-effects can however be quite wide-ranging, depending on the specific drugs used. It is important that patients be warned about what to expect, at least for the most common side-effects, so they can correctly interpret their somatic experience. A recent study (Kaasa and Mastekaasa, 1988) investigated the psychosocial well-being of inoperable NSCLC patients randomized to receive either chemotherapy (cisplatin and etoposide) or radiotherapy. Although the chemotherapy group reported more side-effects, this was not significantly related to psychosocial well-being, in contrast to a clear correlation between disease-related symptoms and well-being. The authors suggest that patients who interpret side-effects as evidence of the treatment working show greater tolerance of chemotherapy toxicity.

The particular side-effects which require to be monitored will vary with the drugs used and the research questions being asked, but in clinical practice it remains important to guard against unwarranted assumptions about their significance to particular patient groups – for example, the potential impact of chemotherapy on sexual function may be overlooked in this age group. The personal significance of particular side-effects may be an important part of the cost–benefit analysis for the individual patient – for example the risks of peripheral neuropathy and hearing loss associated with cisplatin may be unacceptable to a musician or music lover.

Clearly the provision of adequate information about likely side-effects and the opportunity to consider their meaning for the individual are important aspects of supportive care needed by the patient embarking on chemotherapy.

Not all patients' problems related to treatment appear on standard toxicity ratings. Coates *et al.*, (1983) reported that nonphysical side-effects constituted 54 per cent of the most severe complaints of a mixed group of patients undergoing chemotherapy. These included the thought of coming for treatment and being injected. In an unpublished study (Cull and North, 1990) of 50 small cell lung cancer patients we have found boredom a significant problem identified by 20 per cent of patients during chemotherapy.

Alteration of bone marrow function, one of the commonest consequences of treatment, exerts considerable influence on patients' experience of the delivery of treatment. The recovery of leucocyte and platelet levels in peripheral blood has to be monitored prior to each course of treatment. For the patient this means delay until blood test results confirm that treatment can proceed. Where recovery has been insufficient the next course of chemotherapy is postponed. This uncertainty adds significantly to patients' anxiety and in the use of highly emetogenic regimes can be particularly hazardous for the exacerbation of conditioned autonomic responses.

Although patient self-report measures are to be encouraged, some side-effects require improved clinical assessment. There is disappointingly little data available about the impact of cytotoxic drugs on higher mental functions. Silberfarb (1983) found 9 patients in a series of 50 oncology admissions to be cognitively impaired. Memory deficits were associated with the use of chemotherapy but the sample size was too small to identify the specific cytotoxic agents responsible.

Emotional distress associated specifically with chemotherapy has been less clearly identified in lung cancer than in other disease groups (Maguire *et al.*, 1980; Nerenz *et al.*, 1982). Again data are sparse. Hughes (1985b) found patients with inoperable lung cancer generally considered chemotherapy worthwhile in spite of side-effects, whereas patients who had not had active treatment were more likely to be depressed or dissatisfied. The specific drugs used may however be important in determining psychological morbidity. Silberfarb *et al.*, (1983) assessed SCLC patients randomly assigned to one of two chemotherapy regimes. In the absence of differences in tumour response the group receiving vincristine were significantly more likely to suffer fatigue and depression presumably mediated by the effect of the drug on biogenic amines.

Biological Response Modifiers

Interferon is being used increasingly to augment the action of cytotoxic drugs. There have been encouraging results in terms of anti-tumour activity, but neurotoxicity has also been reported (Mattson *et al.*, 1984). CNS side-effects appear dose related and reversible on stopping treatment. Impaired concentration and slowness of cerebration have been observed (Johnson *et al.*, 1983). There is a need for more systematic psychometric assessment of these patients. A study is currently underway in Edinburgh. Interferon also induces a constellation of flu-like symptoms which may be associated with an increased incidence of anxiety and depression (McDonald *et al.*, 1987).

INFORMED CONSENT AND CLINICAL DECISION MAKING

The vast majority of cancer patients are now told their diagnosis, and concern regarding information giving has shifted to issues relating to decision making about treatment options and informed consent. This is particularly relevant to the lung cancer patient given the prognosis and treatment options outlined. Psychological care in this area may need to be as much concerned with support for staff who have to combat feelings of therapeutic nihilism about lung cancer and qualms about randomized clinical trials involving toxic therapies in order to find a balance between their clinical care for individual patients and scientific responsibility to strive to improve prospects for the future.

Slevin *et al.* (1988) found a mixed group of cancer patients more willing than doctors to undergo intensive chemotherapy for very little chance of benefit when faced with a hypothetical question and questioned their ability to make rational decisions about treatment. McKillop *et al.* (1988) investigated the perceptions of a mixed group of cancer patients, including 38 per cent with lung cancer, about their own disease and treatment. He found patients with metastatic disease often believed their disease to be localized and that many incurable patients failed to understand that they were being treated palliatively.

This is a notoriously difficult area to research given the complexities of the information processing involved, from the message the doctor intends to convey to that received, interpreted and recalled by the patient under the influence of all the emotional defence mechanisms at his or her disposal. We asked 61 lung cancer patients about their information preferences following diagnosis and prior to starting chemotherapy (Cull and North, 1990). All had been told and 95 per cent felt they needed to know what chemotherapy and its likely side-effects would involve for them. In spite of apparently excellent forewarning, more than half of those interviewed at the end of their course of chemotherapy said they had experienced unexpected side-effects. One third of the SCLC patients and half the NSCLC patients found side-effects worse than they had expected and it may be that there can be no adequate verbal preparation for the somatic experiences encountered and their impact on the individual.

About 30 per cent of our sample would have preferred not to know whether there was a choice of treatment for them and 40 per cent would have preferred not to know whether the treatment was new or experimental, although all those patients were being treated on clinical trial protocols. These findings confirm the clinical impression of older patients with more traditional attitudes to health care, but it is interesting to note that the proportion expressing a wish to know about treatment choice has risen locally from 28 per cent of a sample of SCLC patients surveyed in 1985 to 70 per cent in this mixed group in 1989.

Modern medical ethics emphasize patients' participation in giving informed consent to medical decisions, but McKillop *et al.* (1988) express the sentiments of many when they point out that mutual participation in medical decisions may not be what every patient wants or needs and that physicians have a continuing responsibility to ensure that the decisions made are balanced. There is also interest in providing patients with the time and opportunity to discuss the issues with someone other than the doctor, particularly when participation in a clinical trial is being suggested.

Information giving and decision making are relevant not only to starting treatment but also to continuing and the decision to stop. Half of our sample of lung cancer patients had felt like stopping treatment at some point during chemotherapy, often because of toxicity but also due to mood disturbance. For 25 per cent of that subgroup morbidity was felt to outweigh benefit and treatment was stopped at that point. The remaining 75 per cent however continued in treatment as planned without conveying their feelings to staff and they emphasized family support in seeing them through this stressful time. In spite of the problems, two thirds of the sample judged that the chemotherapy had been worthwhile. SCLC patients were more positive about the benefits of treatment than NSCLC patients, a realistic reflection of their experience. More and larger longitudinal studies are needed to define lung cancer patients' needs over time but this small study was sufficient to highlight the often neglected issue of the burden on patients' partners. Psychological care for lung cancer should extend to acknowledge the partner's needs.

Impact on Social Function

The peak incidence of lung cancer is the mid 60s when most patients are about to or have just retired. Difficulties may arise for those who find long-cherished retirement plans blocked by illness or treatment. Patients already experience retirement as a loss, for example, of social contact and may find themselves struggling to cope with the added stress of illness at this time. Personal function, activity levels and dependence on others are important parameters for the quality of patients' lives at this stage. Social support is undoubtedly important but this is a stage in life when patients' partners are also becoming less fit and families more scattered. The experience of the European Organization for Research in the Treatment of Cancer studies (Aaronson *et al.*, 1986) warns against the problem of patients giving misleading responses in answer to questions about social relationships in order to appear in a socially desirable light. A more useful assessment can be obtained by asking about the extent to which patients' needs are actually met (for example, questions about emotional closeness, feeling understood etc.). The toll on the care givers providing this support may be high.

Implications for Service Organization

In the current economic climate in health care it is difficult to make a case for the deployment of scarce resources to provide special psychological care for lung cancer patients when data to justify that need are so conspicuously lacking.

Obviously some of the problems outlined are similar to those encountered among patients with malignancies at other sites, thus all professional groups have a contribution to make to the psychological care of lung cancer patients. This begins with an increased awareness of the relevant psychological issues and requires better communication about the patients' subjective experience. Parallel development, again not unique to lung cancer, requires earlier identification of remediable problems which warrant special intervention. Currently this is likely to depend on the sensitivity of the local clinician to psychological problems and the relative accessibility of counselling psychological and/or psychiatric services.

Improved psychological care of lung cancer patients in the future depends on greater investment now in collecting the data needed to inform clinical decision making. Information is required about the use of existing therapies which remain controversial with respect to their impact on morbidity as well as in the evaluation of new treatment modalities. Information is required which will assist in treatment choice for individual patients as well as in policy making as a result of clinical trial data. The role of psychological factors has yet to be tested in the decision as to whether the goal of treatment is curative or palliative or in determining the timing and nature of palliative efforts. Greater attention is clearly required in the assessment of psychosocial morbidity when new treatment modalities are being evaluated but this area of clinical research also needs to consider factors which may predispose patients to adverse effects.

Current service organization needs may thus be best met by investment in clinical research to address these issues.

References

AARONSON, N.K., BAKKER, W., STEWART, A.L., VAN DAM, F.S.A.M., VAN ZANDWIJK, N., YARNOLD, J.R. and KIRKPATRICK, A. (1986) A multidimensional approach to the measurement of quality of life in lung cancer clinical trials. In N.K. Aaronson, J. Beckmann, J. Bernheim and R. Zittoun (Eds) *Quality of Life in Cancer*. New York: Raven Press.

ADAM, K. and OSWALD, I. (1977) Sleep is for tissue restoration. *Journal of the Royal College of Physicians, 11*, 376–388.

ALLAN, S.G., GREGOR, A., CORNBLEET, M.A., LEONARD, R.C.F., SMYTH, J.F., GRANT, I.W.B. and CROMPTON, G.K. (1984) Phase II trial of vindesine and VP16-213 in the palliation of poor prognosis and elderly patients with small cell lung cancer. *Cancer Chemotherapy and Pharmacology, 13*, 106–108.

ANDERSEN, B.L. and TEWFIK, H.H. (1985) Psychological reactions to radiotherapy: A reconsideration of the adaptive aspects of anxiety. *Journal of Personality and Social Psychology, 48*, 4, 1024–1032.

ARONEY, R.S., AISNER, J., WESLEY, M.N., WHITACRE, M.Y., VAN ECHO, D.A., SLAWSON, R.G. and WIERNIK, P.H. (1983) The value of PCI given at complete remission of small cell lung carcinoma. *Cancer Treatment Reports, 67*, 675–682.

ARRIAGADA, R., LE CHEVALIER, T., BALDEYROU, P., PICO, J.L., RUFFIE, P., MARTIN, M., EL BAKRY, H.M., DUROUX, P., LENFANT, B., HAYAT, M., ROUESSE, J.G., SANCHO GARNIER, H. and TUBIANA, M. (1985) Alternating radiotherapy and chemotherapy schedules in small cell lung cancer limited disease. *International Journal of Radiation Oncology, Biology and Physics, 11*, 461.

BACHIOCCO, V., FRANCESCHELLI, N., MORSELLI, A.M., BELELLI, G. and VILLANI, S. (1988) The relationship between post thoracotomy pain and psychological factors. *Lung Cancer 4*. Suppl.4. A182 No. 10.20. (Abstract of paper presented to Fifth World Conference in Lung Cancer 1988, Interlaken.)

BAKKER, W. (1986) *Studies in Lung Cancer Treatment: Impact on survival and quality of life*. (Unpublished doctoral dissertation University of Leiden.)

BAKKER, W., VAN OOSTEROM, A.T., AARONSON, N.K., VAN BREUKELEN, F.J.M., BINS, M.C. and HERMANS, J. (1986) Vindesine, cisplatin and bleomycin combination chemotherapy in non small cell lung cancer: survival and quality of life. *European Journal of Cancer Clinical Oncology, 22*, 8, 963–970.

BECK, A.T. (1979) *Cognitive Therapy and Emotional Disorders*. New York: New American Library.

CANCER RESEARCH CAMPAIGN (1988) *Facts on Cancer Factsheet 5.1*. London: CRC.

CANCER RESEARCH CAMPAIGN (1989) *Facts on Cancer Factsheet II*. London: CRC.

CAPEWELL, S. (1985) Lung Cancer in S.E. Scotland 1981–4. *Thorax, 40*, 209–210.

CELLA, D.F., OROFIAMMA, B., HOLLAND, J.C., SILBERFARB, P.M., TROSS, S., FELDSTEIN, M., PERRY, M., MAURER, H., COMIS, R. and ORAV, E.J. (CALGB) (1987) The Relationship of psychological distress, extent of disease and performance status in patients with lung cancer. *Cancer, 60*, 1661–1667.

CHLEBOWSKI, R.T., HEBER, D. and BLOCK, J.B. (1983) Lung Cancer Cachexia. In

F.A. Greco (Ed.) *Biology and Management of Lung Cancer*. Boston: Martinus Nijhoff Publishers.

COATES, A., ABRAHAM, S., KAYE, S.B., SOWERBUTTS, T., FREWIN, C., FOX, R.M. and TATTERSALL, M.H.N. (1983) On the receiving end – patient perception of the side effects of cancer chemotherapy. *European Journal of Cancer and Clinical Oncology*, 19, 2, 203–208.

COX, J.D., KOMAKI, R., BYHARDT, R.W. (1985) Radiotherapy for non small cell cancer of the lung. In J. Aisner (Ed.) *Lung Cancer*. New York: Churchill Livingstone.

CROMPTON, G.K. (1990) Small Cell Lung Cancer. *British Medical Journal*, 300, 209–210.

CULL, A. and NORTH N. (1990) An investigation of psychological factors relevant to the treatment of lung cancer. (Unpublished data under analysis; Western General Hospital, Edinburgh.)

DEROGATIS, L.R., FELDSTEIN, M., MORROW, G., SCHMALE, A., SCHMITT, M., GATES, C., MURAWSKI, B., HOLLAND, J., PENMAN, D., MELISARATOS, N., ENELOW, A.J. and ADLER, L.M. (1979) A survey of psychotropic drug prescriptions in an oncology population. *Cancer*, 44, 1919–1929.

DI CLEMENTE, C.C. and PROCHASKA, J.O. (1985) Processes and Stages of Self Change: Coping and competence in smoking behaviour change. In S. Stiffman and T.A. Wills (Eds) *Coping and Substance Abuse*. New York: Academic Press.

DOYLE, A.A. and AISNER, J. (1989) Clinical Presentation of Lung Cancer. In J.A. Roth, J.C. Ruckdeschel and T.H. Weisenburger (Eds) *Thoracic Oncology*. Philadelphia: W.B. Saunders Co.

FELLETI, R., SOUTHAMI, R.L., SPIRO, S.G., GEDDES, D.M., TOBIAS, J.S., MANTELL, B.S., HARPER, P.G. and TRASK, C. (1985) Social consequences of brain or liver relapse in small cell carcinoma of the bronchus. *Radiotherapy and Oncology*, 4, 335–339.

FORESTER, B.M., KORNFELD, D.S. and FLEISS, J. (1978) Psychiatric aspects of radiotherapy. *American Journal of Psychiatry*, 135, 8, 960–963.

FORESTER, B.M., KORNFELD, D.S. and FLEISS, J.L. (1985) Psychotherapy during radiotherapy: Effects on emotional and physical distress. *American Journal of Psychiatry*, 142, 22–27.

GEDDES, D.M. (1979) The Natural History of Lung Cancer: A review based on tumour growth. *British Journal of Disease of the Chest*, 73, 1–17.

GINSBERG, R.J., HILL, L.D., EAGAN, R.T., THOMAS, P., MOUNTAIN, C.F., DESLAURIERS, J., FRY, W.A., BUTZ, R.O., GOLDBERG, M., WATERS, P.F., JONES, D.P., PAIROLERO, P., RUBINSTEIN, I. and PEARSON, F.G. (1983) Modern 30 day operative mortality for surgical resections in lung cancer. *Journal of Thoracic and Cardiovascular Surgery*, 86, 654–658.

GLASGOW, R.E. (1986) Smoking. In K.A. Holroyd and T.L. Creer (Eds) *Self-management of Chronic Disease: Handbook of clinical interventions and research*. London: Academic Press.

GLASGOW, R.E. and ROSEN, G.M. (1978) Behavioural Bibliotherapy: A review of self help behaviour therapy manuals. *Psychological Bulletin*, 85, 1–23.

GLASGOW, R.E. and ROSEN, G.M. (1979) Self Help Behaviour Therapy manuals: Recurrent developments and clinical usage. *Clinical Behaviour Therapy Review*, 1, 1–20.

GODDARD, E. and IKIN, K. (1987) *Smoking among secondary school children in 1986*. London: HMSO.

GRECO, F.A. (1988) Chemotherapy for advanced NSCLC. *Advances in Oncology,* 4, 4, 24–29.

GRIFFITHS, D. (1981) Insomnia. In D. Griffiths (Ed.) *Psychology and Medicine.* Leicester: British Psychological Society and Macmillan Press.

HANSEN, H.H., DOMBERNOWSKY, P., HIRSCH, F.R., HANSEN, M. and RYGARD J. (1980) Prophylactic cranial irradiation in bronchogenic small cell anaplastic carcinoma. *Cancer,* 46, 279–284.

HOGBIN, B. and FALLOWFIELD, L. (1989) Getting it taped: The bad news consultation with cancer patients. *British Journal of Hospital Medicine,* 41, 330–333.

HUGHES, J.E. (1985a) Depressive illness and lung cancer. I depression before diagnosis. *European Journal of Surgical Oncology,* 11, 15–20.

HUGHES, J.E. (1985b) Depressive illness and lung cancer II. Follow-up of inoperable patients. *European Journal of Surgical Oncology,* 11, 21–24.

JACOBSON, E. (1938) *Progressive Relaxation.* Chicago: Chicago University Press.

JACOBSON, E. (1964) *Anxiety and Tension Control.* Philadelphia: Lippincott.

JANIS, I.L. (1958) *Psychological Stress: Psychoanalytic and Behavioural Studies of Surgical Patients.* New York: Wiley.

JARVIS, M. (1989) Helping Smokers Give Up. In S. Pearce and J. Wardle (Eds) *The Practice of Behavioural Medicine.* Leicester: BPS Books and Oxford University Press.

JOHNSON, D.H., HANDE, K.R., HAINSWORTH, J.D. and GRECO, J.A. (1983) Neurotoxicity of interferon. *Cancer Treatment Reports,* 67, 958–961.

JOHNSON, B.E., BECHER, B., GOFF, II W.B., PETRONAS, N., KREHBIEL, M.A., MAKUCH, R.W., MCKENNA, G., GLASTEIN, E. and INDE, D.C. (1985) Neurologic, neuropsychologic and computed tomography scan abnormalities in 2–10 year survivors of small cell lung cancer. *Journal of Clinical Oncology,* 3, 1659–1667.

KAASA, S. and MASTEKAASA, A. (1988) Psychosocial wellbeing of patients with inoperable non small cell lung cancer. *Acta Oncologica,* 27, 829–835.

KAASA, S., MASTEKAASA, A. and NAESS, S. (1988a) Quality of life of lung cancer patients in a randomised clinical trial evaluated by a psychosocial wellbeing questionnaire. *Acta Oncologica,* 27, 335–342.

KAASA, S., MASTEKAASA, A. and THORUD, E. (1988b) Toxicity, physical function and everyday activity reported by patients with inoperable non small cell lung cancer in a randomised trial (chemotherapy versus radiotherapy). *Acta Oncologica,* 27, 343–349.

KAASA, S., MASTEKAASA, A. and LUND, E. (1989) Prognostic factors for patients with inoperable non small cell lung cancer limited disease. *Radiotherapy and Oncology,* 15, 235–242.

LEONARD, R.C.F. (1989) Small Cell Lung Cancer. *British Journal of Cancer,* 59, 487–490.

LOOPER, J.D., EINHORN, L.H., GARCIA, S.A., HORNBACK, N.B., VINCENT, B., WILLIAMS, S.D. (1984) Severe neurologic problems following successful therapy for small cell lung cancer. *ASCO Abstracts, C903,* 231.

LUCAS, C.F., ROBINSON, B., HOSKIN, P.J., YARNOLD, J.R., SMITH, I.E. and FORD, H.T. (1986) Morbidity of cranial relapse in small cell lung cancer and the impact of radiation therapy. *Cancer Treatment Reports,* 70, 565–570.

MAGUIRE, G.P., TAIT, A., BROOKE, M., THOMAS, C., HOWAT, J.M.T., SELLWOOD, R.A. and BUSH, H. (1980) Psychiatric morbidity and physical toxicity associated with adjuvant chemotherapy after mastectomy. *British Medical Journal,* 281, 1179–1180.

MARMOR, J. (1958) The psychodynamics of realistic worry. *Psychoanalysis and Social Science*, 5, 155–563.

MATTSON, K., NIIRANEN, A., LAAKSONEN, R. and CANTELL, K. (1984) Psychometric monitoring of interferon neurotoxicity. *The Lancet, Feb 4*, 275–276.

MCDONALD, E.M., MANN, A.H. and THOMAS, H.C. (1987) Interferons as mediators of psychiatric morbidity. *The Lancet*, 21, 1175–1178.

MCKILLOP, W.J., STEWART, W.E., GINSBURG, A.D. and STEWART, S.S. (1988) Cancer patients perceptions of their disease and its treatment. *British Journal of Cancer*, 58, 355–358.

MCNAIR, D., LORR, M. and DROPPLEMAN, L. (1971) *E.I.T.S. Manual for the Profile of Mood States*. San Diego: Educational and Industrial Testing Service.

MCNEIL, B.J., WEICHELBAUM, R. and PAUKER, S.G. (1978) Fallacy of the 5-year survival in lung cancer. *New England Journal of Medicine*, 299, 1397–1401.

NERENZ, D.R., LEVENTHAL, H., LOVE, R.K. (1982) Factors contributing to emotional distress during cancer chemotherapy. *Cancer*, 50, 1020–1027.

NOU, E. and ABERG, T. (1980) Quality of survival in patients with surgically treated bronchial carcinoma. *Thorax*, 35, 255–263.

NUGENT, J.L., BUNN, P.A. and MATTHEWS, M.J. (1979) CNS metastases in small cell bronchogenic carcinoma: Increasing frequency and changing pattern with lengthening survival. *Cancer*, 44, 1885–1893.

PECK, A., BOLAND, J. (1977) Emotional reactions to radiation treatment. *Cancer*, 40, 180–184.

PRASAD, U.S., NAYLOR, A.R., WALKER, W.S., LAMB, D., CAMERON, E.W.J. and WALBAUM, P.R. (1989) Long term survival after pulmonary resection for small cell carcinoma of the lung. *Thorax*, 44, 784–787.

PROCHASKA, J.O. and DI CLEMENTE, C.C. (1983) Stages and processes of self change of smoking: Toward an integrative model of change. *Consulting and Clinical Psychology*, 51, 390–395.

REGISTRAR GENERAL SCOTLAND (1988) *Annual Report 1987*. Edinburgh: HMSO.

ROSEN, S.T., MAKUCH, R.W., LICHTER, A.S., INDE, D.C., MATTHEWS, M.J., MINNA, J.D., GLATSTEIN, E., BUNN, P.A. (1983) Role of prophylactic cranial irradiation in prevention of central nervous system metastases in small cell lung cancer. *American Journal of Medicine*, 74, 615–624.

ROTH, J.A., RUCKDESCHEL, J.C. and WEISENBURGER, T.H. (1989) *Thoracic Oncology*. Philadelphia: WB Saunders Co.

ROYAL COLLEGE OF PHYSICIANS (1962) *Smoking and Health*. London: Pitman Medical.

SCHULTZ, J.H. and LUTHE, W. (1959) *Autogenic Training: A psychophysiological approach to psychotherapy*. New York: Grune & Stratton.

SCOTTISH HOME AND HEALTH DEPARTMENT (1985) *Health in Scotland 1984*. Edinburgh: HMSO.

SILBERFARB, P. (1983) Chemotherapy and cognitive deficits in cancer patients. *Annual Review of Medicine*, 34, 35–46.

SILBERFARB, P.M., HOLLAND, J.C.B., ANBAR, D., BAHNA, G., MAURER, L.H., CHATINIAN, A.P. and COMIS, R. (1983) Psychological response of patients receiving two drug regimens for lung carcinoma. *American Journal of Psychiatry*, 140, 110–111.

SILBERFARB, P.M., HAURI, P.J., OXMAN, T.E. and LASH, S. (1985) Insomnia in Cancer Patients. *Social Science and Medicine*, 20, 8, 849–850.

SILBERFARB, P.M. (1986) Ensuring an optimal quality of life for lung cancer patients: A psychiatrist's perspective. In V. Ventafridda, F.S.A.M. van

Dam, R. Yancik and M. Tamburini (Eds) *Assessment of Quality of Life and Cancer Treatment*. Amsterdam: Elsevier.

SLAWSON, R.G., SCOTT, R.M. (1979) Radiation therapy in bronchogenic carcinoma. *Radiology*, *132*, 175–176.

SLEVIN, M., PLANT, H., STUBBS, L., WILSON, P. and O'SULLIVAN, K. (1988) Balancing the possible benefits against the risk of cytotoxic chemotherapy – patients and doctors decisions. (Abstract of paper presented at meeting of the B.A.C.R. Norwich. 15. 12.)

SMYTH, J.F., FOWLIE, S.M., GREGOR, A., CROMPTON, G.K., BUSUTTIL, A., LEONARD, R.C.F. and GRANT, I.W.B. (1986) The impact of chemotherapy on small cell carcinoma of the bronchus. *Quarterly Journal of Medicine*, *61*, 969–976.

SOLOMON, F., WHITE, C.C., PARRON, D.L. and MENDELSON, W.B. (1979) Sleeping pills, insomnia and medical practice. *New England Journal of Medicine*, *300*, 803–808.

TURNER, E.M., ASCHER, L.M. (1979) A within subject analysis of stimulus control therapy with severe sleep onset insomniacs. *Behaviour Research and Therapy*, *17*, 107–112.

WEISENBURGER, T.H. (1989) Non small cell lung cancer. Definitive radiotherapy and combined modality therapy. In J.A. Roth, J.C. Ruckdeschel and T.H. Weisenburger (Eds) *Thoracic Oncology*. Philadelphia: W.B. Saunders Co.

WILLIAMS, R.L. and KARACAN, I. (Eds) (1976) *Pharmacology of Sleep*. New York: Wiley.

ZWART, C.A. and LISMAN, S.A. (1979) Analysis of Simulus Control Treatment of Sleep Onset Insomnia. *Journal of Consulting and Clinical Psychology*, *47*, 113–118.

BREAST CANCER

Maggie Watson

Each year in the UK 24,500 women are newly diagnosed with breast cancer and 15,000 women die from this disease (CRC, 1988). In the USA these figures are substantially greater with approximately 119,000 new cases per year (Young *et al.*, 1985). Breast cancer accounts for 10 per cent of all new cancer cases and 20 per cent of all female cancers. It is estimated that 1 in 12 women will develop breast cancer some time is their life. The overall five-year survival of patients is 64 per cent on average, although the stage at which the disease is diagnosed is important, with an 84 per cent survival at Stage I (tumour confined to the breast) to 18 per cent at Stage IV (distant metastases present). Overall, about 20 per cent of newly registered cases die within the first year. An examination of survival curves shows little change between two to five years after registration. From these statistics it is clear that breast cancer is not the most lethal of cancers, but the sheer scale of the disease makes it a substantial problem. Generally cancer can be considered a disease of the elderly, with 70 per cent of all new cases occuring in people aged 60 years or over. However, the incidence of breast cancer peaks in the 55–60 age group and it is the commonest single cause of all deaths in women between 35–54 years. Thus it makes a significant impact on the reduction of life expectancy among women.

The cause of breast cancer is not clear although a number of risk factors have been identified (see Table 1). Agreement has not been reached on a number of these; many are still under investigation and some appear to be more strongly related to risk of breast cancer than others. A substantial proportion of these risk factors appear to be hormone based or related to reproductive history and it is considered likely that hormones such as oestrogen may play a part in the development or promotion of breast cancer. However, preventative methods for breast cancer tend to be concentrated on early detection in order to allow treatment before metastasis has occurred.

In summary, breast cancer is the commonest of female cancers which if detected early has a better than 80 per cent five-year survival rate. Given these data it is not unreasonable to expect substantial

TABLE 1   *Possible factors associated with increased risk of breast cancer*

Late childbearing
Nulliparity
Early menarche
Late menopause
Family history of breast cancer
Previous benign breast disease
Oral contraceptives (prolonged uses of high oestrogen pill before first pregnancy)
Increasing age
Obesity
Cigarette smoking
Alcohol use
High-fat diet
Higher social class
Country of origin (higher incidence in western developed countries)
Ionizing radiation exposure
Prolonged use of Hormone Replacement Therapy at high doses
Stress

resources, not only for improving treatment but also for ensuring a good rehabilitation and quality of life for this patient group.

In focusing on the psychological care of women with breast cancer the following will be examined:

– Prevalence and detection of psychological morbidity
– Increased risk of psychological morbidity
– Predominant problems
– A review of psychologically-based treatments
– Service organization

PREVALENCE AND DETECTION OF PSYCHOLOGICAL MORBIDITY

Prevalence

Over a decade has passed since Morris (1979) wrote:

It is clear....that psychological morbidity from mastectomy exists, but its nature and amount, who suffers it and whether it might be reduced are still only hinted at rather than convincingly demonstrated.

Since then treatment for breast cancer has changed somewhat. Within the sphere of surgical treatment there has been a move away from the use of mastectomy towards the more conservative local excision technique. The use of systemic treatments has also changed with cytotoxic drugs and hormone-based treatments being more frequently used now than they were a decade ago. These changes in treatment techniques will, in turn, have contributed to changes in the types of problems breast cancer patients now experience.

Since Morris's original statement there has been a burgeoning literature on psychological morbidity. A recent researcher's bibliography (Burton, 1990) cites more than 600 English-language publications devoted to breast cancer with the vast majority having appeared in the last decade. In the past evidence suggested that the rate of psychological morbidity among breast cancer patients was high (Hughes, 1982; Greer and Silberfarb, 1982; Maguire *et al.*, 1978; Morris *et al.*, 1977), with figures of 20 to 30 per cent being quoted. More recent studies suggest that some of this morbidity is transient and that unremitting and substantial morbidity may be confined to a smaller number of women (Dean, 1987; Hughson *et al.*, 1988; Sensky *et al.*, 1989; Watson *et al.*, 1990). Overall the rates given in the literature vary between 5 per cent (Dean, 1987) and 48 per cent (Derogatis *et al.*, 1983). These figures vary, of course, depending on the method and timing of assessments. Until recently it was usual to find methods of assessing prevalence of depression and anxiety (the most commonly reported psychopathology) which incorporated somatic symptoms. It is now recognized that this introduces a bias which inflates prevalence figures. Such methods pick up treatment and disease-related symptoms as well as known psychiatric symptoms (for example feeling slowed up, anorexia and weight loss, loss of sex drive, insomnia). The development of measures free of these somatic symptoms will remedy this but there is a consensus of opinion (Ganz *et al.*, 1990) that measures developed specifically for this population are needed rather than importing them directly from psychiatric practice. However, taking even the most conservative estimate, the sheer number of patients indicates that there is significant psychological morbidity. This morbidity can also continue long after the diagnosis is known and treatment is completed (Morris *et al.*, 1977; Dean, 1987) and is more common among younger patients (Hughson *et al.*, 1988). Ideally, resources should be available in oncology centres which are directed at reducing levels of psychological morbidity. Within Europe this area of patient care is seriously undersupported and it has been pointed out (Ganz *et al.*, 1990) that few European cancer centres routinely provide the range of psychological services needed, with very few psychiatrists and psychologists being integrated into the medical setting where the cancer treatment is provided. For nurses and doctors, who are most often in the position of trying to offer comfort to breast cancer patients whilst being limited in time and appropriate skills, this is a serious problem.

It could be argued that it is not enough to be able to identify those women who need help if what is actually needed is a greater commitment of resources to this area of patient care. Despite this there is a need to work within the present framework, thus the aim of this chapter is not to provide guidelines for operating a skilled psychological support programme on a 'shoestring', rather the aim is to consider what might be reasonably achieved within the average oncology unit.

Detection

A number of studies have suggested that oncologists fail to detect or inaccurately detect a high proportion of patients with significant psychological morbidity (Derogatis *et al.*, 1976;. Maguire *et al.*, 1978; Maguire, 1983; Sensky *et al.*, 1989). However, it has been pointed out (Sensky *et al.*, 1989) that this may not be a failure in recognition of symptoms but rather a failure to acknowledge them. This is an important distinction and may explain some of the low recognition figures quoted. To a certain extent what Sensky and colleagues have highlighted are the problems which arise when psychological morbidity is recognized but it is not clear how it should be dealt with because of poor referral services. Nevertheless recognition skills can and should be improved and two approaches are described.

Screening interviews. Maguire (1983) has given a number of very sensible screening questions to be used at follow-up clinics which are worth repeating. These questions can be asked selectively within the context of an informal consultation at the clinics:

- *How have you been feeling since the operation?*
- *How have you been sleeping?*
- *Have you found it easy to adapt to everyday life?*
- *Do you often feel especially miserable or worried?*
- *Are you as active socially as you were before surgery?*
- *What about your relationship with your husband (partner); has that been affected?*
- *Have you resumed love-making yet?*
- *How do you feel about your breast?*
- *How do you feel when you catch sight of your chest?*
- *Have you had any...pain?*
- *Are there any other problems?*

Brief training in psychiatric interviewing techniques has been shown to improve detection rates vastly (Maguire *et al.*, 1980). Patients can be monitored routinely at outpatient clinics when they attend for follow-up appointments. In some instances specialist nurses have been trained in this monitoring function and have been shown to recognize nearly 80 per cent of patients needing further help (Maguire, 1980).

Screening questionnaires. Although a variety of questionnaires (often borrowed from work with psychiatric samples) have been used to detect symptoms of depression and anxiety, most contain somatic symptoms. This introduces the bias described earlier which only a separation of physical functioning from the emotional symptoms will avoid.

The development of the Hospital Anxiety and Depression [HAD] Scale (Zigmond and Snaith, 1983), however, has provided a reliable and brief screening instrument which has been validated on a cancer patient sample (Razavi *et al.*, 1989). This scale has been developed specifically for medical patients and excludes somatic symptoms, with the exception of one item ('I feel as if I am slowed down'). Because it is brief, has good face validity, can be easily completed and scored, and is one of the few scales appropriate for medical rather than psychiatric patients, it has been overwhelmingly embraced by many working in the area of psychosocial oncology. Its reputation as a good swift measure of depression and anxiety is probably well deserved although more recent studies (Ibbotson *et al.*, 1987; Razavi, *et al.*, 1989) suggest that it might have a high false positive rate. It has also been suggested by Razavi and colleagues that the depression and anxiety scales are not distinct and ought to be combined for the purpose of scoring. However, a separate examination (Moorey *et al.*, 1990) of the structure of this scale suggests that the depression and anxiety subscales are distinct but related and should be scored separately as in the original form.

It is important to emphasize that the HAD is a rough-and-ready screening method and, as it covers only the preceding week, may need to be repeated at regular intervals. The detection of symptoms using this method should *always* be followed by a more detailed assessment interview. The advantage of the HAD screening is that the more time-consuming assessment interview can then be confined to those patients who score above the thresholds for significant morbidity. With its high false positive rate this scale will tend to pick up some patients who are not true 'cases' but it is better to pick up a few inappropriate patients than miss those with significant symptoms of depression and anxiety. Further refinement in this scale may take place as more data from cancer patients becomes available. For the present is seems a worthwhile method that clinicians, nurses and mental health professionals might use to enable them to select patients who need a more detailed assessment.

More recently a questionnaire measure of coping, the Mental Adjustment to Cancer [MAC] Scale (Watson *et al.*, 1988b) has been developed which might also act as a screening device, assessing as it does feelings of helplessness or a positive 'fighting spirit'. This method has the advantage that it was developed specifically for cancer patients and could be used in conjunction with the HAD.

When to screen. It is not always appropriate to use a screening questionnaire – the MAC Scale for instance is not appropriate for patients in the terminal phase of their illness, and such patients should be monitored through less formal techniques. Perhaps the obvious time to avoid screening is at diagnosis of primary disease or relapse. Assessments made at this time tend to show that high levels of morbidity exist (Derogatis *et al.*, 1983). Routine support for patients is often concentrated in these periods anyway. Much of this psychological morbidity, as a response to the 'crisis' of diagnosis, will remit spontaneously without any specialized or skilled intervention by a mental health professional, as patients muster their resources and begin to cope. The crisis intervention literature suggests that important adaptation takes place during the four to six weeks following the crisis, after which there is a return to normal functioning. It is important to detect those patients who are not returning to their former level of functioning, so that appropriate help can be offered and a proper rehabilitation initiated. Patients are therefore best screened after this period of adaptation and certainly such screening would appear to be inappropriate during the first month after being told the diagnosis if the primary aim is to detect those who continue to fail to adjust.

INCREASED RISK OF PSYCHOLOGICAL MORBIDITY

There are a number of factors which have been associated with increased risk of psychological morbidity among women with breast cancer. It is possible to be sensitive to these patients 'at risk' and monitor them more closely at follow-up clinics. The identification of 'at risk' patients is in the best tradition of preventive medicine because not only does it allow early formulation of a management policy but early psychological intervention has an improved chance of reducing psychological morbidity (Gordon *et al.*, 1980; Watson *et al.*, 1988a). Using an informal interview method it should be possible to identify not only those patients presently experiencing a significant level of morbidity but also those who are 'at risk' and require close and more frequent monitoring. Factors which have been associated with increased risk of psychological morbidity are given in Table 2.

TABLE 2 *Factors associated with increased risk of psychological morbidity*

Psychiatric history
Lack of support from family or friends and no opportunity to confide worries
Pre-existing marital problems
Cancers and cancer treatments associated with visible deformity
Inability to accept the physical changes associated with the disease or its treatment
Younger patients are more susceptible
Tendency to suppress or contain negative feelings
Low expectation for efficacy of treatment
Lack of involvement in satisfying activities or occupation
More physical symptoms reported when cancer is diagnosed, regardless of the actual stage of the illness
An adverse experience of cancer in the family
Treatment by aggressive cytotoxic drugs
Additional concurrent stress

It was pointed out, quite some time ago by Cobliner (1977) that:

> Patients who frequently shared worries and confided intimacies with close friends appeared to make the best adjustment.

and that:

> None of the patients who had confidantes experienced prolonged episodes of emotional disability directly related to her illness.

In summarizing the findings relating to increased risk, age, support systems and level of pre-diagnostic functioning appear to determine level of adjustment to a large extent (Bloom, *et al.*, 1982; Cobliner, 1977; Dean, 1987; Gordon *et al.*, 1980; Hughes, 1982; Jamison *et al.*, 1978; Lehmann *et al.*, 1978; Weisman, 1976; Weisman *et al.*, 1980). Increasingly breast cancer treatment units now use a specialist nurse to cover much of the routine counselling provided pre- and post-operatively. At the point where primary treatment ends there is usually an opportunity to see patients and discuss any outstanding issues and this is often a good time at which to establish the need for monitoring the 'at risk' patients. Lack of a confiding relationship, previous problems with 'nerves', marital difficulties etc. may point to a need to *monitor* more closely even if there is no evidence of distress at that time. This type of informal interview can be incorporated into the routine care of the breast cancer patient and requires little in the way of additional resources.

PREDOMINANT PROBLEMS

The predominant problems for breast cancer patients are not dissimilar from other diagnostic groups but the focus may be shifted somewhat. Essentially problems can be broken down into a chronological sequence, namely: communication of diagnosis or relapse; treatment-related problems; and long-term consequences of diagnosis and treatment.

Communication

Problems for the breast cancer patient begin with the detection of the breast lump and women often comment that this was the worst time because of the uncertainty. The introduction of more widely available breast-screening services should provide an opportunity for effective communication with the patient at this early stage. Ideally breast cancer screening services should include a counsellor and/or specialist nurse who can see patients at this early stage, deal with any questions and provide adequate information to help allay fears and misconceptions. Where appropriate, patients should be given the opportunity to ventilate worries and feelings.

Communication of a definitive diagnosis of breast cancer raises other sorts of issues. Doctors still have difficulties with this themselves, as one patient's comment aptly illustrated when she was describing what she had been told about her diagnosis: 'I asked him [the doctor] if I had cancer and he said I had a "tumour". He just couldn't seem to bring himself to say it was cancer.' An atmosphere of openness and honesty has become more usual over the last decade but a reluctance to disclose the diagnosis still exists among some doctors. (This situation is somewhat different in the USA where legal pressures have contributed to more frank and open discussion between doctors and patients regarding the diagnosis and any treatment options.) Feldman (1984) quotes one doctor who refused permission for a patient to take part in a cancer research study saying:

> I never use that word and I don't want anyone else to use it with my patients and for them to think of themselves as cancerous.

This is done seemingly to protect the patient, but by so doing perpetuates the idea that:

> cancer can be likened to an unspeakable plague, secretly ravaging the body which gradually wastes away until the inevitable agonizing death (Parr, 1989).

Patients can and do come to terms with the diagnosis but they need accurate information aimed at demystifying cancer that is given in a supportive environment. At this point the treating physician must be aware that he or she is the key figure from whom the patient needs support. As Holland and Jacobs (1986) point out, the doctor must be prepared to accept, in a supportive manner, the patients' distress and sometimes hostility.

Treatment-Related Problems

The treatment modalities used in breast cancer bring problems specific to each type of treatment. Problems arising from surgical treatment not only appear to be the most frequently documented but much debate has been generated regarding the merits or otherwise of mastectomy versus more conservative techniques (Hall and Fallowfield, 1989). The effects of mutilating surgical techniques, such as mastectomy, are well known and disturbances in body image and psychosexual functioning have been commonly reported (Dean, 1987; Hughes, 1982; Hughson *et al.*, 1988; Maguire, 1978; Morris, 1977). The more conservative local excision technique also brings some degree of mutilation. It is easy to fall into the trap of assuming that there will be no body image or psychosexual problems where the less mutilating local excision has been used. Each woman is different and the impact of either mastectomy or conservative surgical treatments upon body image needs to be ascertained on an individual basis. The nurse and/or mental health professional can play an important role here by gently exploring the degree of distress or deterioration in sexual functioning linked to mutilating surgical treatments. For mastectomy patients the restoration of external body image is often linked with the ability to cope and adjust to breast cancer (Denton and Baum, 1982). Helping to restore the patient's appearance through the successful fitting of a breast prosthesis is an integral part of any help offered to assist patients in coping with surgery.

For radiotherapy, again, clear information can help patients to cope with and anticipate the side-effects of this treatment. It is also important to explain the need for radiotherapy, as some patients still harbour the idea that it is used *only* for palliation. For some patients, being told that radiotherapy is needed is an automatic 'death sentence'. The process of treatment can also be made easier for patients in a very practical way by paying attention to the environment of the radiotherapy suite. Treatment environments do not have to be cold and clinical and treatment can be made easier by providing an informal and comfortable environment. This applies to both treatment and waiting areas. Some patients are very uncomfortable with the claustrophobic effect of the radiotherapy treatment room and in a few cases may experience panic attacks or extreme anxiety during the radiotherapy preparation and treatment. Making the radiotherapy treatment room look more pleasant and providing music and/or relaxation tapes are very simple ways of helping to reduce some of this anxiety and make the procedure more comfortable for the patient.

Systemic treatments for breast cancer involve the use of hormones or cytotoxic drugs. Hormone-based treatments such as Tamoxifen can have side-effects and coping with these is easier if they can be anticipated. Cytotoxic drugs have a number of well-documented side-effects including, alopecia, nausea and vomiting, and in some cases weight gain. It is also known that certain cytotoxic agents can cause depression and this should be closely monitored as it is often treatable (see Hughes, this volume). A substantial proportion of patients develop conditioned nausea and vomiting or treatment-related phobias (Burish and Carey, 1986) which are treatable using psychological techniques. Simply giving patients a relaxation tape is not adequate, however, as there is some skill involved in successfully implementing these techniques and this is described by Black and Morrow in this volume.

It is not always clear to breast cancer patients why chemotherapy treatment is being used and when offered as an adjuvant treatment this needs to be clearly explained so that patients may, where desired, play some role in determining the treatment choice. Being told that the adjuvant chemotherapy is being used to 'mop it up' in no way communicates the basis for this treatment or the benefits it might offer in terms of reducing relapse rates. Of course, not all patients want to make treatment decisions or to know the details of treatment, but time should be taken to explore with the patient the amount of information they would like to have. It has been clearly shown in numerous studies that where patients are adequately prepared for treatments by being given clear information they tend to cope better.

Long-term Consequences of Diagnosis and Treatment

Tumours of the breast are known to be generally slow-growing and relapse may occur quite some time after the original diagnosis of primary disease. Thus for breast cancer patients there is the long-term issue of when they might consider themselves 'cured', if at all. This continuing uncertainty may to some extent explain why rates of psychological morbidity remain high long after the initial diagnosis. Ventilation of worries about relapse may therefore need to be encouraged long after primary diagnosis. Psychosexual difficulties also appear to persist long after treatment is finished (Dean, 1987). In Dean's study the major area of morbidity was in the deterioration of sexual relationships which was linked to the mutilation caused by mastectomy. The author also noted that this sexual morbidity was not reduced by immediate breast reconstruction. Long-term follow-ups of patients should therefore pay some attention to psychosocial functioning. Where a return to pre-diagnostic sexual functioning has not occurred, help can be offered in the form of counselling or referral to a psychosexual clinic.

If recurrence of breast cancer is diagnosed at a later date the process of psychological care and support must begin anew. It should not be assumed that patients who coped well with their primary diagnosis will also cope with the news of relapse. Patients' feelings, needs and problems should be reassessed in the same way as after diagnosis of primary disease. In the terminal phase of the illness the issues for breast cancer patients are similar to other diagnostic groups and an optimal model for terminal care is described by Cassidy in this volume.

A REVIEW OF PSYCHOLOGICALLY-BASED TREATMENTS

In the literature relating to the efficacy of psychological intervention, breast cancer patients are notably the most frequently investigated group. It should be possible, therefore, to find out whether psychologically-based treatments work, and which techniques work best.

Overall, the evidence suggests that intervention is beneficial (Massie *et al.*, 1989; Watson, 1983) thus the question is no longer, 'should we provide psychosocial care?' but instead relates to what model of care might be adopted and what framework ought to be used. Within the literature a wide range of techniques has been described but because of methodological difficulties comparisons across outcome studies are extremely limited. It is not possible, at this stage, to say that one therapeutic model is better than another. There is, indeed, an argument in favour of an eclectic approach with models of treatment being utilized according to individual patient need. An overview of studies of psychological intervention is given in Table 3. This does not cover the whole range of intervention studies but is confined to those where a control group was included in the outcome study and where the intervention was confined to breast cancer patients.

Because the techniques have been quite varied, a more straightforward way of categorizing the approaches is to divide studies up on the basis of whether individual or group therapy was used.

Group Programmes

Group programmes tend to fall into two categories. In the first the patient and her family are offered a 'drop-in' group. This is available on an informal basis with patients attending when they come to the outpatient clinics. These are usually not very highly structured or

TABLE 3 *Selected studies of psychological intervention with breast cancer patients*

Reference	Outcome
	Group Therapy Method
Blake (1982)	0 Depression, anxiety, locus of control
Ferlic *et al.* (1979)	↑ Confidence in medical staff
Golonka (1977)	0 Anxiety
Kriss & Kraemer (1986)	↑ Positive affect, sexual adjustment
Spiegel *et al.* (1981)	↓ Mood disturbance
Spiegel & Glafkides (1983)	↓ Negative affect
	Individual Therapy Method
Baum & Jones (1979)	↓ Pre-operative anxiety level
Bridge *et al.* (1988)	↓ Mood disturbance
Burton & Parker (1988)	↓ Anxiety
Capone *et al.* (1980)	0 Mood disturbance
Christensen (1983)	↓ Depression
	↑ Sexual satisfaction
Clacey *et al.* (1987)	↓ Depression
Gordon *et al.* (1980)	↓ Negative emotional disturbance
Linn *et al.* (1982)	↑ Quality of life
	↓ Depression
Maguire *et al.* (1980)	↑ Anxiety
Watson *et al.* (1988a)	↓ Depression
	↑ Locus of control
Weisman *et al.* (1980)	↓ Distress

KEY: ↑ = Increase
↓ = Decrease
0 = No Difference

directive and often serve to provide patients with an opportunity to ventilate emotions and discuss any current practical problems. The second type of group programme has tended to be more educational, providing patients with information and advice during particularly critical periods, such as primary diagnosis or relapse.

Groups have the advantage that patients can share worries with others in the same situation and provide a social comparison function. They have the disadvantage that less vocal members may have limited opportunities to ventilate concerns – although a skilled group leader will deal with this difficulty. Groups allow a more effective use of the therapist's time. However, for patients with well-entrenched problems needing in-depth psychotherapy individual sessions may be more appropriate.

Individual Programmes

Although groups can play an important role in alleviating some of the psychological morbidity experienced, there appears to be a trend toward the individual approach being used more often. The literature seems to bear this out, as there appear to be more outcome studies relating to individual rather than group therapy (see Table 3). This individual approach seems to be beneficial for patients who use inappropriate or ineffective methods of dealing with stress and who therefore have difficulties resolving illness-related problems. The most obvious advantage to the individual approach is that therapy is tailored to the patient's needs and the pace of therapy can be adjusted according to requirements.

Despite the difficulties in deciding upon what might be optimal therapeutic techniques there are some general principles which apply and these are:

- that support should be tailored to individual needs;
- that the therapeutic methods be developed to pay particular attention to cancer patient problems and not simply be borrowed from other areas of psychiatry or psychology;
- that continuity be maintained with the same therapist seeing the patient throughout, thereby facilitating an effective relationship between therapist and patient;
- that information be given to demystify the cancer treatments and dispel the myths surrounding the illness;
- that the patient's choice of avoidance as a way of coping should be respected;
- that successful therapy involves encouraging patients to develop active coping strategies to overcome feelings of helplessness and bring a more positive attitude to their illness.

As a recent review pointed out:

> the emphasis in therapy should be not on psychopathology but on fostering personal strengths, raising self-esteem and finding the most effective ways of coping with cancer. (Greer, 1987)

Over the last five to ten years there has been a gradual shift in attitudes, with far more attention being paid to the issue of how to improve quality of life for women with breast cancer. As a result some progress has been made in providing psychosocial care for breast cancer patients. However, further progress is still needed and a good model of care might involve the following:

- The provision of information and counselling at breast-screening clinics.

- The availability of a specialist breast nurse at diagnosis of primary disease or relapse to provide emotional support and practical advice. Monitoring of emotional status and 'at risk' patients could be included, with appropriate referral to psychological and/or psychiatric services for those patients with more difficult and entrenched problems.
- The availability of skilled mental health professionals who are able to deal with the unremitting psychological morbidity and problems which are beyond the skills of the physician or nurse counsellor.

SERVICE ORGANIZATION AND CONCLUSIONS

Psychological morbidity at the time of diagnosis of breast cancer appears to be quite high (Derogatis *et al.*, 1983). Specialist nurses have an important role to play in supporting patients through a crisis and there is some evidence that providing a nurse counsellor at this stage speeds up the rate of adjustment (Watson *et al.*, 1988a). Physicians also have an important role. Both nurses and doctors need to have the skills to recognize psychological morbidity and the acquisition of these skills should be incorporated into their training. For the specialist nurse counsellor there is a need for training in counselling techniques and, in the UK at least, this is a serious deficit in the training of specialist nurses (Roberts and Fallowfield, 1990) with only about one quarter having any formal training in counselling. Where more serious psychological morbidity exists doctors and nurses need to be able to recognize this morbidity and be able to refer patients appropriately to skilled mental health professionals. It is just as important to recognize limitations in one's skills and to know when to refer on. It is possible to be sensitive to women who are vulnerable and use the techniques described earlier to monitor their progress. The counselling process which specialist nurses might use has been described in more detail elsewhere (Denton and Baum, 1983; Watson *et al.*, 1988a) but covers three areas:

(i)   emotional support and facilitation of adjustment;
(ii) information about physical state;
(iii) practical advice on breast prostheses, where required.

Within Europe, and especially the UK, there is a serious lack of skilled mental health professionals operating within the centres where medical treatment takes place. This means that at the present time the psychosocial care of patients is still inadequate. The multidisciplinary ward round can play an important role in providing a channel of communication and a mental health professional should be encouraged to be part of this meeting. The idea of improving recognition

and monitoring skills is fine but must be accompanied by a commitment of resources aimed at providing referral services. Oncologists
may play an important role here by being more vociferous in their
demands for services which provide total patient care. To a certain
extent patients have taken their own action as a result of the lack of
hospital-based psychosocial oncology services and the burgeoning
self-help movement bears witness to this dissatisfaction. Increasingly
however it is being acknowledged that quality of life is as important
as quantity of life and this may bring a more holistic approach to
patient care over the next decade.

The aim here has been to provide some guidelines for the psychosocial care of women with breast cancer. The skills needed to do this
should not, as so often happens, be underestimated. The 'anybody
can do it' attitude needs to be dispensed with so that a more skilled
and professional psychosocial support service can emerge. The patient
deserves a well-trained professional to deal with the different aspects
of psychosocial care. This training need has been neatly summarized
by Hall and Fallowfield (1989):

> it is important to remember that the stress of caring for women with
> breast cancer is emotionally distressing for health carers. Any efforts
> to improve the psychological well-being of patients must include
> appropriate training and support for the whole of the oncology
> team.

In times of limited financial resources (when is there not such a time!)
it is difficult to expand or introduce new services. In an era of high
technology medicine the patient's emotional well-being often has a
low priority. Yet it is possible to make a cold financial argument in
favour of introducing psychosocial services. There is some evidence
that investment in such services has long-term financial benefits
(MAS, 1989; Schlesinger *et al.*, 1983). Massie and colleagues (1989)
have made the point that:

> results might be found in cancer patients that would support not
> only reduced emotional distress but fewer medical visits for control
> of symptoms.

Thus it would appear that expanded psychosocial services for breast
cancer patients might have both short- and long-term benefits both
financially and in terms of improving quality of life. There is a clear
need for further training in the techniques needed for good psychosocial care of breast cancer patients. This chapter provides some
guidelines but in no way supercedes the need for further training.

References

BAUM, M. and JONES, E.M. (1979) Counselling removes patients' fear. *Nursing Mirror, 8*, March, 38–40.

BLAKE, S.M. (1982) *Group psychotherapy with breast cancer patients: A controlled trial.* (Unpublished MSc thesis: Department of Psychiatry, University of Manchester.)

BLOOM, J.R. (1982) Social support, according to stress and adjustment to breast cancer. *Social Science and Medicine, 16*, 1329–1338.

BRIDGE, L.R., BENSON, P., PIETRONI, P.C. and PRIEST, R.G. (1988) Relaxation and imagery in the treatment of breast cancer. *British Medical Journal, 297*, 1169–1172.

BURISH, T.G. and CAREY, M.P. (1986) Conditioned aversive responses in cancer chemotherapy patients: Theoretical and developmental analysis. *Journal of Consulting and Clinical Psychology, 55*, 42–48.

BURTON, M. (1990) *A Researcher's Bibliography.* (Unpublished, private communication.)

BURTON, M.V. and PARKER, R.W. (1988) A randomized controlled trial of pre-operative psychological preparation for mastectomy: A preliminary report. In M. Watson, S. Greer, and C. Thomas (Eds) *Psychosocial Oncology.* Oxford: Pergamon Press.

CANCER RESEARCH CAMPAIGN (1988) Factsheet 6.1. London: Cancer Research Campaign.

CAPONE, M.A., GOOD R.S., WESTIE, S. and JACOBSON, A.F. (1980), Psychosocial rehabilitation of gynaecologic oncology patients. *Archives of Physical Medicine and Rehabilitation, 61*, 128–132.

CHRISTENSEN, D.N. (1983) Post mastectomy couple counselling: An outcome study of a structured treatment protocol. *Journal of Sex and Marital Therapy, 9*, 266–275.

CLASEY, R., THOMAS, C. and PEARSON, H. (1988) Does counselling by nurses for mastectomy patients work? In M. Watson, S. Greer and C. Thomas (Eds) *Psychosocial Oncology.* Oxford: Pergamon Press.

COBLINER, W.G. (1977) Psychosocial factors in gynaecologic or breast malignancies. *Hospital Physician, 10*, 38.

DEAN, C. (1987) Psychiatric morbidity following mastectomy: Preoperative predictors and types of illness. *Journal of Psychosomatic Research, 31*, 385–392.

DENTON, S. and BAUM, M. (1982) Can we predict which women will fail to cope with mastectomy? *Clinical Oncology, 8*, 375.

DENTON, S. and BAUM, M. (1983) Psychosocial aspects of breast cancer. In R. Margolese (Ed.) *Breast Cancer.* Edinburgh: Churchill Livingstone.

DEROGATIS, L.R., ABELOFF, M.D. and MCBETH, C.D. (1976) Cancer patients and their physicians in the perception of psychological symptoms. *Psychosomatics, 17*, 197–201.

DEROGATIS, L.R., MORROW, G.R., FETTING, J., PENMAN, D., PIASETSKY, S., SCHMALE, A.M., HENRICKS, M. and COUNICKE, C.L. (1983) The prevalence of psychiatric disorders among cancer patients. *Journal of the American Medical Asociation, 249*, 751–757.

FELDMAN, F.L. (1984) Wellness and work. In C. Cooper (Ed.) *Psychosocial Stress and Cancer.* Chichester: Wiley & Sons.

FERLIC, M., GOLDMAN, A. and KENNEDY, B.J. (1979) Group counselling in adult patients with advanced cancer. *Cancer, 43,* 760–766.

GANZ, P.A., BERNHARD, J. and HURNY, C. (1990) Quality of life and psychosocial research in Europe: State of the art. (Submitted for publication.)

GOLONKA, L.M. (1977) The use of group counselling with breast cancer patients receiving chemotherapy. *Dissertation Abstracts International, 37* (10-A), 6362–6363.

GORDON, W.A., FREIDENBERGS, I., DILLER, L., HIBBARD, M., WOLF, G. and LEVINE, L. (1980) Efficacy of psychosocial intervention with cancer patients. *Journal of Consulting and Clinical Psychology, 48,* 743–759.

GREER, S. (1987) Psychotherapy for the cancer patient. *Psychiatric Medicine, 5,* 267–279.

GREER, S. and SILBERFARB, P.M. (1982) Psychological concomitants of cancer: Current state of research. *Psychological Medicine, 12,* 563–573.

HALL, A. and FALLOWFIELD, L. (1989) Psychological outcome of treatment for early breast cancer: A review. *Stress Medicine, 5,* 167–175.

HOLLAND, J.C. and JACOBS, E. (1986) Psychiatric sequelae following surgical treatment of breast cancer. *Advances in Psychosomatic Medicine, 15,* 109–123.

HUGHES, J. (1982) Emotional reactions to the diagnosis and treatment of early breast cancer. *Journal of Psychosomatic Research, 26,* 277–283.

HUGHSON, A.V.M., COOPER, A.F., MCARDLE, C.S. and SMITH, D.C. (1988) Psychosocial consequences of mastectomy: Levels of morbidity and associated factors. *Journal of Psychosomatic Research, 32,* 383–391.

IBBOTSON, T., MAGUIRE, P., SELBY, P., PRIESTMAN, T. and WALLACE, L. (1989) Validation Self-Rating Questionnaires . Paper presented to the Annual Conference of the British Psychosocial Oncology Group.

JAMISON, K.R., WELLISCH, D.K. and PASNAU, R.O. (1978) Psychosocial aspects of mastectomy: I. The woman's perspective. *American Journal of Psychiatry, 135,* 432–436.

KRISS, R.T., and KRAEMER, H.C. (1986) Efficacy of group therapy for problems of postmastectomy self-perception, body image and sexuality. *The Journal of Sex Research, 22,* 438–451.

LEHMANN, J.F., DELISA, J.A., WARREN, C.G., DELATEUR, B.J., SANDBRYANT, P.L. and NICHOLSON, G.G. (1978) Cancer rehabilitation: Assessment of need, development and evaluation of a model of care. *Archives of Physical Medicine and Rehabilitation, 59,* 410–419.

LINN, M.W., LINN, B.S. and HARRIS, R. (1982) Effects of counselling for late stage cancer patients. *Cancer, 49,* 1048–1055.

MAGUIRE, G.P. (1983) Psychiatric problems of mutilating surgery. *Readings in Psychiatry and Neurology,* 20–22.

MAGUIRE, G.P., TAIT, A., BROOKE, M., THOMAS, C. and SELLWOOD, R. (1980) Effects of counselling on the psychiatric morbidity associated with mastectomy. *British Medical Journal, 281,* 1454–1456.

MAGUIRE, G.P., LEE, E.G., BEVINGTON, D.J., KUCHEMANN, G.J. CRABTREE, R.J. and CORNELL, C.E. (1978) Psychiatric problems in the first year after mastectomy. *British Medical Journal, 1,* 963–965.

MAS (1989) *National Review of Clinical Psychology Services.* Cheltenham: Management Advisory Service to the National Health Service.

MASSIE, J.M., HOLLAND, J.C. and STRAKER, N. (1989) Psychotherapeutic interventions. In J.C. Holland and J.H. Rowland (Eds) *Handbook of Psychosocial Oncology.* Oxford: Oxford University Press.

MOOREY, S., GREER, S., WATSON, M., GORMAN, C., ROWDEN, L., TUNMORE, R., ROBERT-SON, B. and BLISS, J. (1990) The factor structure and factor stability of the Hospital Anxiety and Depression Scale in patients with cancer. *British Journal of Psychiatry*. (In press.)

MORRIS, T. (1979) Psychological Adjustment to Mastectomy. *Cancer Treatment Reviews*, 6, 41–61.

MORRIS, T., GREER, H.S. and WHITE, P. (1977) Psychological and social adjustment to mastectomy: A two year follow-up study. *Cancer*, 40, 2381–2387.

PARR, M. (1989) Work-related stress in oncology. (Unpublished dissertation, Brunel University.)

RAZAVI, D., DELVAUX, N., FARVACQUES, C. and ROBAYE, E. (1990). Screening for adjustment disorder and major depressive disorders in cancer in-patients. *British Journal of Psychiatry*, 156, 79–83.

ROBERTS, R. and FALLOWFIELD, L. (1990) Letter in the British Psychosocial Oncology Group Newsletter, Spring issue.

SCHLESINGER, H.J.E., MUMFORD, G.V., GLASS, C.P., SHARFSTEIN, S. (1983) Mental health treatment and medical care utilization in fee-for-service system: Outpatient mental health treatment following the onset of a chronic disease. *American Journal of Public Health*, 73, 422–429.

SENSKY, T., DENNEHY, M., GILBERT, A., BEGENT, R., NEWLANDS, E., RUSTIN, G. and THOMPSON, C. (1989) Physicians' perceptions of anxiety and depression among their outpatients: Relationships with patients' and doctors' satisfaction with their interviews. *Journal of the Royal College of Physicians*, 23, 33–38.

SPIEGEL, D., BLOOM, J.R. and YALOM, I. (1981) Group support for patients with metastatic cancer. *Archives of Group Psychiatry*, 38, 527–533.

SPIEGEL, D. and GLAFKIDES, M.C. (1983) Effects of group confrontation with death and dying. *International Journal of Group Psychotherapy*, 33, 433–474.

WATSON, M. (1983) Psychological intervention with cancer patients: A review. *Psychological Medicine*, 13, 839–846.

WATSON, M., DENTON, S., BAUM, M. and GREER, S. (1988a) Counselling breast cancer patients: A specialist nurse service. *Counselling Psychology Quarterly*, 1, 23–32.

WATSON, M., GREER, S., YOUNG, J., INAYAT, Q., BURGESS, C. and ROBERTSON, B. (1988b) Development of a questionnaire measure of adjustment to cancer: The MAC Scale. *Psychological Medicine*, 18, 203–209.

WATSON, M., GREER, S., ROWDEN, L., GORMAN, C., ROBERTSON, B., BLISS, J.M. and TUNMORE, R. (1990) Relationships between emotional control adjustment to cancer and depression and anxiety in breast cancer patients. (Submitted for publication.)

WEISMAN, A.D. (1976) Early diagnosis of vulnerability in cancer patients. *American Journal of the Medical Sciences*, 271, 187–196.

WEISMAN, A.D., WORDEN, J.W. and SOBEL, H.J. (1980) Psychosocial screening and intervention with cancer patients. Project Omega, Department of Psychiatry, Harvard Medical School Publication.

YOUNG, J.L., PERCY, C.L. and ASIRE, A. (Eds) (1985) Surveillance epidemiology and end results: Incidence and mortality data, 1973–1977. *Cancer Institute Monograph*, 57, 81–2330.

ZIGMOND, A.S. and SNAITH, R.P. (1983) The hospital anxiety and depression scale. *Acta Psychiatrica Scandinavica*, 67, 361–370.

TESTICULAR CANCER

Clare Moynihan

Testicular tumours are relatively rare. However, they are the most common malignancy in men between the ages of 15 and 35 years. The incidence in the UK is 2–3:100,000 and appears to be rising. North American incidence is 2.1:100,000. The aetiology is unknown. There is an increased incidence of testicular germ cell tumours in patients with a history of testicular maldescent.

Major advances in treatment have taken place during the past decade which are largely due to the introduction of effective chemotherapy, although new methods of diagnosis such as computed tomography and monitoring of disease with specific tumour markers have contributed. The current cure rate is now more than 90 per cent – a spectacular contrast to the results of 40 years ago when more than half of men with metastatic testicular cancer died within three years of diagnosis.

Outline of Management

The majority of testicular tumours are malignant and arise from germinal cells. They can be histologically classified into two groups: seminomas and non-seminomatous germ cell tumours of variable histology described as teratomas. Seminomas usually present in men in their 40s and 50s and have a more indolent course. The majority of patients present with localized disease. In contrast, teratomas present in younger men commonly with disseminated disease. The treatment depends on tumour histology and extent of spread at presentation.

Patients usually present with a gradually enlarging, painless testicular mass. When a tumour is suspected the testis is removed through the inguinal approach (inguinal orchidectomy). The extent of disease is subsequently assessed through a number of staging investigations. They include CT scanning of chest, abdomen and pelvis and measurement of serum markers, alphafetoprotein and beta human chorionic gonadotrophin, as well as baseline investigations such as full blood count, biochemical profile and chest x-ray. Specific treatment is decided on the basis of tumour histology and stage of disease.

Chemotherapy regimens are used in the majority of patients with disseminated testicular tumours and result in high cure rates. The use of radiotherapy is largely confined to localized presentations of seminoma.

Seminoma. The majority of patients with seminoma present without evidence of metastases (stage 1) and are treated by orchidectomy and radiotherapy to potential sites of spread in the para-aortic region, with cure rates approaching 100 per cent.

Patients with small volume metastatic disease confined to para-aortic lymph nodes (stage IIA and IIB) are treated with radiotherapy to para-aortic and pelvic nodes. More extensive disease, which is detected in a minority of patients at presentation, is treated with chemotherapy. This results in high cure rates.

Relapse. Relapse post radiotherapy has an excellent salvage rate (90 per cent) with chemotherapy. Those who have undergone chemotherapy and relapsed are now treated with second-line intensive regimes. The salvage rate is, as yet, unknown because of short follow-up.

Teratoma. Approximately half of patients with testicular teratomas present with disease in the testis alone (stage 1). The treatment approach used to involve irradiation of para-aortic and pelvic lymph nodes, although in a proportion of patients there was still recurrence with metastases outside the irradiated area. As chemotherapy is effective in eradicating small volume metastases and clinical staging procedures are highly accurate in detecting metastatic disease, it has now become possible to defer treatment in patients in this group; curative chemotherapy is instituted when necessary. This policy of close surveillance for stage 1 testicular teratomas was introduced at the Royal Marsden Hospital in 1979 and the overall survival for this group is 99 per cent. Such a policy relies heavily on good patient compliance and close observation at regular intervals.

Patients with metastatic disease at presentation are treated with a highly effective combination of drugs, with cure rates approaching 90 per cent. Chemotherapy usually necessitates hospitalization for six-day periods every three weeks. The majority of patients receive four three-weekly cycles of treatment. Side-effects include hair loss, nausea, vomiting and soreness of the skin, and less commonly peripheral neuropathy and a degree of lung damage.

Relapse. Salvage post chemotherapy for metastatic disease is difficult: the present rate is 20 per cent.

Retriperitoneal lymph node dissection (RPLND). RPLND is a surgical procedure performed in the USA and parts of Europe. It entails a

ection of the retreperitoneum which, in its classical form, sacri-
ed the sympathetic nerve plexus. Normal sexual function is jeop-
rdized as it can lead to impotence or retrograde ejaculation causing
infertility. However, the latter does not effect libido and sensation of
orgasm. Classical RPLND techniques have recently been modified. A
new nerve-sparing operation helps to maintain ejaculatory function
and reduces the risk of impotence.

Fertility. Approximately 50 per cent of men will have abnormally
low sperm counts prior to excision of the affected testis. Chemotherapy results in temporary sterility, with a return to normal within
an average time of two years. There is no evidence of increased risk of
congenital malformation of children born after aggressive treatment.

Patients with a testicular tumour have a low probability of recurrence if in complete remission two years after completion of chemotherapy. A patient in remission can think of himself as 'cured'.

While spectacular medical progress bodes well, survival itself may
harbour its own problems which are, in many instances, unique to a
young testicular cancer patient and his partner or relative. For this
reason I will describe those problems in some detail by locating them
in research findings from Europe and the USA. Thus a firm basis of
current knowledge will put any suggestions for a psychological intervention (counselling) into its proper context. As yet, we in this
field of research are not able to make definitive pronouncements as to
the efficacy of psychological support. However, it has been established that psychological intervention is beneficial in other cancer
groups (Massie *et al.*, 1989). A systematic evaluation of Adjuvant
Psychological Therapy (see Moorey and Greer, 1989 and this volume)
with testicular cancer patients is currently in progress at the Royal
Marsden Hospital. Thus preliminary and anecdotal evidence will be
submitted as guidelines for providing psychological support for these
patients and their relatives.

PREDOMINATING PSYCHOSOCIAL PROBLEMS

Psychosocial Morbidity

At diagnosis. Men who have been told their diagnosis have low
rates of severe psychological morbidity one month post diagnosis and
before treatment has commenced (Moynihan *et al.*, in preparation) as
measured by the Hospital Anxiety and Depression Scale (Zigmond
and Snaith, 1983) which is discussed by Watson, this volume. Anecdotal evidence and retrospective data (Moynihan, 1987) indicate that

the actual diagnosis is a time of uncertainty and fear of death. Subsequent uncertainty due to ongoing staging procedures and unresolved treatment decisions are recounted as times of fear and anxiety (Moynihan, 1987).

During treatment. Both retrospective (Gritz *et al.*, 1989a) and prospective (Trump *et al.*, 1985) data show that levels of anxiety and depression are elevated during treatment. Few studies have shown the specific effects of differing treatment regimens on patients' psychological state. Tiredness and exhaustion are recounted by patients especially amongst those in the surgery and radiotherapy groups and in patients receiving vinblastine (Aass *et al.*, 1989).

Post treatment. A picture of psychological well-being is reported in the majority of men (Cassileth and Steinfeld, 1987; Gritz *et al.*, 1989a; Moynihan, 1987; Rieker *et al.*, 1989; Schover, 1987; Tross *et al.*, 1984; Trump *et al.*, 1985). In many cases, a more enhanced view of life is experienced (Gritz *et al.*, 1989a; Rieker *et al.*, 1989). A significant minority, however, suffer psychological symptoms, even years after treatment has ended (Cassileth and Steinfeld, 1987; Gritz *et al.*, 1989a; Moynihan, 1987; Rieker *et al.*, 1989).

The incidence of moderate to severe psychological morbidity in patients who have survived one to twenty years post treatment is 10 per cent to 23 per cent. Distress may be related to sexual impairment, a pessimistic outlook on life, low self-esteem, diminished personal relationships, unemployment, financial difficulties, a fear of relapse or death and low socio-economic status (see Table 1). Time since diagnosis and treatment type are not predictive of distress, although there is an indication that symptom levels decline six months post treatment (Trump *et al.*, 1985), and those men in the surveillance group suffer as much psychological morbidity as those who undergo aggressive treatment regimes (Moynihan 1987).

TABLE 1   *Patients' risk factors for psychological distress*

Age
Low socio-economic and educational status
Unemployment
Financial difficulties
Fear of relapse/death
Diminished personal relationships
Low self-esteem
Sexual dysfunction
Infertility distress

...e most important areas of dysfunction centre around sexual
...ivity (including infertility), body image and social upheaval, and
...re described in some detail below.

Sexual Function

Diagnosis and pre-treatment. Sexual dysfunction is minimal both
prior and post diagnosis and does not differ from a sample of age-
matched men (Fossa *et al.*, 1988). Post-surgery discomfort may account for the little sexual dysfunction reported after orchidectomy
(Gritz *et al.*, 1989a).

During treatment. A curtailment of sexual activity and a loss of
sexual drive is reported (Fossa *et al.*, 1988; Trump *et al.*, 1985) and is
more pronounced in radiotherapy and chemotherapy groups (Gritz *et
al.*, 1989b). However, it is temporary in many cases: median duration
2.3 months. A decrease in the quality of orgasm has been reported by
men in all treatment groups, but the highest rate has been observed
in those groups who have undergone RPLND (median duration 3.4
months) (Gritz *et al.*, 1989b).
  Surgical scarring and hair loss effect a man's self-esteem (Gritz *et
al.*, 1989b; Schover 1987). This in turn, causes sexual anxiety and
further sexual dysfunction (Schover 1987).

Post treatment. Sexual function and activity is not unduly com-
promized in survivors of testicular tumours (Cassileth and Steinfeld
1987, Fossa *et al.*, 1988; Gritz *et al.*, 1989b; Moynihan 1987; Trump *et
al.*, 1985). However, some patients report significantly more dysfunction than comparison groups even years after treatment has ended
(Rieker *et al.*, 1989; Schover and von Eschenbach, 1985; Tross *et al.*,
1984).
  The overall incidence of the nature of dysfunction varies between
10 per cent and 50 per cent and lies in the following areas: erectile
dysfunction, difficulty in reaching orgasm, a decrease in its intensity,
sexual dissatisfaction, an inability to ejaculate, a decline in semen
volume, a loss of libido, and a decrease in sexual frequency. Teratoma
patients with RPLND report a greater decline in semen volume
compared with seminoma patients treated with radiotherapy alone.
Within a non-seminomatous group, those men who received lymphadenectomy and radiotherapy have significantly higher rates of erectile dysfunction, difficulty in reaching orgasm, reduced orgasmic
intensity (Schover and von Eschenbach, 1985) and retrograde ejaculation (Nijman *et al.*, 1987a) than those men who have lymphadenectomy or lymphadenectomy plus chemotherapy (Nijman *et al.*, 1987b;

Schover and von Eschenbach, 1985). In seminoma patients, higher dose irradiation to the para-aortic field is predictive of erectile and orgasmic problems (Schover *et al.*, 1986).

Evidence strongly suggests that sexual dysfunction is related to treatment types. It is especially evident in those men who have undergone RPLND (with concomitant ejaculatatory dysfunction) plus or minus additional treatment (Gritz *et al.*, 1989b; Rieker *et al.*, 1989; Schover, 1987). RPLND is not a routine procedure in the UK and may account for low levels of sexual dysfunction amongst English patients. Interestingly, those men who had been 'treated' by close surveillance report fewer sexual problems when compared to comparison groups (Blackmore 1988).

Time since diagnosis, perceived sexual problems prior to diagnosis and participation in sperm-banking programmes, do not effect sexual function post treatment or the distress it may cause (Moynihan, 1987; Rieker *et al.*, 1989). However, differences in rates of sexual malfunction may represent ageing. The younger teratoma patients have fewer sexual problems than their older seminoma counterparts when they were compared to the same control group (Schover *et al.*, 1986; Schover 1987).

The concealment of emotions, elevated mood, and lower income and educational status are related to sexual performance distress (Rieker *et al.*, 1989). Orgasmic difficulties and erectile dysfunction have been found to be more common in men worried about sexuality (Schover and von Eschenbach, 1984). Men with sexual dysfunction (including infertility distress), have reported a greater propensity to report negative changes in the following areas: self-respect, relaxation, a fear of death, outlook on life and personal relationships (Rieker *et al.*, 1989).

Infertility Distress

At diagnosis. Little information is available on the distress caused by what may subjectively be regarded as a major side-effect of testicular disease. Anecdotal evidence suggests that there are minimal levels of infertility distress one month post diagnosis and before the start of treatment. A diagnosis of cancer appears to eclipse other considerations.

Post treatment. Overall rates of distress range from 7 per cent (Schover, 1987) to 31 per cent (Rieker *et al.*, 1985) and appear to be related to treatment procedures. The lowest rates of infertility distress are found in seminoma patients treated with radiotherapy (Rieker *et al.*, 1985; Schover and von Eschenbach, 1985) and the highest among those who have RPLND and chemotherapy (Rieker *et al.*, 1989; Schover and von Eschenbach, 1985).

However, the older seminoma patients are more likely to have completed their families, substantiating the consensus that younger, childless men are more likely to suffer distress (Gritz *et al.*, in press; Rieker *et al.*, 1989; Schover and von Eschenbach, 1985), regardless of time elapsed since treatment (Rieker *et al.*, 1985) or whether sperm is banked (Moynihan, 1987; Rieker *et al.*, 1985), although childless men have been shown to be more likely to do the latter (Gritz *et al.*, in press).

Distress is significantly associated with low socio-economic and educational groups (Rieker *et al.*, 1985), a conflicting marriage at an early stage of a man's cancer experience (Schover and von Eschenbach, 1985), negative changes in close interpersonal relationships (Rieker *et al.*, 1985) and low self-esteem (Schover *et al.*, 1986).

Body Image

The loss of a testicle does not appear to have an overt effect on patients (Moynihan, 1987; Gritz *et al.*, 1989a). Few English men (when offered) accept a prosthesis at initial surgery regardless of age or marital status. Rates of acceptance are slightly higher in the USA. Perceived diminishment in overall attractiveness is not negligible among these men, however. Patients indicate that surgical scarring most adversely effects their body image, followed by the aftereffects of chemotherapy, such as hair loss (Gritz *et al.*, 1989b).

SOCIAL ISSUES

Employment Experience

The majority of men continue with career goals and educational plans (Edbril and Rieker, 1990; Moynihan, 1987; Rieker *et al.*, 1989; Trump *et al.*, 1985). A significant minority, however, experience a negative impact in their work lives (Edbril and Rieker, 1990; Moynihan, 1987; Rieker *et al.*, 1989). General worries about job maintenance, a lack of confidence to handle strenuous work and general dissatisfaction help to contribute to a negative impact in this area.

Evidence strongly suggests that a man's well-being is greatly enhanced by his employment status (Moynihan, 1987). However, a simple return to work is not necessarily a useful indicator of psychosocial stability (Edbril and Rieker, 1990). While dissatisfaction at work is associated with anxiety, depression and fatigue, 'satisfied' workers also exhibit distress, especially when they conceal their emotions and uphold traditional masculine ideals. This suggests a need to over-compensate for physical and psychological loss through an overt expression of job satisfaction and job security (Edbril and Rieker, 1990). Job satisfaction does not, however, preclude the *fear* of job loss or discrimination at work (Moynihan, 1987).

Unemployment is more likely to be experienced by those in lower socio-economic groups who, in turn, are more prone to psychological distress as a consequence of financial difficulties, especially when there are children in the family (Moynihan, 1987).

Political and cultural factors may have a strong impact on the lives of working men. During and preceding one study the rate of unemployment was high (Moynihan, 1987). Rates of unemployment were low at the time of another (Rieker and Edbril, 1990; Rieker *et al.*, 1989). This highlights the importance of considering the dynamic of culture and change in all aspects of research that seeks to establish the grounds for psychological intervention.

Marital Relationships and Social Support

Divorce rates have been found to be similar to those in the general population (Moynihan, 1987; Gritz *et al.*, 1989a; Rieker *et al.*, 1989). Marriages are often perceived as strengthened (Cassileth and Steinfeld, 1987; Gritz *et al.*, 1989b; Gritz *et al.*, in press; Rieker *et al.*, 1989), although lover relationships may become strained. Conflict is attributed to sexual dysfunction and other cancer-related anxieties (Rieker *et al.*, 1989; Schover and von Eschenbach, 1985).

The influence of cancer on relationships appears to be related to histological differences. Short marriages between teratoma patients are found to be more vulnerable: conflict is attributed mainly to infertility or sexual problems (Schover and von Eschenbach, 1985) although a loss of the expected role in a partnership is shown to cause strain (Schover and von Eschenbach, 1984; Schover and von Eschenbach, 1985). Unhappy relationships among seminoma patients are more prone to disruption, although the length of marriage is not a predictor of conflict (Schover *et al.*, 1986).

Support from relatives during and post treatment is of special benefit (Gritz *et al.*, in press; Moynihan, 1987) as is support derived from hospital staff and the camaraderie of other patients (Moynihan, 1987). While good communication and 'bonding' is reported between patients and spouses, significant correlations between their scores of anxiety and depression are known to exist rendering it difficult for those couples who are vulnerable to support one another. Although the quality of partner support is perceived as stable, diligence in its administration is felt by patients to diminish with time (Gritz *et al.*, in press).

Families' Psychological Morbidity

The psychosocial consequences of cancer on the relatives of patients remains a relatively neglected area of research. It is likely that the stability of this group has a beneficial effect on patients (Gritz et al., 1989b). Thus it is important that morbidity in the former is systematically documented in order that a policy for psychological support for both parties may be obtained.

While relatives are relied upon to provide an ambiance of 'normality' and to be generally supportive both during and after illness (Gritz et al., in press; Moynihan, 1987), their brave façade often masks a high degree of bewilderment, helplessness and fear, especially at the time of diagnosis and during treatment (Moynihan, 1987). Moreover, while relatives strive to conceal emotions and to 'cope', the tension experienced is often inadvertently transmitted to the patient who, in turn, is unable to reveal his own fears and anxieties to his close family for fear of provoking anxiety (Moynihan, 1987). A vicious circle of unexpressed emotion sets in as both parties become locked in a drama of superficial well-being.

At diagnosis. Partners have significantly higher levels of anxiety and depression than patients do one month post diagnosis and before treatment has commenced (Moynihan et al., in preparation). This may be due to feelings of exclusion in a clinical setting (Moynihan, 1987), a need for general support, but especially as worry centres around a lack of patient–relative communication (Gritz et al., 1989b), the fear of the possibility of having to bring up a child alone (Gritz et al., in press), an inability or reluctance to articulate worries to medical staff and a general feeling that 'intrusion' must be avoided (Moynihan, 1987).

During treatment. Relatives spontaneously reported the months during treatment and soon after it to be the most difficult time (Moynihan, 1987). While partners' levels of anxiety and depression remain high during the four months post diagnosis, this especially applies to those who suffer severe morbidity at base line (Moynihan et al., in preparation).

Post treatment. Levels of distress are known to decrease at follow-up (Gritz et al., 1989b). However, a rate of 22 per cent morbidity is found amongst relatives post treatment (Moynihan, 1987). Relatives' status *per se*, time and proximity to patients during diagnosis and treatment have no bearing on distress. However, when wives are analysed separately, childlessness is associated with anxiety and depression, especially in women over thirty. Neither sperm banking, nor a husband's perception of his fertility alter this finding (Moynihan, 1987) (see Table 2).

TABLE 2   *Relatives' risk factors for psychological distress*

Age
Feelings of exclusion
Childlessness
Fear of widowhood

Sexual Function

Sexual function distress is not an obvious manifestation amongst partners (Gritz *et al.*, 1989b; Moynihan, 1987). Wives perceive increased sexual satisfaction after diagnosis (although their spouses experience reduced sexual pleasure) (Gritz *et al.*, 1989b). A decrease in sexual activity up to four years post treatment is reported by couples with high concordance between the two (Gritz *et al.*, 1989b). However, a loss of sexual drive is perceived as a relatively short-term problem by both man and wife (median 2.3 months) usually following a surgical procedure. Avoidance by wives of sexual relationships during treatment, while brief, and with no lasting effects, is found to be more frequent than patients realized, suggesting that a protective strategy is mobilized by wives to shield their husbands from adverse reactions (Gritz *et al.*, 1989b). The physical depletion of the patient as a result of chemotherapy is thought to be the cause of this short-term aversion to sexual intimacy (Gritz *et al.*, 1989b), but may also be due to fear of venereal contagion (Moynihan, 1987; Schover and von Eschenbach, 1985).

Partners' Perception of Patients' Body Image

Changes in a man's body have little effect on a wife's attraction to her husband in the long term (Gritz *et al.*, 1989b, Moynihan 1987), although a few spouses feel the need for their husbands to look as much as possible as they did prior to orchidectomy (Gritz *et al.*, 1989b).

Marital Relationships and Support

As described above, marital relationships are known to be strengthened as a result of cancer. However, while the patient acknowledges the importance and existence of partner support during the illness, this is the very time when spouses feel that communication decreases between couples (Gritz *et al.*, in press). Although communication resumes its status quo, certain issues such as fertility, a concern for the patient's emotional status, fear of a partner's recurrence, sexual difficulties, a need for emotional reassurance and a general lack of communication and distancing between partners become and remain potent issues in a small but significant minority (Gritz et al., in press).

At present we have little idea about relatives' support systems. Do they 'use' their close families during difficult times and if so what is the content of their 'supportive communication'? Prospective data may highlight these issues and provide a firmer basis for policy making with regard to a formal intervention of psychological support for this group.

PSYCHOLOGICAL SUPPORT

Counselling is advocated for those men who suffer adverse psychosocial sequelae as a result of diagnosis, treatment and survival (Moynihan, 1987; Rieker et al., 1989; Schover and von Eschenbach, 1984). However, a systematic evaluation of a psychological therapy has not been completed.

It is recognized that men do not normally seek counselling services to deal with their distress (Edbril and Rieker, 1985) and that within this cancer group there is evidence of a propensity to conceal emotions (Fossa et al., 1988; Moynihan, 1987; Rieker et al., 1989). My experience shows that, contrary to widespread belief, many men will express their thwarted feelings if and when they are invited to do so (Moynihan 1987). Although approximately 48 per cent declined entry to my Adjuvant Psychological Therapy (APT) trial, agreement to participate does not depend on high levels of anxiety or depression. An in-depth analysis may reveal certain characteristics of men who comply. My impressions are that late stage disease, an anxious preoccupation with the cancer and an acceptance of counselling as being other than a sign of weakness or masculine failure contribute to the acceptance of support when it is offered. (See Moorey, this volume, for further details of APT.)

Although partners' scores of anxiety and depression are high soon after diagnosis, this group do not readily take up an offer of therapy. Not only do domestic factors prevent regular attendance at the hospital, but this group find it important that they should be seen as coping. Often relatives will ask for support on a 'one-off' basis and find it reassuring to know that it is available.

Preventative Strategies by Health Care Staff

It is known that those men who are least likely to disclose problems to their physicians are at greater risk of negative outcomes (Rieker et al.,

1985). Clinicians and other health care staff can therefore perform an extremely useful preventative measure by initiating discussions and by giving accurate and simple information in lay language about the patient's disease at all stages of his cancer experience. Justified reassurances can greatly help to quell initial fears and may be reiterated as time goes on.

Anecdotal evidence suggests that men are particularly distressed to find that a surgeon has, for example, removed a testicle without prior warning and without explicit explanation of the reasons for having done so. However, there is evidence to suggest that patients do not necessarily 'hear' what is told to them, especially at times of crisis (Cassileth and Steinfeld, 1987). Thus, it is useful to include a close family member in the consultation. Feelings of ostracism on the part of the family can be eliminated and information given but forgotten by either one or other can be re-established. At the same time open communication is promoted between family members and hospital staff.

The majority of patients recount a preference for 'straight talk': a need to be told that it is 'cancer' they have (Moynihan *et al.*, in preparation.) Gentle probing by the doctor such as 'Is there anything else you would like to know at this stage?' will ascertain whether the patient is ready to take on more details of his disease. All too often it is assumed that patients understand the meaning of, for example, 'malignancy' or 'tumour'. This is not necessarily the case and patients are left to cope with their own fantasies in isolation as they include either outright denial or an exaggerated horror of what may lie ahead for them. (Cassidy, and Bluglass, this volume, give detailed advice on breaking bad news.)

During these early encounters it is appropriate for the doctor to provide cues which will demonstrate the patient's need to talk to someone in an unhurried setting, Questions such as 'How are you feeling?'; 'Would you like to talk about your problems if you have any?' or 'How has the loss of your testicle worried you?' will provide a means of knowing whether the patient should be referred to a counsellor who may then proceed with a more in-depth assessment of a man's psychological state. It is at this time that patients' myths specific to urologic cancers need to be addressed (Cassileth and Stenfield, 1987). They include the idea that testicular cancer is sexually transmitted, that surgery spreads tumour cells, that a testicular cancer in the lung or abdomen is tantamount to a primary cancer in those sites and that a normal life especially in terms of infertility and sexual activity, is not possible as a result of urologic surgery.

A diagnosis can bring a sense of relief with it. Many men have procrastinated in presenting, fearing 'the worst'. Thus, feelings of guilt and shame may be transformed when responsibility is placed in reassuring medical hands. For many men however, cancer is perceived as a self-induced death sentence; for others, whose doctors have delayed in diagnosing, a time of bitter reproach and ensuing anger. Thus, this time may represent chaos and disorder only to be followed by further clinical procedures compounding feelings of uncertainty.

Cassileth and Steinfeld (1987) point out that uncertainty is one of the most difficult feelings to endure, but can be managed providing that clinicians designate a meeting in the near future. This will give the patient and family time to organize fears, to prepare questions and will help to restore order and control.

It is my impression that the manner in which the doctor–patient interaction is conducted can have an effect on patients' psychological and social adjustment both in the short and long term. As Cassileth and Steinfeld (1987) point out, an environment conducive to ongoing communication is not only important in terms of information gathering and psychological adjustment, but is also related to patient compliance. It is during early encounters that the patient will gauge how possible it is for him and his family to acquire knowledge and how open the doctor is to issues which lie outside the medical aspects of disease but are of paramount importance to the patient. Such issues would include the impact of treatment on his ability to perform at work and sexual and family adjustment. Thus, the doctor–patient relationship is an intrinsic part of the psychological preparation of the patient and cannot be perceived as separate from the formal intervention made by a counsellor or psychologist (Cassileth and Steinfeld, 1987).

Transient states of emotional distress which occur at diagnosis are thought to be healthy (Greer, 1985) and may not require *formal* psychological intervention. However, some patients continue to feel anxious and in a few cases depressed, at a level that warrants an intervention by skilled mental health personnel (See Watson, this volume, pages 6–7.)

Cognitive Techniques

A young man may be anxious because he thinks that cancer will ruin his life. He may believe, for example, that he will lose his job, sexual function will be impaired, his leisure pursuits hampered or his girl-friend may leave him as a consequence of his diagnosis and possible infertility. A prognosis of 'cure' may be treated with scepticism. For such problems APT may be used. The main aim of APT is to help to alleviate psychological distress by identifying and correcting underlying errors in thinking that may have become habitual (Moorey and Greer, 1989). It can be pointed out that the way we construe a situation will determine our reactions to it. A recording of negative automatic thoughts together with the situation in which they occur and the anxiety felt at the time will help patients to learn that thoughts are connected to emotional distress. The following negative thoughts were recorded by Mr X as he lay anxiously awake in the early hours of the morning.

'My girlfriend looked sad. She must be planning to leave me because I am infertile.'

A challenging intervention pointed to distorted and unrealistic thinking which, in turn, was responded to in a personally meaningful way by the patient himself. He found this easier to do by asking the following questions:

1. What is the evidence?
2. Are there alternative ways of looking at it?
3. If it is true, is it as bad as I think?
   (Moorey and Greer, 1989)

Mr X found that infertility was not a certainty and if it became so, there were other alternatives such as artificial insemination or adoption to consider. Furthermore he found that there were certain things he could do to distract himself during anxious times and he was able to respond to his negative thoughts in the following way:

'My girlfriend's usual expression is one of sadness. She has told me before and she tells me again that she loves me for myself and not for the children we may or may not have.'

This is not to presume that facing up to infertility is not a painful process and may have far reaching consequences of a negative kind, but encouraging the open expression of anger or sadness or both and dealing with them in cognitive terms will help to overcome negative emotions.

Men are often anxiously preoccupied with their disease (and may continue to be so for some time following diagnosis and treatment). In many cases these anxieties extend to the threat of recurrence or the notion that they are 'cancer prone'. Thus every symptom experienced is registered as a sign of disaster. The patient is out of control and uncertainty may cloud all rational thinking as he seeks reassurance. This is very often through the gauging of blood marker levels, of which the patient, more often than not, has no true understanding. To produce cognitive change in these circumstances, not only can the techniques described by Moorey and Greer (1989) contribute to patient management, but education or 'fact finding' is a powerful tool in regaining equilibrium. Explanations may also help to illustrate how control can be lost. For example the therapist can point to the 'spiralling effect' created by the patient's own sensitivity to the possibility of recurrence. His close surveillance of every little ache or pain is mistakingly noted as a recurrence of cancer. Ensuing anxiety can produce more physiological symptoms, confirming anxieties and causing more painful reactions both physically and psychologically (Moorey and Greer, 1989).

Behavioural Techniques

Behavioural techniques, such as visualization and relaxation, can be useful in combating, for example, anxiety, anticipatory nausea and needle phobia (Moorey and Greer, 1989). However, many men find it difficult to learn these techniques, often ridiculing the procedures. A commercial relaxation tape spoken by Neil Fiore (1984) himself a testicular cancer survivor, can, on occasions, convince even the most cynical patient, as it provides the added therapeutic effect of listening to someone who has come through the same, often harrowing, ordeal. Many men have recounted the usefulness of, for example, shaving their heads before the onset of alopecia. This, apart from practical reasons, gives a man a sense of control during a difficult time.

Those men who are 'treated' by surveillance may have to be helped to surmount the 'Sword of Damocles' syndrome. Apart from giving simple and comprehensive details to the patient (which will also enhance follow-up compliance), cognitive strategies may be applied to exaggerated notions of possible relapse.

Ventilating Feelings

In many cases, men do not require cognitive therapy *per se*. The fact that counselling is offered is reassuring in that it allows a patient or his partner to bring up subjects such as sexual dysfunction or infertility. A reiteration of facts is often all that is needed. However, 'fact-finding missions' may be a cover for a need to ventilate feelings which have hitherto remained veiled for fear of appearing unmanly or because of an inability to voice apprehensions to medical staff. A skilled counsellor will attempt to elicit such feelings when appropriate.

While gathering information about his future treatment (which was already giving the patient a sense of control), Mr Y looked particularly unhappy as he spoke of the possibility of future surgery. The counsellor gently probed his feelings and thoughts about his initial orchidectomy and the possible effects of that operation. A Pandora's box of emotions was exposed as the patient recounted his loss of self-esteem and helplessness which were inextricably entwined with his fear of job loss. The latter would, in itself, be an indication of impotency, not only to himself but to others too. *Mr Y had been invited to tell his story*: the personal *meaning* that cancer held for the patient, causing him secret anxiety, was out in the open and could be dealt with. A course of cognitive therapy enabled him to work through his loss and to deal with his related negative thoughts accordingly.

Practical Considerations

Men such as Mr Y may, (1) positively respond to the suggestion that a letter is sent from the clinician in charge to the employer explaining the patient's diagnosis and good prognosis. While many men explain their situation clearly to employers, a few find it difficult to do so for fear of being discriminated against or even ridiculed; (2) find that a testicular prosthesis helps to restore lost confidence. Physicians sometimes underestimate a man's psychological discomfort over such loss and may not inform him that one is available, either at orchidectomy or later when the cancer is in remission.

Counselling for fertility problems. Despite the potential of infertility many patients and their partners require contraceptive counselling, especially one to two years post treatment (Schover *et al.*, 1986). While banking sperm does not appear to enhance psychological well-being, this finding may mask untapped anxieties about infertility only superceded by the cancer experience itself. Young and childless men and those undergoing aggressive treatment regimes may benefit from counselling in this area. Older childless women may be in particular need of support. When infertility is inevitable, alternative options such as artificial insemination or adoption can be explored. Such decisions are often initially met with negative reactions by men and their partners (Schover, 1984). Men may feel jealous: women guilty of manipulation and a sense of betrayal.

Men of low socio-economic and educational groups are vulnerable in this area (as in others) and this should be borne in mind. This may be a result of disease as it damages self-esteem, confidence and masculine self-image. As Rieker *et al.* (1989) point out, these are the constant concerns of testicular tumour survivors, but men in these groups may have restricted chances and fewer options for accomplishing goals that would help to enhance the real and existential losses brought about by cancer.

Counselling for sexual difficulties. Sexual difficulties, experienced at an early stage and during treatment, may result in future dysfunction of a more serious kind. Thus early intervention is advocated. Evaluating the cause of sexual dysfunction in those who have had testicular cancer is a complex task. Attention should be paid to both organic and psychological factors.

As in all areas of sexual rehabilitation amongst cancer patients, close attention should be paid to medication (both current and past) which would include alcohol intake and non-prescribed drugs. While there is strong evidence to suggest that sexual dysfunction in this group is related to type of treatment, at least some of the adverse impact on sexual function may reflect the emotional trauma of experiencing a life-threatening disease in young adulthood, the loss of fertility and/or the symbolic aspects of losing a testicle. Loss of self-esteem (which may be closely linked to sexual dysfunction), may have been brought about by all these factors, as well as the many fears experienced by patients and/or their partners. Ideally, both partners should be encouraged to accept joint and individual counselling. Not only will the counsellor gain useful insights into a couple's relationship, but areas such as fear of contagion and guilt arising out of a belief that past 'misdemeanours' have caused the onset or relapse of cancer and an aversion to sexual activity at certain times may be major concerns which can be brought out into the open and dealt with.

If psychosexual difficulties arise, it is crucial to compare sexual frequency and function before and after treatment. Questions such as 'Did your sexual problems coincide with your diagnosis and/or treatment?'; 'Does it occur in certain places, with certain people and/or at a particular time?'; 'Are there other stresses in your life that may be causing the sexual distress you are experiencing?' will help to decipher the cause of the problem and subsequent management. I have found that those sexual problems that preceded the onset of diagnosis may need a prolonged course of sexual therapy, and may be best dealt with in a specialized clinic. When psychosexual dysfunction has arisen as a result of diagnosis and treatment the techniques of sexual therapy, especially in the form of cognitive behavioural interventions may be readily applied to, for example, impotence, loss of libido and orgasm problems (Schover, 1984).

Men with bilateral orchidectomy may experience a low level of testosterone and should be screened accordingly. This group do not necessarily experience more sexual problems than men with unilateral testicular loss (Moynihan *et al.*, forthcoming) but the symbolism entailed should not be underestimated in either group.

Homosexual men have their own problems. A link between cancer and sexuality is sometimes made and the loss of a testicle and a lack of semen at ejaculation can be hard to explain. Anxiety and loneliness experienced by homosexuals in a 'straight' society may be exacerbated by the added loss of surgery and treatment (Schover, 1984). The encouragement of open expression and communication between partners is important, especially in areas such as fertility and sexuality.

Counselling couples and their families. Counselling is required for those couples whose relationships have become strained. Role changes cause confusion and/or resentment (Schover and von Eschenbach, 1984). A career women may have had to become a nurse figure; a man to relinquish his role as decision maker and breadwinner. Open discussion, patience, appreciation and compromise may help to reinstate lost self-esteem. In a very few cases couples seek the help of marriage guidance. While support from relatives is an acknowledged bonus, some patients have recounted their intermittent need to be alone during treatment. Feelings of rejection can be confusing and painful: not only do relatives make every practical effort to be with the patient but their own need to be present is important. Explanations that the patient's behaviour is 'normal' may help to eliminate misunderstandings.

The potential disruption amongst children of this group should not be forgotten. Simple but truthful explanations and easy access to fathers at all stages, will help to dissipate distorted fantasies. Involvement of a child's teacher may help to put possible reactive behaviour into perspective and will give a child an alternative emotional outlet. Counselling of a more formal nature is seldom requested, but the offer is reassuring.

Counselling at relapse. Patients and relatives find that disease relapse is particularly difficult to deal with. Whether or not a patient adjusted well to his initial diagnosis, support may be needed to combat the feeling of a profound sense of loss of control often brought by the belief that the patient has 'failed', either through an inability to stave away a stressful situation or because of individual characteristics that have not been conducive to 'cure'. Again, a full appraisal of the facts can be presented. Often, hope may be given in the form of additional aggressive treatments which may help to 'salvage' the patient or palliate the disease. Side-effects (including psychosocial factors) should be explained so that patients and relatives can, if desired, participate in the management of their recurrence.

Counselling at the terminal stage. When a patient has received all effective treatments and active disease persists, I have found that many men accept their prognosis with remarkable equanimity. Perhaps the relatively long time span and the treatment options that have been put forward have given the patient time to come to terms with his destiny. However, some men will need the support of a psychological intervention (Moorey and Greer, 1989). It is difficult for therapists at this point to suspend their emotions while they use empathy to deal with feelings such as young men may have at this time. In my own work with dying testicular cancer patients I have found that it can be effective to share some of that grief with the patient in a way that is explicit but does not detract from the needed sense of the therapist's strength. It may allow the patient to express his feelings in greater depth and to share them with his own relatives. Often it is the latter who find this time more difficult to come to terms with. Counselling should be offered both before *and* after the death of the patient.

Many young men find that while they can cope with a bad prognosis, the imparting of that information to parents or partner is particularly difficult. An offer by a member of the psychological support team and/or doctor to intercede and explain the details of the patient's prognosis is usually gratefully accepted. This facilitates open communication between the patient and his family with the added benefit that the latter may establish contact with those who can provide more medical information or support when needed. It also lifts the enormous onus of false bravado from a young man, enabling him to proceed with his life in as normal a way as possible.

IMPLICATIONS FOR SERVICE ORGANIZATION

It has become increasingly obvious that a small but significant minority of patients require psychological support. However the optimum timing and duration of this support is not yet clear. Evidence suggests that diagnosis and treatment are difficult times, but patients also feel bereft of support after treatment has ended (Moynihan, 1987). Thus a protracted intervention may be required. In my experience, patients prefer an individual therapy, although group methods should not be discounted, especially where funding is scarce and trained personnel are few and far between. The sex of the therapist appears to be an irrelevant factor; their approach and willingness to give these young men time to come to terms with their feelings and the meanings they may bring to their disease are important and will reap greater benefits than the well-voiced belief that it is *only* men who can talk to men.

Certain practical considerations affect treatment planning. While psychological treatment is carried out under the auspices of the hospital, 'on the spot' response to referrals can be made and problems can be identified and dealt with immediately. However therapy planned for the duration of in-patient treatment can be problematic as the patient often feels too tired and sick to respond. Routine follow-up appointments provide a good opportunity for psychological treatment to continue. Difficulties arise either because of protracted clinical procedures and long waits in out-patient departments or because the patient may live beyond commuting distance. Regular attendenance for counselling can be jeopardized. There are no easy solutions, but if both clinicians and patients perceive the need for psychological support as an intrinsic part of patient management, these difficulties may be overcome to some extent.

Clinicians and nurses are in an excellent position to 'pick up' distress in patients, who should then be referred (with consent) to either specialist nurses or other skilled mental health workers. The latter become appropriate when a patient exhibits symptoms which require a psychiatric intervention or when problems are beyond the scope of a counsellor. A multidisciplinary meeting is the ideal place to pass on information so that referrals may be made to appropriate personnel.

It is important that when cognitive therapy becomes the elected treatment it is administered by trained therapists. This applies equally to psychodynamic therapists and counsellors. A 'kind' person cannot undertake what is often an extremely difficult and onerous task without training and the supervision and support of experienced parties. Many men request the help of 'cured' patients. Extreme caution should be taken; 'helpers' may not have worked through their own feelings of distress and may be in need of counselling themselves.

The current state of health care may not be conducive to the allocation of resources for psychological treatment. However, funding may become a reality if clinicians are aware of the extent of potential psychosocial morbidity amongst testicular cancer patients and a recognition that psychological support is seen to be beneficial both financially and in terms of a patient's psychological health (Massie *et al.*, 1989). While the triumphs of medicine have enabled testicular cancer patients to live their lives, the triumphs of the patients themselves warrant our efforts to help them to attain the best possible quality of life that embraces all aspects of psychosocial well-being.

References

AASS, N., FOSSA, S., OTTO, F. and OSE, T. (1989) Acute subjective morbidity after cisplatin based combination chemotherapy in patients with testicular cancer: A prospective study. *Radiotherapy and Oncology, 14*, 27–33.

BLACKMORE, C. (1988) The impact of orchidectomy upon the sexuality of the man with testicular cancer. *Cancer Nursing, Vol 11*, 33–40.

CASSILETH, B., STEINFELD, A. (1987) Psychological preparation of the patient and family. *Cancer, 60*, 547–552.

EDBRIL, S. and RIEKER, P. (1985) Fertility issues facing testis cancer survivors.

(Paper presented at the meeting of the American Psychological Association, Los Angeles. Available from Dr P. Rieker, Dana Faber Cancer Institute, 44 Binney Street, Boston, MA02115, USA.)

EDBRIL, S., RIEKER, P. (1990) The impact of testicular cancer on the work lives of survivors. *Journal of Psychosocial Oncology*, 7, 3, 17–20.

FIORE, N. (1984) *The Road Back to Health*. New York: Bantam Books.

FOSSA, S., AASS, N., KAALHUS, O. (1988) Testicular cancer in young Norwegians. *Journal of Surgical Oncology*, 39, 43–63.

GREER, S. (1985) Cancer: Psychiatric aspects. In K. Granville-Grossman (Ed) *Recent Advances in Clinical Psychiatry*. London: Churchill Livingstone.

GRITZ, E., WELLISCH, D., SIAU, J. and WANG, H. (in press) Long-term effects of testicular cancer on marital relationships. *Psychosomatics*.

GRITZ, E., WELLISCH, D. and LANDSVERK, J. (1989a) Psychosocial sequelae in long-term survivors of testicular cancer. *Journal of Psychosocial Oncology*, 6, (3/4), 41–63.

GRITZ, E., WELLISCH, D., HE-JING, W., SIAU, J., LDANDSVERK, J. and COSGROVE, M. (1989b) Long-term effects of testicular cancer on sexual functioning in married couples. *Cancer*, 64, 7, 1560–1567.

MASSIE, M.J., HOLLAND, J.C. and STRAKER, N. (1989) Psychotherapeutic interventions. In J.C. Holland and J.H. Rowland (Eds) *Handbook of Psycho-Oncology*. Oxford: Oxford University Press.

MOOREY, S. and GREER, S. (Eds) (1989) *Psychological Therapy for Patients with Cancer: A new approach*. London: Heinemann Medical Books.

MOYNIHAN, C. (1987) Testicular cancer: The psychological problems of patients and their relatives. *Cancer Surveys, Vol 6*, 3, 477–510.

MOYNIHAN, C., BLISS, J. and HORWICH, A. (forthcoming) Bilateral orchidectomy: psychosocial aspects.

MOYNIHAN, C., GARDNER, R. and HORWICH, A. (in preparation)

NIJMAN, J., SCHRAFFORDT KOOPS, H., OLDHOFF, J., KREMER, J. and JAGER, S. (1987a) Sexual function after bilateral retroperitoneal lymph node dissection for non seminomatous testicular cancer. *Archives of Andrology*, 18, 255–267.

NIJMAN, J., SCHRAFFORDT KOOPS, H. and OLDHOFF, J. (1987b) Sexual function after surgery and combination chemotherapy in men with disseminated non-seminomatous testicular cancer. In J. Nijman (Ed) *Some Aspects of Sexual Gonadal Function in Patients With a Non-Seminomatous Germ Cell Tumour of the Testis*. Groningen: Drukkerij van Denderen B.V.

RIEKER, P., EDBRIL, S. and GARNICK, M. (1985) Curative testis cancer therapy: Psychosocial sequelae. *Journal of Clinical Oncology*, 3, 8, 1117–1126.

RIEKER, P., FITZGERALD, E., KALISH, L., RICHIE, J., LEDERMAN, G., EDBRIL, S. and GARNICK, M. (1989) Psychological factors, curative therapies and behavioral outcomes: A comparison of testis cancer survivors and a control group of healthy men. *Cancer*, 64, No 11, 2399–2407.

SCHOVER, L. (1987) Sexuality and fertility in urologic cancer patients. *Cancer*, 60, 553–558.

SCHOVER, L., GONZALES, M. and VON ESCHENBACH, A. (1986) Sexual and marital relationships after radiotherapy for seminoma. *Urology*, 27, 2, 117–123.

SCHOVER, L. and VON ESCHENBACH, A. (1984) Sexual and marital counseling with men treated for testicular cancer. *Journal of Sexual and Marital Therapy*, 10, 1, 29–40.

SCHOVER, L. and VON ESCHENBACH, A. (1985) Sexual and marital relationships after treatment for nonseminomatous testicular cancer. *Urology*, 25, 3, 251–255.

TROSS, S., HOLLAND, J., BOSL, G. and GELLER, N. (1984) A controlled study of psychosocial sequelae in cured survivors of testicular neoplasms. *Association of the Society of Clinical Oncology*, 3, 74 (abstr C-287).

TRUMP, D., ROMSAAS, E., CUMMINGS, K. and MALEC, J. (1985) Assessment of psychologic and sexual dysfunction in patients following treatment of testis cancer: A prospective study. *Proceedings of the American Society of Clinical Oncology (abstr C-975)*.

ZIGMOND, A.S. and SNAITH, R.P. (1983) The hospital anxiety and depression scale. *Acta Psychiatrica Scandinavica*, 67, 361–370.

GYNAECOLOGICAL CANCER: A PSYCHOTHERAPY GROUP

Gerjanne Bos-Branolte

Amongst women the incidence of gynaecological cancer is second only to that of breast cancer (which is not included amongst the gynaecological cancers in The Netherlands). In the USA 49 per cent of genital malignancies originate in the endometrium, 20 per cent in the cervix, 25 per cent in the ovary and 6 per cent in the vulva and vagina (American Cancer Society, 1984). (The respective figures for The Netherlands are 39 per cent, 24 per cent, 27 per cent and 10 per cent (Dutch Society of Gynaecologic Oncology, 1985).) Progress in the treatment of gynaecological cancer has dramatically increased the number of those cured. In 1960 only 25 per cent of patients in the USA survived five years or longer, whereas more recent figures indicate that nearly 50 per cent will survive (Silverberg and Lubera, 1986).

Treatments for gynaecological cancers vary according to the site and stage of disease. For cancers of the cervix and endometrium for instance, surgical treatment may range from a simple hysterectomy (followed by radiotherapy) to a radical hysterectomy which includes the removal of the upper third of the vagina, parametria and a pelvic lymphadenectomy. The surgical treatment for ovarian cancer may range from simple oophorectomy to total hysterectomy and bilateral salpingo-oophorectomy including omentectomy and cytoreductive surgery in more advanced disease. Surgical treatment may be followed by radiotherapy and/or chemotherapy.

The side-effects of treatment invariably cause some loss of function such as cessation of menstruation, infertility and hormone imbalance. These changes may in turn influence sexual functioning; for example, when a Wertheim's hysterectomy is performed the vagina is shortened and scarring may cause decreased vaginal elasticity. If an oophorectomy is performed, decreased production of oestrogen may reduce vaginal lubrication. For women with vaginal or pelvic cancer, vaginal intercourse is no longer possible due to loss of the vagina. Additional problems may be brought about where treatment involves an ileostomy and/or colostomy. In addition to these specific effects patients may experience a general feeling of malaise.

TABLE 1   *Effects of gynaecological cancers*

PHYSICAL	PSYCHOLOGICAL	SOCIAL/CULTURAL
Assault on organs	*Assault on identity*	*Assault on image*
uterus, ovaries, tubes, vulva, vagina, cervix, clitoris	self-esteem body image self-respect	health ideal beauty ideal motherhood ideal
Loss of female functions	*Loss of identity*	*Loss of value*
menstruation fertility hormonal equilibrium	devalued as woman feeling not 'whole'	feminine status social status feminine mystique
Disturbances in sexual functioning	*Disturbances of sexual identity*	*Disturbances caused by sexual norms*
sensory perception uterine contractions lubrication orgasm capacity	devalued as sexual partner insecure inhibited anorgasmic (also male impotence) anxious about being contagious	genital cancer seen as punishment for sexual 'sins' sexuality is taboo for sick people sexuality is taboo for mutilated/castrated people ambiguity about non-coital sex

The possible effects of the disease and treatment are wide-ranging, affecting physical, psychological and social/cultural functioning, as illustrated in Table 1. Rehabilitation and restoration of quality of life thus becomes an important goal for women treated for gynaecological cancers.

Psychological and Social Effects

Generally psychological effects differ depending on age, personal history, phase of life and characteristic coping methods (Derogatis, 1980). When comparing three groups of women patients with breast cancer, gynaecological cancer and a 'healthy' group Anderson and Jochimsen (1985) found that 82 per cent of the gynaecological cancer patients reported a poor body image compared to 38 per cent of the healthy women and, surprisingly, 31 per cent of the breast cancer patients. Gynaecological cancer may therefore be experienced as a serious assault on female identity. Gynaecological cancer may also have a connotation leading to feelings of shame, embarrassment, or ignorance (Bos, 1984). Negative feelings about body image and self-esteem may also affect a woman's sexual identity. Some women feel devalued as a sexual partner and, because of inhibitions and fears of contagion, they fear that they will lose their partner. Therefore sexual dysfunction is not uncommon, as illustrated by Dennerstein *et al.*'s (1977) study where the incidence rate for sexual disorders following hysterectomy and oophorectomy was found to be 37 per cent.

At a socio-cultural level gynaecological cancers may threaten the female image. Loss of female organs and functions can be perceived as a loss of feminine value. Traditional sexual values and norms can add to the heavy burden experienced by patients and their partners (Bos, 1986). Taken together, the physical, psychological and socio-cultural effects of gynaecological cancer may have an important influence on the patient's reactions to her losses as well as the way she copes with them (Schain, 1981).

Quality of Life

After being treated for gynaecological cancer, many women are left with unanswered questions. Some questions deal with physical consequences like: 'My body has betrayed me, how can I trust it again?', or: 'I have become infertile, menopausal, how can I ever cope with that?' Other questions deal with the psychological effects, like: 'I am weary and tired of everything, how can I regain my vitality?', or: 'I feel insecure, how can I achieve harmony with myself?'. More sensitive questions relate to the sexual and partner relationship: 'My husband does not understand me', or: 'My husband does not want to make love with me any longer. How can I regain my self-esteem and feel attractive?'. Finally, key questions relate to reactions of women's social network: 'I am lucky that the cancer could be removed, but why don't my family and friends understand that I am unhappy?'.

In their usual surroundings, these cured patients are not entitled to grieve for their handicaps and mutilations, let alone mourn about emotional losses. Most people who have not had cancer, or who have not experienced any other serious life event, cannot understand the mourning process related to cancer. Moreover, they are misled by the patients themselves. In the beginning, most of the cured patients are glad they are alive. It is, however, a misconception to assume that once that wish is fulfilled, there is nothing left for them to desire for the rest of their life. Only after survival has become a reality does the patient realize the extent to which the quality of her life has been affected and what a high price she has paid. Patients may feel that they are not allowed to mourn, and suffer silently.

The Coping Process

According to psychodynamic (Horowitz, 1976) and modern stress theories (Kleber, 1982; Taylor, 1983; Wortman, 1983) traumatic experiences are characterized by three components: extreme powerlessness, acute disruption and confrontation with death, or extreme discomfort. Such experiences must be coped with and integrated into everyday behaviour and thinking. The majority of cancer patients in remission are able to cope with this trauma with the help of people close to them. For a minority of them however the coping process either does not develop or is disturbed. A number of studies have shown that about one third of patients have psychological morbidity with chronic associated symptoms (Worden, 1983; Cohen, 1982; Kennedy *et al.*, 1976; Maguire, 1985; Morris *et al.*, 1977; Derogatis, 1980; Lehmann *et al.*, 1978).

Patients' inability to cope adequately with the aftermath of cancer must not be seen as negative or stigmatizing. We are concerned here with normal individuals who are forced to face abnormal circumstances. Life rarely provides adequate preparation for confronting life-threatening situations whilst still young. Undergoing radical and long-lasting medical treatment, and having to accept physical changes while in the prime of life goes against all our expectations. Martin (1982) has commented that:

> Five-year cure rates and long remissions are of little consequence if the patient's quality of life and state of well-being are less than optimal.... . In order to place the psychosocial needs of the cancer patient in perspective, there is a need for greater understanding and treatment of his emotional and social problems.

The aim of psychotherapy with cancer patients, like that of traditional psychotherapy, is to teach people in distress to reduce suffering and get more pleasure out of life. In my opinion patients who have, or have had, cancer need a form of treatment that differs to some extent from that needed by non-cancer patients. The difference lies mainly in the cause of the psychological problems: in the former group we are concerned with the psychological consequences of a life-threatening somatic disease, whereas for the latter it is more often a psychological dysfunction not associated with a serious disease. Thus, psychotherapy for cancer patients is directed not so much at neurotic problems but predominantly at problems related to reality: facilitation of the coping process, integration of the consequences of the disease and treatment, and stimulation of the patient to improve their quality of life in spite of the losses experienced.

LONG-TERM EMOTIONAL EFFECTS OF GYNAECOLOGICAL CANCERS AND POSSIBILITIES FOR SHORT-TERM PSYCHOTHERAPY

A research project to identify patients with psychological morbidity or poor quality of life, and then to improve their quality of life by short-term psychotherapy, was carried out at Leiden University Hospital's Department of Gynaecology between 1984 and 1988 (Bos-Branolte, 1987). Some results of this study are reported here, along with a description of the group therapy programme that was evaluated, in order to provide the reader with a workable model of the psychosocial care of gynaecological and, with slight adaptations, breast cancer patients.

Materials and Methods

Patients. All patients were selected from the files of the Department of Gynaecology at Leiden University Hospital in consultation with the medical staff. In 1985 and 1986 119 patients were invited to participate, and 90 patients (76 per cent) agreed. The sites of their malignancies were: ovaries (41 cases), cervix (29 cases), corpus uteri (16 cases) and vulva (4 cases). The forms of treatment were: surgery (29 cases), combined surgery and chemotherapy (31 cases), combined surgery and radiotherapy (22 cases), and combined surgery, chemotherapy, and radiotherapy (8 cases).

At the time of entry to the study, their ages ranged from 14 to 70 years, with a mean age of 49 years.

The duration of remission ranged from 6 to 86 months with a mean of 35 months.

Selection criteria. Weisman and Worden (1976–77) found that during the first hundred days of being a cancer patient concern is predominantly existential in nature and is centered around death and life. In this early post-treatment period, worries about physical symptoms and health are dominant. Only after the patient recovers and gains some trust in the idea that she has a future and that her body seems likely to survive do psychological problems gradually become more noticeable. This is often six to nine months after treatment (Mantell and Green, 1978; Lamont *et al.*, 1978; Krant, 1981; Bloom and Ross, 1982). Patients therefore had to be in remission at least six months. This delay also eliminated euphoric reactions or denial so often encountered in the first six months following medical treatment.

The following selection criteria were also applied: the patient had to be (a) aged 70 or under; (b) Dutch-speaking; (c) informed of the cancer diagnosis; (d) without any other type of cancer; (e) free of manifest psychiatric disturbance.

Instruments. The method of assessment used was the Basic Oncology Scale (BOS), designed specifically for use with gynaecological cancer patients in remission. It focuses on anxiety, depression, body image, self-esteem, partner relationships, and general well-being. (Questions about anxiety and depression relate specifically to affective states, in order to avoid any confusion with physical symptoms.) Further details of this scale are reported in Bos-Branolte (1987). Information about demographic variables was also collected. The questionnaire took about 30 minutes to complete and was administered individually in our consulting room in the hospital.

Study design. Psychotherapy was offered during the first three months following the initial assessment. Follow-up measurements using the same methods were made six and nine months later.

Data analysis. The scores for the main variables were dichotomized: scores 0.50 standard deviation below the mean were labelled as severe problems as against moderate or slight problems. On the basis of these scores patients were assigned to either the 'severe problems' or 'moderate/slight problems' categories prior to calculating what percentage of them had a negative score on the variables assessed. (A more detailed description of these analyses is given in Bos-Branolte, 1987.)

Results

Psychological morbidity. The percentage of patients considered to have severe problems is shown in Table 2.

Scores across the six variables were averaged to provide an indication of the degree of psychological morbidity. Using this averaging method, 28 per cent showed some morbidity.

TABLE 2 *Severe problems experienced by oncology patients*

Variables	% ($n = 90$)
Anxiety	34
Depression	28
Body image	22
Self-esteem	36
Partner relationship	26
Well-being	21

The psychological morbidity was also assessed in two control groups of patients with a cervical intraepithelial neoplasia (CIN) ($n = 59$), and patients who underwent a hysterectomy for non-malignancies (HYS) ($n = 58$). (For detailed discussion of the control groups see Bos-Branolte and Duivenvoorden, 1989.)

The relationship between severe psychological morbidity and different organ sites is shown in Table 3.

TABLE 3   *Severe problems in ovarian, cervical, CIN and HYS groups*

	%
Ovarian	36
Cervical	21
CIN	21
HYS	22
Endometrial	17
Vulva	46

The percentages of patients considered to have severe problems related to the six variables are shown in Table 4.

TABLE 4   *Percentage of patients with severe problems in each diagnostic group**

	Ovary	Cervix	CIN	HYS
Anxiety	46	31	25	29
Depression	37	17	20	24
Body image	22	21	10	19
Self-esteem	42	24	17	22
Partner relationship	32	17	25	12
Well-being	34	14	29	28

*The number of patients with cancer of the vulva and endometrium was too small to include in the analysis given in Table 4.

An analysis of the frequency of negative scores for two or more variables according to the duration of remission gave important results. About 40 per cent of the patients developed severe problems on two or more variables during the first two and a half years of remission, and a year later this was the case for more than half of them (57 per cent). This percentage was always the highest for the ovarian cancer patients. In general, a decrease did not occur until the magical limit of five years had been reached, although even then nearly one fifth (19 per cent) still continued to have problems.

Psychotherapy was accepted by 27 patients (30 per cent), six choosing individual psychotherapy (IPT) and 21 group psychotherapy (GPT). The psychotherapy (PT) and nonpsychotherapy patients (NPT) were compared at baseline with respect to their medical characteristics. The groups showed no significant difference as to the type of cancer or medical treatment, or with respect to age. The only difference was that patients receiving psychotherapy had a significantly shorter remission than the non-psychotherapy patients (means 27 and 40 months, respectively).

However comparison of these groups with respect to the six variables showed that those patients who accepted psychotherapy suffered significantly more frequently from severe anxiety and depression and had a more negative body image than patients who refused such treatment. Self-esteem and well-being showed a similar, albeit non-significant, trend. When seen over a period of nine months, the results indicated that, of the patients who had severe problems, those who accepted therapy were considerably better off than those who did not. The majority (two thirds) of the therapy patients had improved and less than one third remained unchanged. With minor exceptions, there was no deterioration. Almost two thirds of the PT patients with severe problems improved with respect to anxiety and depression and more than half had a better body image. The best and most important result related to self-esteem: nearly 75 per cent of the patients improved significantly on this variable. Only 40 per cent of the patients who had severe relationship problems with their partner improved, although in individual therapy the results were considerably better, probably because here we had the opportunity to organize therapy sessions with the partner alone and/or with patient and partner together.

In contrast with the favourable results obtained in treated patients, the untreated patients with severe problems did less well: one third improved on anxiety and 13 to 14 per cent on the other variables. Overall, about two thirds had not changed for the better after nine months; only a minority improved and the remaining patients' problems had worsened.

Finally, an attempt was made to compare the extent to which patients improved with respect to the six variables in group and individual therapy. With GPT the average improvement of all six variables was 61 per cent; the greatest improvement was for well-being (93 per cent), followed by self-esteem (64 per cent). IPT patients improved more than GPT patients, although the number of patients in IPT was too small to permit unequivocal conclusions concerning differences in the effectiveness of IPT and GPT. Improvement of problems after 9 months was significantly higher in patients who accepted therapy than for patients with severe problems who did not. It can be concluded from these results that psychological intervention should be offered to gynaecological cancer patients in remission, and that it has a beneficial effect on their quality of life.

GROUP PSYCHOTHERAPY

Over a period of some years we have developed a short psycho-therapy programme for patients treated for gynaecological cancers. What follows is a description of the specific components of the programme. It may be possible that some elements can be adapted for other patient groups.

Organization

Liaison.   Before any programme is started it is essential to establish consultation with medical and nursing staff, as without their coopera-tion it is impossible to build up a psychosocial unit. It is necessary to have access to patients' medical files and to be informed about their medical history and possible changes in their medical state (for example recurrence or death). Patients' general practitioners should also be kept informed. It is also important to realize that the overall impact of the disease and treatment on the patient's perceived well-being tends to be underestimated by physicians. Furthermore, psychological problems are rarely apparent to the hospital staff. Patients and their relatives are reluctant to disclose their difficulties to those involved in their physical care; they give few verbal clues and perceive doctors and nurses as being primarily concerned with their physical well-being (Morris *et al.*, 1977; Maguire *et al.*, 1978).

Recruitment and composition of the group.   An important finding in our study was that although one third of the patients were in need of psychotherapy, very few of them would have been referred to us for help outside the context of this investigation. So it is an illusion to expect sufficient referrals if general practitioners and oncologists are not specifically trained in psychosocial oncology. Moreover, to de-pend on patient-initiated requests for help is to underestimate the strength of social forces which discourage self-confrontation. Para-doxically, many patients only accept help which is kindly offered and fully explained to them. Increasing referrals and recruiting patients is difficult. So far, only volunteer networks of cancer patients seem to be successful in increasing an awareness of emotional problems and of the effectiveness of psychosocial help.

The composition of our groups was heterogeneous as patients with different kinds of gynaecological cancers and treatments were en-rolled in the same group. The reason for this was that we did not want to place patients on a waiting list – some patients had already waited more than seven years for help! These mixed groups were successful and enabled patients to compare their different cancer sites with others and judge the relative severity of their own situation.

They nearly always felt 'better off'. Only very young patients and patients with unwanted infertility due to cancer treatment sometimes regretted that they could not share their feelings of grief, anger and sorrow about their infertility.

It is disturbing for a group's dynamic to enroll two participants who know each other. We prefer rather small groups with a minimum of four and a maximum of eight participants. Group cohesion and safety within a group tends to heighten participants' motivation and commitment, so we decided not to have open groups where patients might enter and leave at different times.

Group leaders. If a group leader is experienced in group work in general and with cancer patients in particular, then it is reasonable for them to lead a group alone. In this case it is essential to ensure that they are supervised and that they have the opportunity to ventilate their own feelings. If there are two group leaders, the tasks have to be divided according to preference and degree of education and experience. It is also possible to train co-therapists – volunteers who have had cancer and want to become active in group work with patients. Their motivation and endeavour in having coped reasonably well with their own cancer must be initially screened. They should also be trained and supervised. As trained group leaders are scarce in the psychosocial oncology field the possibility of training co-therapists should be seriously considered.

Group leaders (psychotherapists, clinical psychologists, psychiatrists, social workers or volunteers) need to be experienced in group therapy. They should have adequate knowledge of the psychosocial aspects of cancer and the impact of different treatments and their side-effects and a specific knowledge of the participants' type of cancer. Furthermore, they should be able to share their own feelings, to have a tolerant attitude and to respect other people's defence mechanisms.

The role of the therapist includes eliciting, clarifying, interpreting, 'confronting' and recapitulating patients' feelings as well as offering an opportunity to express negative feelings. The success of such treatment depends to a high degree on what are called the Rogerian therapist variables: empathic understanding, positive regard, and genuineness.

Practical details

The group's *name* has to be chosen. We found that 'talking group' was not sufficiently accurate a description and that 'discussion group' had a negative connotation. We opted for 'Live-Your-Life group', which proved to be a therapeutic concept in itself.

Place.   The room – preferably your own – should have a nice, friendly atmosphere. Easy chairs should be placed in a circle without a table in the middle. If possible, coffee or tea should be served. The group leader should position their own chair so that they can observe the participants' face and posture. Make sure no outsiders can enter the room, and take the phone off the hook.

Time.   Because our treatment was part of a research project we had to select eight 90-minute sessions spaced over ten weeks. So patients were carefully questioned about whether they were willing to come eight times and told that if they were not their place would have to be given to other patients. In establishing a therapeutic contract with participants the need for openness and willingness to disclose feelings was emphasized. (Interestingly, after the third session three quarters of the participants spontaneously asked for the number of sessions to be increased, although they had originally thought that eight would be too many.)

Because continuity is necessary for the therapy to be successful, and because participants must be able to count on each other, no one should be allowed to stay away. It is therefore necessary to devise a suitable schedule. We sent patients a card on which they could choose three out of six possible dates.

In some cases it may be necessary to include some individual sessions or sessions with the participant's partner or the couple together.

Letters should be sent out, inviting patients to participate and confirming the place, date and time of the meetings.

Structure of the group therapy sessions. A rather fixed structure was adopted. Each session consisted of: an opening round; a main theme; individual experiences, and a closing round.

Opening round.   This is a relatively quick round. Patients are asked to talk about their feelings during the past week, especially in relation to the main theme. Other questions relate to their quality of life and their relaxation exercises.

Main theme.   Each session covers a different theme. In order to encourage patients to talk openly, the group leader starts by giving some short examples of other patients' emotional experiences in relation to the session's theme. It is important not to distance the group by overusing jargon and statistics.

The eight sessions covered: medical background; anxiety and depression; body image and self-esteem; support; partner relationships; coping; well-being, and consolidation.

Individual experiences. The individual experiences of the participants are related to the main theme. The group leader invites one of the participants to talk about her experiences and feelings and then moves on to the other participants, preferably one at a time. The group leader should try to ensure that everyone participates. He or she should also try to clarify, interpret and compare experiences. The participants are encouraged to comment to one another, to support and to reassure each other.

Relevant questions are: 'What do you think?' or 'Is your experience the same, or different?'. Questions which may give patients a feeling of control over their situation are: 'What did you do to solve the problems, to feel better?'; 'Did it work?'.

Be enthusiastic and encourage hope and belief in the benefit of the treatment so as to keep up their motivation. Many participants will encounter criticism about their attendance at the group with questions like: 'Why do you go there so often just to repeat all your problems?' and 'Why can't you talk about it with me?' Rhetorical questions like these from family and friends who feel threatened by psychotherapy are very burdening and tiresome and they should be anticipated and discussed.

Concluding round. In order to stop in time, about ten minutes before the end of the session the group leader asks the participants how they feel about the session and if they have any questions about it. A reminder is given about the date and time of the next session. The group leader then closes the session by giving a maxim that is related to the session's main theme.

Methods. The treatment plan we used included progressive relaxation training (each patient was given a tape to practise this method at home), role playing, and learning by imitation. Since the majority of cancer patients have little idea of what to expect from psychotherapy they may feel ill at ease or even frightened. We therefore recorded two 30-minute video films, to show to new patients, in which cancer survivors who had already been through group therapy acted as participants in the therapy and talked openly about their emotions and experiences.

Implementing Treatment

After thorough organization of the group therapy treatment plan along the lines described above, the 'real' work can start. The patients arrive!

Session 1

Opening Round

Once everyone has sat down the group leader welcomes his or her patients and tells them that they are glad they are all there. 'You all have (had) cancer – a serious disease – which also has many emotional consequences which we want to open up and share with each other. We are here to learn how to improve our quality of life; this will be a recurring theme in all our sessions.' He or she explains that it will be necessary to start and stop each session on time and that 'As you need each other and it is disturbing if you cannot count on each other, in principle nobody should stay away. Should you have an important reason for not attending please inform us at least one day before the session'.

The group leader then explains that 'All members in the group should guarantee each other's privacy. You should not therefore mention each other's names outside the group. As members of this group, we have to respect each other, accept each other as we are, feel free to express our feelings and support each other without being critical. There is always the possibility that your sorrow will be brought to the forefront in the first few sessions and that you want to talk about it in between the sessions. I will give you my telephone number, but I trust that you only will use it in an emergency. In other cases you may ask one of the other participants to listen to you. It is also our experience with other groups that in the beginning patients may feel "worse", have headaches, become more tired, cry, or are more anxious and experience their medical background more vividly. However, this is an unavoidable part of the coping process so do not worry! And if your family and friends advise you to stop attending, tell them that it is only temporary.

I will introduce each session's main theme and you will then have the opportunity to tell us about your own experience. As we are interested in all of you, we have to take care that each of you has enough time to talk. Sometimes it may be necessary to ask you to continue another time. We hope we have a good time together and that you learn to improve your quality of life.

I will tell you something about myself. Then I will invite you each to tell us your name, age, family situation and diagnosis.'

Medical background

'We will now show you a video of another group of patients in which they talk about their medical background, their diagnosis, hospital stay and their first time back at home.'

Individual experiences

'Who's brave enough to start us off?' One at a time the participants talk about their disease experiences. Relevant interventions by the group leader can be made.

Concluding round

Relaxation exercises are explained, and tapes given for practice at home. The date and time of the next session are mentioned. You can chat to people about what they thought of the session, and might point out a coffee shop around the corner.

Don't forget the relaxation exercises. *Maxim*: Live your life!

Session 2

Opening round

Questions to be asked: 'How did the preceding week go? Did you do the relaxation exercises? Who had difficulties? Why?'

In our experience, it is very difficult for many women to have time to themselves. If this is the case, tell them that this often happens and has to do with female role patterns. If one patient is able to be independent she should be asked to explain how she manages to do this so as to give her and the others the message that it is all right to take time for oneself. Any feelings of guilt are destructive and of no use.

Anxiety and depression

Explain that the diagnosis of cancer nearly always provokes anxiety and depression – anxiety about recurrence, about pain, about loss and death. It also brings fear of losing others, fear about children or about not having children. Mention how a patient in one of the other groups felt extremely anxious, unsafe and tense. After practising her relaxation exercises and learning how to relax, she was more able to control her anxiety and her quality of life improved considerably.

'Cancer also elicits depression: sadness, feeling low, desperate, lonely and powerless. However you can *choose* your emotions, although this is not easy. You don't have to stay depressed. As one patient told me: "In the morning I was always hunched at the breakfast table, gloomy and reluctant to do anything. Since coming to the 'Live-your-life group' where I realized that I can choose my emotions, I have managed – with some difficulty – to pull myself together and have started swimming, having saunas, and walking with my dog".'

Individual experiences

Ask a different person from the one that began last week to share her feelings in connection with anxiety and depression and then move on to the other participants. Questions which can be asked include: 'What did you do to feel less anxious, less depressed? Did it work?'

Do not give the message that it is 'wrong' to have negative emotions, but that, after such a serious disease, it is a pity. Explain that they should feel free to cherish their precious life. Use the positive experiences of others. Be aware of victims' roles and powerlessness.

Concluding round
Note the time of the next session. Ask participants to remember their exercises and to keep negative feelings under control. *Maxim*: Look after your quality of life!

Session 3

Opening round
Open the session as before.

Body image and self-esteem
Explain that after treatment for gynaecological (or breast) cancer, many women feel less attractive. They have negative feelings about their body which has changed considerably. They dislike scars, regret mutilations and disabilities. The physical consequences of cancer are often considerable, and each site has specific physical effects in terms of loss of organs, functions and disturbances. In the case of a colostomy or clitoridectomy their body image will be even further threatened. Moreover, many women have to face general feelings of malaise and tiredness. Cancer may also lead to disturbances of sexual functions. All in all, a woman's positive feelings about her body are often changed into a negative body image. It is clear that loss of (female) organs and functions is therefore damaging to a woman's self-esteem, making her feel insecure, worthless, inferior and lacking in self-respect.

Individual experiences
Start up the discussion. Remind participants that physical activities such as swimming and walking are good for their physical and mental well-being. Ask if they happily touch their scars and their body. 'Do you ever soothe your body with a scented body lotion? Do you love yourself? Do you respect yourself? You have (had) cancer, so you have earned the right to this! Give yourself permission to be selfish – make your own decisions; pay attention to your own needs.'

Concluding round
Close the session as before. *Maxim*: 'Love your body, love yourself'.

Session 4

Opening round
Open the session as before.

Support
'From past experience we know that many of you need emotional

support, comfort and acknowledgement when coping with your disease and its long-term consequences. In our culture cancer is seen as an assault on one's health and body ideal and many of you may therefore experience cancer as a loss in social status because you may feel inferior to healthy women. You may gain friends, but you may also lose them. Critical remarks, especially from your mother or mother-in law, may hurt you. And others close to you may tell you that now everything is normal again you should behave as you did before your cancer.' Explain that during the disease many women find out for the first time who they really are and that these processes do not end once they are cured. Explain that there is positive and negative support. If they experience any negative support they should refuse it, and learn to rely on themselves.

Individual experiences
Encourage participants to discuss each other, especially if a woman does not allow herself to be angry or disappointed about negative support because it was 'well-meant'. Tell them that it is not necessary and can even be dangerous, to respond to such support as if you are grateful. Ask them if they appreciate the support given to them. Sometimes it may be worthwhile to mention experiences of other people in general, outside the context of cancer, and refer them to Sartre's play *Huis Clos* in which one of the characters says: 'Hell is other people'.

Concluding round
Close the session as before. *Maxim*: 'Beware of negative support'.

Session 5

Opening round
Open the session as before.

Partner relationships
Introduce the second video in which women talk about their general and sexual relationship with their partner. In our video one woman talks about the problems she's experienced in relation to her infertility, while a divorced woman asks for advice on what to do when she meets a possible future lover. Explain that after a traumatic illness such as cancer the way individuals express affectionate and sexual feelings often changes. Usually their need for emotional support and open communication increases. Many women feel a need to talk about their fears and uncertainties – even years after their recovery. The need for physical closeness and intimacy also increases, whereas the need for intercourse decreases considerably. Patients with cervical cancer especially often fear that intercourse will lead to the

recurrence of cancer. This can become a source of tension between the patient and her partner. For others, intercourse becomes painful or overtiring or unsatisfying.

Individual experiences
Stress the fact that, although some of the participants may feel that it is disloyal to talk about their partner, this is a special occasion and that we are not sitting here to gossip, but to ventilate and share feelings and learn from each other. Be alert if a patient feels guilty when she abstains from sex. There is always a reason. Ask whether her partner does not want to make love any longer, whether he has become impotent. Many partners themselves fear intercourse and avoid physical contact as well.

Questions: 'What is intimacy? What is sexuality? When does it enhance your life and when does it make it worse? How does it do this? What can you do yourself to improve it?'

Mention other non-coital possibilities and suggest that stimulation of the clitoris might be more in accordance with their needs.

Patients' partners also deserve attention. If you can talk to them separately or form a 'partners' group' in which they can share their experiences, this could be an excellent supplement to the patients' groups. I am not in favour of combined groups.

Concluding round
Close the session as before. *Maxim*: Embrace your partner.

Session 6

Opening round
Open the session as before.

Coping
Explain that cancer is a disease of loss: the physical, psychological and social effects all intermingle and influence reactions to these losses, as well as the way one copes with them. 'After this session, we only have two left. We must prepare ourselves to part, which is a loss too, and to talk about our feelings connected with this. Most people have difficulties leaving, whether they leave freinds, a school, or, ultimately, life itself. Perhaps we can use these last sessions to talk about this.'

Individual experiences
Questions: 'How is it possible to cope with your disease in spite of your losses? Which problems did you encounter? How did you solve some of them? Why didn't you solve others?' You could introduce

role playing. Patients like it; it is funny and they learn quickly without feeling criticized.

Concluding round
Conclude the session as before. *Maxim*: Cope with your partner, look after your quality of life.

Session 7

Opening round
Open the session as before.

Well-being
'Many people have not learnt how to get much out of life. On the contrary, they are not taught to choose for themselves and to live their own life, nor to look after their mental well-being. Women in particular have often been taught to sacrifice themselves for others and to neglect their own needs. I am convinced that after cancer, the time has come to choose for yourself, to try to live your own life and to live happily. For many women this is difficult. But it is essential!'

Individual experiences
Ask whether it really is selfish to choose for yourself. 'If you say "I am selfish" out loud ten times the word loses its negative connotation. Many women have learnt not to be selfish. That lesson was misguided, because there is only one of you, and you only live once.'

Concluding round
Conclude the session as before. *Maxim*: Enjoy life and feel pleased with yourself.

Session 8

Opening round
Open the session as before. Ask participants what they want to discuss.

Consolidation
'This is the last session, but we will have some reunions later on. I hope you have learnt a lot, and I know that even after this last session, the learning process will continue. You will remember important topics and will remember the group and what we discussed. If you have difficulties an inner voice will give you an answer or idea about how to solve these and how to feel better. Feel the richness of sharing your emotions and sorrows with others, the warmth, the precious moments and individuals' valuable experiences. You learnt to feel less anxious and depressed, to feel better about your body and yourself. You made changes in your relationships with others, and

you allowed yourself to put yourself first. And finally, you learnt that life is precious and that you want to enjoy it and suffer less.

Individual experiences
Participants may worry that they cannot continue alone, that they feel sad, and that they will miss you. Your response to this might be: 'Do not feel helpless, because this will destroy your energy. Make full use of your capacity for a positive outlook on life. Be confident that you can fight negative feelings and that you can *choose* to feel better. Do not forget all your personal resources. It is also all right to feel sad now – I think we are all sad, and want to cry because we have to say goodbye to each other. I will miss you and I also feel sad. We don't have to hide these feelings.'

Concluding round
Arrange a day for the reunion. 'You may feel the need to phone or see each other or to share activities. It is also possible that you will want to ask for help, comfort or support. Find the courage to ask one of the group members for support and companionship. Thank you all for giving me your trust and sharing your feelings with me. I have learnt from you; thank you.'
Maxim: Love yourself.

Checklist

Listed below are some practical do's and dont's that relate to the treatment plan.

ALWAYS:
- Look at the patients' history to try to find a learning goal for them. Seek out the patient's personal resources and enable her to 'own' them.
- Teach them how to say 'no'.
- Use role playing if a patient feels shy with her doctor.
- Make it clear that a partner can be a man or a woman.
- Recognize and explain survival guilt. Survival must be seen as a responsibility to make life worthwhile.
- Stop your programme if a patient announces a recurrent cancer. Ask the group to share their feelings and to comfort the ill patient. Ask the patient whether, and in what way, she needs the group's help.
- Find moments to laugh together.

NEVER:
- Tell patients that they need not be anxious.
- Allow a patient to act as your co-therapist.
- Criticize patients.

- Leave it unnoticed when a patient is disloyal to herself.
- Attack defence mechanisms.
- Let myths and misconceptions pass unspoken.
- Answer medical questions.
- Allow patients to believe that cancer is a punishment for sins.

Conclusion

Our treatment plan covers the main points that will help patients in remission to cope better and to improve their quality of life. It is a pragmatic approach in which patients learn to take responsibility for their own well-being. The informational part of the sessions aims to give advice, suggestions and education about mental health and psychological functioning. For patients with gynaecological cancers and breast cancer (as well as patients with testicular and prostate cancer) it is particularly important to discuss their relationship with their partner and other issues such as the need for intimacy and open communication, and changes in their sexual relationships. This chapter has focused on the patients themselves, but their partners' situation also deserves attention. Love is a powerful source of strength for coping with cancer, and when it is absent the quality of a patient's survival is seriously limited. Cancer can be a turning point in life, enabling individuals to change their life for the better. Finally, remember that the effective therapist is the person who risks making mistakes and loves their patients.

References

AMERICAN CANCER SOCIETY (1984) *Cancer Facts and Figures 1985.* New York: American Cancer Society.
ANDERSEN, L. and JOACHIMSEN, P.R. (1985) Sexual functioning among breast cancer, gynecologic cancer, and healthy women. *Journal of Consulting and Clinical Psychology*, 53, 25–32.
BLOOM, J.R. and ROSS, R.D. (1982) Measurement of the psychosocial aspects of cancer: Sources of bias. In J. Cohen, J.W. Cullen and L.R. Martin (Eds), *Psychosocial Aspects of Cancer*. New York: Raven Press.
BOS, G. (1984) Psychological aspects of gynaecological oncology surgery. In A.P.M. Heintz, C.T. Griffiths and J.B. Trimbos (Eds), *Surgery in Gynecological Oncology*. The Hague: Martinus Nijhoff.
BOS, G. (1986) Sexuality of gynecological cancer patients: Quantity and quality. *Journal of Psychosomatics, Obstetrics and Gynecology*, 5, 217–224.
BOS-BRANOLTE, G. (1987) *Psychological problems in survivors of gynaecologic cancers. A psychotherapeutic approach.* Oegstgeest: De Kempenaer.
BOS-BRANOLTE, G. and DUIVENVOORDEN, H.J. (1989) Psychological problems in

280   Gerjanne Bos-Branolte

survivors of gynecological cancer. A controlled psychosocial study. *Advances in Gynecology and Obstetrics*, 3, 203–212.

DENNERSTEIN, L., WOOD, C. and BURROWS, G. (1977) Sexual response following hysterectomy and oophorectomy. *Obstetrics and Gynecology*, 49, 92–96.

DEROGATIS, L.R. (1980) Breast and gynecologic cancers. *Frontiers of Radiation Therapy and Oncology*, 14, 1–11.

DUTCH SOCIETY OF GYNECOLOGIC ONCOLOGY (1985) Gynecologic cancer morbidity and mortality. (Leiden: internal report)

HOROWITZ, M.J. (1976) *Stress Response Syndromes*. New York: Jason Aronson.

KLEBER, R.J. (1982) *Stressbenaderingen in de Psychologie*. Deventer: Van Loghum Slaterus.

KRANT, M.J. (1981) Psychosocial impact of gynecologic cancer. *Journal of Cancer*, 48, 608–612.

LAMONT, J.A., DE PETRILLO, A.D. and SARGEANT, E.J. (1978) Psychosexual rehabilitation and exenterative surgery. *Journal of Gynecologic Oncology*, 6, 236–242.

MAGUIRE, G.P., LEE., E.G., BEVINGTON, D.J., KUCHEMANN, C.S., CRABTREE, R.J. and CORNELL, C.I. (1978) Psychiatric problems in the first year after mastectomy. *British Medical Journal*, 1, 963–965.

MANTELL, J.E. and GREEN, C. (1978) Reducing post-mastectomy sexual dysfunction: An appropriate role for social work. In A. Comfort (Ed.) *Sexual Consequences of Disability*. Philadelphia: Stickley.

MARTIN, L.R. (1982) Overview of the psychosocial aspects of cancer. In J. Cohen, J.W. Cullen and L.R. Martin (Eds) *Psychosocial Aspects of Cancer*. New York: Raven Press.

MORRIS, T., GREER, H.S. and WHITE, P. (1977) Psychological and social adjustment to mastectomy: A two-year follow-up study. *Journal of Cancer*, 40, 2381–2387.

SCHAIN, W.S. (1981) Role of the sex therapist in the care of the cancer patient. *Frontiers of Radiation Therapy and Oncology*, 15, 168–183.

SILVERBERG, E. and LUBERA, J. (1986) Cancer Statistics. *CA*, 6, 5–21.

TAYLOR, S.E. (1983) Adjustment to threatening events: A theory of cognitive adaptation. *American Journal of Psychology*, 38, 1161–1173.

WEISMAN A.D. and WORDEN J.W. (1976-77) The existential plight in cancer: Significance of the first 100 days. *International Journal of Psychiatric Medicine*, 7, 1–15.

WORTMAN, C.B. (1983) Coping with victimization: Conclusions and implications for future research. *Journal of Social Issues*, 39, 195–221.

WORTMAN, C.B. (1984) Social support and the cancer patient: Conceptual and methodologic issues. *Journal of Cancer*, 53, 2339–2360.

Recommended Reading

YALOM, I.D. (1975) *The theory and practice of group psychotherapy*. New York: Basic Books.

LEUKAEMIA: BONE MARROW TRANSPLANTATION

Nicole Alby

The global incidence rate for the leukaemias is approximately 1 per 40,000 of the population, with the three major diagnostic categories being acute myeloblastic leukaemia (AML), acute lymphoblastic leukaemia (ALL) and chronic myeloid leukaemia (CML). Worldwide some 5,000 allogenic bone marrow transplantations (BMTs) are performed every year. This treatment method is increasingly used, and at present approximately 75 per cent of transplants are performed on patients with leukaemia. The use of BMT as a treatment for leukaemia varies widely from country to country because of differences in the availability of transplantation facilities, haematologists' attitudes, patients and the stage of their disease and, of course, the existence of donors (Gluckman, 1989). Autologous BMTs are increasing in number but are still far less frequently performed as a treatment for leukaemias than allografts.

The USA, France and the UK have the largest treatment programmes and 25 per cent of patients diagnosed with leukaemia will receive BMT. Such figures show that BMT has developed from being an experimental procedure to become an important treatment method of acute and chronic leukaemias. It has transformed the prognosis of fatal diseases such as chronic or acute leukaemias, aplastic anaemias and congenital diseases such as Fanconi anaemia. Today more than 50 per cent of these patients will survive (Gluckman, 1989). The development of bone marrow banks will allow more transplants, enabling patients without family donors to receive BMT.

However specific aspects of BMT are very demanding for patients, families and staff and the treatment always has a psychological cost (Patenaude, 1979). To survive is not enough: cured patients' quality of life is now an essential concern for their care takers. Psychological assessment and support are necessary because of the demands of the BMT procedure. In our unit, close collaboration between haematologists and psychologists is a routine part of the patients' daily care. The decision to proceed with BMT is always taken within the stressful context of a fatal disease. It involves the choice of a healthy donor who in most cases is a sibling. Whatever the statistical chances of a given patient, uncertainty will dominate for a lengthy period. The treatment includes isolation, painful medical procedures and severe limitations for at least six to eight weeks, as well as changes in body image and body functioning. These factors always threaten the patients' psychological equilibrium. Graft versus host disease (GVHD) is a severe complication in both its effects and treatments. Whatever the circumstances, recovery always takes time after BMT.

But the miracle is real: patients successfully cured of leukaemias or aplastic anaemias enjoying their new life after BMT are a priceless reward for their families and care takers. However, this miracle occurs after a long period which I will now explore.

DECIDING ON BMT

Deciding on BMT is always a dramatic choice for patients or the families of paediatric patients. Where there are known risk factors such as age, nature and stage of disease, there remains a large degree of uncertainty and individual hazard. As a last hope, BMT is often accepted or begged for while its risks or side-effects are minimized. Giving information is as essential as it is arduous. BMT is an aggressive treatment with long-term side-effects, and its technical phases, consequences and risks must be discussed precisely. Very often however patients and families enter a stressful situation where good decision making is impossible. As stated so well by Pot-Mees (1989) it is a paradoxical situation. Parents have to balance the immediate risks of submitting their child to a life-threatening procedure against the prospect of losing their child anyway. This dilemma is discussed in two thorough papers by Lesko et al. (1989) and Patenaude et al. (1986), who conclude that patients' and parents' feelings of stress are most effectively reduced by the physician's conviction that BMT is the best treatment. For the clinician there is always the problem of how much information to give and in some instances where too much information has been given, with the patient then feeling overwhelmed. The usual procedures of informed consent raise specific problems here. Once the conditioning treatment has been given there is a point of no-return and the patient cannot withdraw consent.

In my experience the very specific and sophisticated world of the complex immunological processes involved in BMT paradoxically encourages a sense of magical omnipotence in patients. This feeling becomes a useful defence mechanism which may replace the desperate feeling of helplessness and loss of control many patients experience. It is within this stressful situation that the psychologist or psychiatrist working in a BMT unit is asked to assess the patients' and the families' coping abilities, their emotional responses and the risks of psychopathological reactions. Support begins in this period and the mental health professional's role is to interpret patients' and parents' anxiety, seeing their problems not as paradoxical reactions but as defence mechanisms.

LOOKING FOR A DONOR

Most donors are siblings, even if nowadays marrow banks allow some patients without family donors to undergo BMT. If there is a donor, most often the risks are forgotten, denied or exaggerated – anything but faced objectively. Human Leukocyte Antigen (HLA) typing will present a true haematological family picture and it arouses many anxieties and may reveal family secrets. HLA identity can often change the relationship of the siblings. There is always an intrusion of the biological dimension in the family. The role of the donor is not easy due to the uncertainty of the outcome. It is important to explain the hazards of BMT and limit the role of the donor to a normal act of solidarity and, especially with child donors, to explain that failure is possible. This helps to prevent any identification with the role of a hero or saviour. Transplantation facilitates identification between donor and recipient. It can explain some refusals to be a donor. They are rare and may occur not only because of family conflicts or the more logical fear of anaesthesia but because being identified as 'identical' can lead to a fear of becoming identically sick. After a transplant, the donor's concern for the recipient often reveals their concern for their own health and bone marrow. One donor, the older brother of a leukaemic boy said, 'I am afraid of becoming sick myself. In our family we only have bad luck, so I wonder – why not me?'. He thought that his biological similarity with his sick brother increased the chances of another life-threatening disease occurring in their family. The support team and the haematologist can prevent much of this anxiety by discussing these points with the donor and helping the family to prepare the child for the boost. Here again, understanding their subconscious fears and fantasies helps more than repeating logical information. An essential point is children's consent. Allowing the child donors to make their own decision faces them with an impossible dilemma. Even if children understand the explanations, and they usually do, their decision is most often determined by imaginary fears and unconscious reactions (Alby, 1987). Refusal, if it occurs, would be traumatic for both patient and sibling. The decision should therefore be presented as a family matter, handled by the parents, asking for the donor's cooperation but giving the child no real choice in case of refusal.

The most painful situations occur when there is a conflict between the parents or a preference for one or the other child. Counselling donors, both adults and children, will help them to express these difficult feelings. Fears about graft failure are often linked to the normal guilt induced by sibling conflicts and rivalry. With adults, donation may cause conflict between the spouse or spouse's family, with the donor being asked to choose between them and the sick sibling. Support given to the donors can be indirectly helpful to patients if it relieves or explains family situations or conflicts.

In what is a very scientific and high-tech procedure, it is fascinating to observe all the myths and fantasies about blood and donation. Titmuss (1971) suggests that attitudes towards blood are indicative of societies' beliefs: 'The very thought of individual blood touches the deepest feelings in man about life and death; even in modern times mystical and irrational group attitudes to blood have sharply distinguished certain western societies'. So bone marrow donation will never be the simple harvesting of a human organ. Unrelated donors present new problems which we are currently studying.

HOSPITALIZATION

Patients and families need to be carefully prepared for hospitalization, so:

(1) Apart from emergency cases, patients and families should visit the unit, see a laminar air-flow or isolation room, and talk to another patient. We have a booklet explaining medical and practical aspects of BMT and a video is shown on the very day the decision for BMT is taken. Patients are relieved to have seen the unit, their fears often being worse than the very difficult reality. But the most effective preparation is to observe how inpatients cope.

(2) Psychosocial assessment is another important step. While social or psychosocial distress is rarely seen as a sufficient obstacle to BMT, this is not always the case with psychiatric disorders which cannot be controlled. Psychiatric evaluation must be available with a psychiatrist being well-integrated into the transplant unit.

Transplantation demands patients' compliance and cooperation, and families' involvement. The psychologist or psychiatrist has to assess patients and families' past psychosocial history, previous psychiatric or psychological disorders, level of understanding and usual defence mechanisms. Their religious and cultural environment is of course also taken into account. Clearly, their past medical history and stage of disease are important factors that affect their coping abilities. There is a great difference between a patient suddenly affected with aplastic anaemia, and a patient who has relapsed with acute leukaemia reaching BMT often exhausted and with little confidence. Distance from home is another disruptive factor as many patients come from far away or foreign countries.

Assessing each of these points is essential as they represent variables in patients' coping abilities. They help:

(1) To gain a better understanding of patients' reactions, needs and fears;

(2) To allow the nursing and medical staff to prepare the best conditions of care, and

(3) To prevent psychopathological disorders.

It is important at this point to prepare patients for unknown and painful feelings and emotions and to present psychological intervention as a way to help normal people to adjust to an abnormal environment. Patients are often afraid of being unable to cope or of being confronted by a totally unknown situation.

Hospitalization will last at least six to eight weeks and is a break from the familiar external world. Figure 1 illustrates the usual pattern of hospitalization and follow-up.

During treatment patients are confined to a limited space, under their plastic curtains, a fragile barrier that they never pass, thus reflecting how vulnerable they feel. After chemotherapy and total body irradiation they can experience severe fatigue, nausea and anorexia. Some patients bitterly resent the conditioning treatment as it makes them even more sick. Their somatic condition, loss of

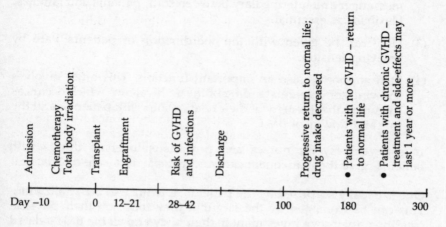

FIGURE 1 *Pattern of BMT hospitalization and follow-up*

autonomy and bodily closeness with the nurses facilitate regression or excessive demands. Patients form intense links with their care takers which explains their tolerance of isolation. The balance between the necessary regression and patients' struggle for some autonomy is difficult. Reality testing and interest in the outside world is hampered as their only concern is with the progress of the transplantation. Even the notion of time is altered and all days seem the same. Life is only lived through BMT-related events such as conditioning, and BMT infusion.

Throughout this period family visits should be unlimited. Families or friends may feel like outsiders and need to be helped to understand patients' attitudes.

There is evidence that the patients' physical status has an important influence on their state of mind. GVHD and immunosuppressive treatments impose special diets and create cushingoïd face, body image changes and mood instability. Some very anxious or obsessional personalities cannot adjust whatever their condition and want to control every medical or nursing activity.

The BMT unit is a group at risk of psychological disorders (such as burn-out) which is always seeking equilibrium, so the mental health professional must be a closely integrated member of the unit. As stated by Patenaude *et al.* (1979), the usual techniques need to be modified in such a specific setting. The mental health professional needs to:

(1) Assess coping strategies in an abnormal situation where abnormal reactions may have different meanings.

(2) Modify the usual rules of confidentiality in order to act as a messenger and intermediary between staff, patients and families. Flexibility is essential.

(3) Help can be given with the coordination of patients' care by relieving tension.

(4) Staff support is also an important function. This often involves showing some understanding of the ambivalence which occurs as a result of the intensity of their relationship with patients, and the ups and downs of BMT.

It is never easy for nurses and physicians to share things with patients, give them adequate care and yet stay at a safe distance.

One is usually surprised by the patients' tolerance to hospitalization. This can be explained by the fact that they focus on their physical condition, their own investment in their body and all the BMT-related events, such as blood counts. Patients obsessionally organize their life according to nursing schedules and rely on care takers, their physical condition being their primary focus and, of course, the main cause of psychological ups and downs. A small number of patients will cope only through refusal and aggressiveness.

DEATH IN A BMT UNIT

In such units, intensive care of patients in a critical state is part of the daily routine and training of the physicians and nurses. Patients and families are immersed in the same fighting spirit. With the exception of some rare sudden deaths, staff and patients share a long battle and period of intense mutual involvement. Patients' severe physical status increases their dependency and their anxiety. They rely entirely on their care takers. Families may feel as if they are helpless spectators of the patients' worsening condition. Because they had hoped for a miracle and put their faith in such a powerful treatment, they cannot hear the truth and will suddenly move from hope to despair or belligerence. The aggressive treatment regimen so often questioned by the family becomes a miracle that has failed.

Medical and nursing staff may resent feelings of professional impotence, and failure and guilt are easily experienced as they are faced with iatrogenic complications. Patenaude *et al.* (1989) described the intensity of the staff's emotional experiences. Personal investment in patients for long weeks, with only a 50 per cent chance of survival, is a costly experience. 'Burn-out' is common, particularly in younger professionals. Support for staff and families must therefore be available on a daily basis.

Families also need to be helped to stay beside their very sick relative and to be allowed to express their anxieties, questions, anger and their very ambivalent emotions. They often cannot talk with physicians about the death they fear, so it can look as if they have accepted it.

As the psychologist or other mental health professional has no direct medical role, psychological intervention enables families and staff to be supported and understood without medical issues being involved. During this painful period it may be the best form of support. The patient's first need, apart from pain control, is to feel that they are not abandoned. A peaceful environment, including an alliance between families and staff, if not always simple, is essential. The mental health professional then acts as an interpreter of the different and sometimes opposing needs of the patient and those caring for him or her. Death will always mean rupture and suffering but one can prevent unnecessary distress.

Death is especially painful in BMT units, where powerful medical procedures can be seen to produce 'miraculous' results for other patients. Of course the death of any patient is a terrible blow to the other patients and their families. BMT units are very close-knit settings with highly emotional interactions between all their lay and professional members. A death in the unit therefore can potentially affect others outside of the patient's immediate family. Encouraging patients, families and staff to talk about their feelings at this time is an important part of the mental health professional's role.

DISCHARGE FROM THE BMT UNIT

Discharge is feared just as much as it is wanted. It is the model of the ambiguous situations BMT patients so often face. In our unit patients used to be so anxious when all the curtains of the laminar air-flow room were opened on the same day that now the policy is to open them progressively one by one.

All patients, including children, experience:

(1) Fear of leaving the protected environment of the unit and being without the staff's skills and support.

(2) Fear of facing their changed body image (including baldness, loss of strength, weight loss, or, in the case of GVHD, cushingoïd face and modified skin) and fear of infection. Although temporary, these changes are the most important obstacle to their return to a normal life.

(3) Constraints of treatment and diet. Drug intake may last for some time and close medical follow-up is necessary for many months. Noncompliance can be very dangerous and adolescents are specially vulnerable.

Sterility and sexual problems also need to be discussed. All patients who have undergone BMT for leukaemia become sterile. Women experience induced menopause. The difference between sterility and impotence should be clearly explained, especially with male adolescents. It is never easy for haematologists to discuss these issues with their patients. Information should be adjusted according to individual needs and different stages of BMT. Hormonal treatment must be offered to women, as well as information about artificial insemination (AIDS) and adoption. It is often useful to introduce newly transplanted patients to ex-patients who have adopted children or taken part in AIDS. Once they have the relevant medical information patients may need to discuss their anxieties and fears regarding their sexual life and their future as parents.

Infertility is often unconsciously linked with the absence of life –

i.e. with death. It is one of the most painful consequences of BMT, as shown in many post-BMT quality of life evaluations. The mental health professional's role is important in facilitating doctor–patient dialogue, explaining the specific anxieties and losses due to infertility and sexual problems.

Leaving the unit also means facing the world of the healthy. Patients often complain of communication problems and their experience of BMT is difficult for them to put into words. During the period after discharge, patients often experience more distress, anxiety and even depression than when they were supported by the BMT environment, where there was no choice or autonomy.

Restoration of identity takes time and is related to appearance, weight change and effective psychological defences. The role of a caring family environment is as essential as support by the staff, and much is demanded of families in terms of affective, social, financial and vocational sacrifices. Not all families are equally able to make these sacrifices. Therefore social and psychological support for families must be readily available (Alby, 1986).

At this point anxiety and depression need to be reassessed and can often be relieved through therapeutic sessions. Fatigue may also be related to a hidden depression. Guilt, because of all the demands on their family, is often hidden and has to be discussed. It is during this period that close psychological follow-up of patients is essential. This needs to occur in collaboration with a psychiatrist in order to treat depression or anxiety and in some rare cases acute psychiatric disorders quickly and effectively. These reactions most often occur after discharge when patients are faced with problems they cannot manage, or, in some cases, physical complications. Adjustment can be achieved in all patients with proper psychiatric treatment. Families need psychological and social support in parallel. After discharge parents or spouses may feel exhausted and resent being responsible for a vulnerable patient. So families are also at risk of depression.

The most demanding aspect of BMT is the continuing *uncertainty* that follows treatment: patients fear infectious or viral disease relapse in the case of the leukaemias. The smallest symptom may cause a panic attack. The Damocles syndrome described by Koocher and O'Malley (1981) is a most appropriate term here. It is a true pathology of uncertainty facilitated by the physicians' double talk 'You are well but don't forget any of your drugs'; 'You are fine but I want to check you next week'. As Lesko (1989) points out, discharged patients express their concern about developing 'from living as a patient to living as a survivor'. For some obsessional or fragile personalities it is very demanding. One patient said 'I don't know if I am sick or cured, I am neither one nor the other, who am I?' Change in appearance, fatigue, loss of weight, communication problems with the healthy increase their identity problems. As one patient said: 'When I looked at my reflection in the mirror, I wondered, is that a half or three-quarters of my usual self?'

Patients speak of a new life, of a rebirth, they know that BMT saved their life. It is also in this period that they can speak of their fears and emotions during transplant, elaborate on their feelings and take measure of the risks they went through. They can speak of their confused feelings about being changed and of living through some-one else's organ. Others may fear having received more than the blood characteristics of their donor: 'I am not surprised about being depressed, my sister has always been so, and she gave me her blood'. Families also have many fantasies about mood changes or risks linked to psychological differences. A mother was convinced that the patient would suffer from Graft versus Host Disease because 'My two sons may be biologically identical, but in real life they are opposite, so their marrows must fight'. Incidentally, the patient did suffer from a life-threatening GVHD.

It is not that easy to accept being alive because of someone else's organ, albeit a diffused organ without clear representation or loca-tion. Fantasies are different from those aroused by solid organ trans-plantation and the debt to the donor is different, as is the donor–recipient relationship. Patients experience various feelings of pos-session by the donor's bone marrow and of threat to their own identity.

I do not agree totally with Lesko (1989) when she says that patients do not experience any fear of change in sexual identity when they are not the same sex as their donor. In fact they often dare not discuss their feelings.

Patients have to go through all these conscious and unconscious experiences and through the medical ups and downs of the post-transplant period. Psychological sessions help to put names to their fantasies and emotions and restore some continuity between their life before and after BMT. The therapist can also help families, and interpret their problems in dealing with patients' needs.

GRAFT VERSUS HOST DISEASE

There are two categories of patients after BMT: those suffering from severe or chronic GVHD and the others. GVHD affects approximately 40 per cent of patients and produces a group of symptoms expressing the immunological conflict between donor- and recipient-competent T-cells. It can be a life-threatening complication and it always threatens the patients' quality of life. Although some cases respond easily to treatment it often imposes a long therapeutic battle. First, the risks of GVHD have to be constantly balanced against the treatment's risks by the immunosuppressive drugs and this is a very demanding task for the physician. Second, GVHD symptoms are in themselves distressing; skin rash and abnormalities, painful contractures, dryness of mouth and eyes, diarrhoea, anorexia, weight and muscle loss and liver problems are often very debilitating and require long-term management. Body image is especially affected by GVHD and its treatment and patients may suffer from symptoms including cushingoïd face, general modification of appearance and fatigue. It increases infectious and viral risks and imposes dietary restrictions. GVHD after the acute phase turns into a chronic disease. Some patients will achieve complete recovery with little or no sequelae but a small number will have to adjust to the limited life of a chronic patient. Treatment may cause motor limitations due to necrosis of the hips or shoulders and surgery is often necessary. It demands a *very* long period of medical follow-up, and uncertainty continues as GVHD may disappear and reappear.

Patience is the most needed virtue for patients, families and staff, and one can never emphasize this enough. A good doctor–patient relationship is essential as noncompliance is a temptation when drug side-effects may seem more distressing than the GVHD. Of course, medical progress gives hope that in the future this painful aspect of BMT will be better controlled.

The psychological consequences may be great, with anger and aggressiveness or, on the other hand, depression and passivity. There is also a tendency for patients to segregate themselves from the outside world. Muscular atrophy due to corticosteroids is another very incapacitating symptom. During this period the support of the multidisciplinary team is necessary. Changes in mood may also be caused by some drugs (mainly corticosteroids) and sleep and eating disorder are frequent.

Patients are again committed to a close relationship with the staff and they become dependent and disease-centred. The mental health professional is not responsible for their medical treatment, not involved in their family problems and, as an integrated member of staff, is able to have a global and more distant appreciation of the patients' situation and problems.

Families can become exhausted, experiencing the limits of their resistance to the disease and treatment demands. Often patients feel guilty for what has been imposed on their parents, spouses and children. The balance between each family member's needs during this period is not easy. The financial, social and vocational consequences of such a long treatment are always heavy and should never be underestimated.

Conflicts and aggressive reactions by family or staff are not uncommon, but it is often useful to interpret them as consequences of the disease rather than true aggressive reactions, and to understand the different types of suffering for each person involved, whether they are patients or carers. Recovery occurs after a long process during which the support of patients and families is often difficult. Staff meetings and family group sessions with patients are types of help available to deal with these difficulties.

THE CURED PATIENT

Time is a most important factor in post-BMT adjustment. Children usually return to school after six months, and are not allowed to do so before then. Adults take on average a year or more to resume normal life. There may be large differences in adjustment which relate to their pre-diagnostic circumstances. Manual jobs are more difficult to resume, while people with sedentary occupations and the self-employed can make compromises more easily in order to allow for the constraints fatigue imposes and can adjust work schedules appropriately. All patients need understanding and help from their employers.

Here again there may be confrontations with those who are healthy, and this is illustrated by one patient's comment that 'They cannot understand, one cannot explain BMT'. Problems of body image, fatigue and muscular problems may persist and patients need to be very motivated to resume work.

Some patients may be determined never to accept the disease, BMT, and even mild sequelae. Some make constant emotional demands, as if they need to show staff either directly or indirectly that they will never be well again. This behaviour is often explained by a previous history of early frustrations and affective or social losses. It may also depend on family reactions to disease and transplantation. There is not always a close relationship between the importance of somatic sequelae and patients' adaptation. Some patients need to resume work early, to prove to themselves as well to others that they are doing well. Others explicitly state that they feel they have won the right to a long leave of absence; as one patient said: 'I need to be economical with myself'. Most patients feel vulnerable, even years after transplant and their anxiety can be aroused by any symptoms, a TV programme, or the death of another patient. They usually maintain close links with a physician or a nurse in the unit, as if they need a guarantee of their own safety. We have also seen patients discovering the value of their own life, as a result of their relationship with their care takers. They accept and prepare for positive changes in their life.

This is often the point when those with vulnerable personalities have their first contact with a psychologist or a psychiatrist and are offered psychological and even psychotherapeutic support.

As with any severely stressing situation, BMT brings out the worst and the best of the patients' defence mechanisms, affective and social resources. 'I never imagined that my parents cared so much for me' said one adolescent. A woman who had been in very a masochistic marriage for 15 years was able to ask for a divorce after BMT. As she said 'without my disease and what I experienced with you I would never had dared to get divorced but at least I now know that I can take care of myself'. Some patients feel omnipotent because they have gone through such a dangerous experience and survived and the vulnerability of such defence mechanism must be recognized. Others need to help science, raise money, organize support for other patients in a close identification with physicians.

One should not have a model of the ideal patient: some patients need to please doctors, others need to complain. Both positions are misleading. Care takers should therefore be flexible, and tolerant of the wide variety of defence mechanisms patients need. Psychological sessions must be similarly flexible and easily available. They can vary from a ten-minute checkup to a thorough interview and it is not predictable when a patient may need to talk about his or her long-lasting experience, fears and fantasies. Such sessions form the basis of recovery.

During their child's treatment parents must be encouraged and helped to be present and to share the daily care. Where possible continuity in school work must be preserved. In our unit, teachers are available on an everyday basis. Children with no previous school problems usually return eventually to their normal class. Although children make a faster physical recovery they often resent fatigue, muscular atrophy and appearance problems caused by chronic GVHD. They need a great deal of support to resume their normal social life. It is notable that children's coping abilities are largely dependant on their parents' ability to preserve normal life and normal goals.

As Pot-Mees (1989) says, most children show a remarkable adjustment one year after BMT, but more must be done as regards support services during and after transplantation. Prospective studies and thorough evaluation are especially needed for children. One has to care not only for their physical recovery but also their affective, social and educational recovery and their right to a full and satisfactory return to normal life. Much can be said about siblings (see Lansdown and Goldman this volume) who are also at risk of psychosocial disorders and suffering. Psychological support ought to be available for them too and a good preventative model advocates early counselling for both parents and siblings of BMT patients.

STAFF SUPPORT

Staff burn-out has been studied by many authors, as highlighted by Lederberg (1982). All staff members experience ups and downs and periods of uncertainty as a result of BMT. Intimacy with patients is emotionally draining. Psychological support should include recognition of the staff's needs. Staff meetings, as well as informal discussions, provide an opportunity to interpret patients' reactions, discuss communication problems and accept any failures and losses. Some staff fear an intrusion on their relationship with patients and may see the mental health professional as critical of their professional role. They may think that any expression of emotions is a dangerous sign of vulnerability. It takes time to achieve a trusting relationship between staff members and the psychologist or psychiatrist, and a period of mutual assessment is often necessary. Only then can the psychologist and the psychiatrist act as intermediary between the contradictory needs of patients and staff.

Discussions enable staff to recognize dangerous situations and the problems associated with a desire to cure patients. This will facilitate a better understanding of their own reactions, reduce their need to make moral judgements and help maintain a better distance between themselves and their patients. Such discussions also help relieve guilt and allow conflicts to be resolved. Staff may also appreciate better their own role in the patients' care and cure, the true gratitude of families and the stimulation of belonging to a scientific and advanced medical team.

SERVICE ORGANIZATION

I have already emphasized that psychosocial support for BMT patients must be available from the day transplant is decided upon, during hospitalization and throughout the long process to recovery. It demands conviction and the full participation of staff members and mental health professionals.

Before transplant:

— In our unit, patients are invited to visit the unit and talk to an inpatient who is recovering from their transplant.

— A video is shown to the patient, the donor, and their family which gives explanations and details on the transplant procedure. Their questions are then answered by a member of the nursing staff.

— A leaflet written by the BMT nurses is given to them which covers the different stages of the transplant, and gives precise information on everyday life in the unit, including visits, hospital rules and facilities.

— Accommodation for parents of transplanted children is available at the hospital.

— Social workers and chaplains give their specialist support. An initial interview with adult patients (or with the families of young patients) is organized with the psychologist to evaluate patients' and families' specific psychological problems and needs.

After admission:

— The medical and nursing staff meet with the psychologist (or other mental health professional) to discuss the patient's level of understanding and communication, their level of anxiety, past medical and psychological status and available family support.

— Some patients may require more specific help, such as regular sessions of psychotherapeutic support. Collaboration with a psychiatrist who is closely involved with the unit must be available if patients present psychopathological disorders.

Preparing discharge:

— A thorough interview with patients (or with younger patients' families) when discharge is decided is needed in order to evaluate their present psychological status. Psychological preparation is one of the important parts of the discharge process.

— Another video is shown to patients and their families. It explains the stages of recovery and necessary precautions during the first months after BMT. Patients are clearly informed that they will undergo close medical and psychological supervision. Meetings with the families are available, as are visits from members of a patients association.

After discharge:

— As I have already said, there is a long period of fear and uncertainty after discharge. Psychotherapeutic sessions are easily available on a flexible basis with the psychologist or psychiatrist who is already in charge of the patients. The psychologist or psychiatrist regularly sees patients and families during their weekly outpatient visits. Their role is one of intermediary, involving discussions with the haematologist in charge of the patient and with families. It also involves liaison with school, or other mental health professionals if aftercare is needed. Family sessions may be especially helpful to interpret and deal with problems between patients and family care givers (see also Bluglass, this volume). Early intervention prevents severe disorders and unnecessary suffering. Because one is usually dealing with normal individuals facing a stressful and abnormal situation, the usual techniques of psychopathological care may have to be modified.

— Some patients or families may prefer to cope without professional support: their right to do this must be accepted. There must be no obligation for them to accept help.

— Some severe psychopathological disorders may occur after discharge, but in my experience early intervention by a psychiatrist is effective in dealing with these problems.

Conclusions

BMT is always a stressful event. Patients and families need psychological and social support and it ought to be an integral part of their total care. It must begin before transplantation and last until a total physical and psychological recovery is achieved. Staff also need the opportunity for support.

Transplantation is a distressing, long-lasting medical procedure, and patients', families' and staffs' needs change with its different stages. One often has to recognize and interpret psychopathological disorders as normal reactions to an abnormal situation and slowly to follow patients' recovery. Clinical research is necessary in order to understand and prevent the psychological consequences of transplantation. Then the real miracle of how these high-risk patients are cured can be appreciated as something of priceless value.

References

ALBY, N. (1986) Difficultés psychologiques de la période post-greffe de moelle osseuse. *Revue Soins*, 483–484, 6 August, 38–40.
ALBY, N. (1987) Trapianto di midollo osseo. In *Pediatria Problematiche Etico-giuridiche e Scientifiche*. Pisa: Industrie Grafiche della Pacini Editore.
ALBY, N., DEVERGIE, A., GLUCKMAN, E. and BOIRON, M. (1983) Role of collaboration between the haematologists and the psychologists for a better follow-up of patients after BMT. (Communication XV annual conference SIOP, New York 20–24 Sept. 1983.)
GLUCKMAN, E. (1989) *Recent trends in Allogenic Bone Marrow Transplantation*. In P. Terasak (Ed.), *Clinical Transplants*. Los Angeles: UCLA Tissue Typing Laboratory.
KOOCHER, G.P. and O'MALLEY, J.E. (1981) *The Damocles Syndrome: Psychosocial consequences of surviving childhood cancer*. New York: McGraw Hill.

LEDERBERG, M.S. (1982) Support groups to prevent burnout. In J.C. Holland (Ed.) *Current Concepts in Psychosocial Oncology*. New York: Memorial Sloan Kettering Cancer Center.

LESKO, L. (1989) Bone marrow transplantation. In J. Holland and J. Rowland (Eds), *Handbook of Psycho-Oncology*. New York: Oxford University Press.

PATENAUDE, A., RAPPEPORT, J. and SMITH, R. B. (1986) The physician's influence on informed consent for bone marrow transplantation. *Theoretical Medicine*, 7, 19, 165–179.

PATENAUDE, A., SZYMANSKI, L. and RAPPEPORT, J. (1979) Psychological costs of bone marrow transplantation in children. *American Journal of Orthopsychiatry*, 49, 3.

POT-MEES, C. (1989) *The Psychological Effects of Bone Marrow Transplantation in Children*. Delft: Eburon.

TITMUSS, R. (1971) *The Gift Relationship From Human Blood To Social Policy*. New York: Pantheon Books.

CHILDREN WITH CANCER

Richard Lansdown and Ann Goldman

'I could cope if I knew that my daughter was going to die and I could cope if I knew that she would live; what I can't cope with is uncertainty'.

The thread of uncertainty runs through departments of oncology and haematology wherever they are. Even after children have been in remission for years there remains what two authors have called 'The Damocles Syndrome' (Koocher and O'Malley, 1981): a constant background feeling that events are, or might easily become, out of control. Here we write not only of parents and children but of staff as well. Anyone working with families of a child with a life-threatening disease must be prepared for personal pain, must be prepared at times for it to show and must develop ways of coping with emotion other than denying it.

One cannot generalize about families. One can talk legitimately about 'most' or perhaps 'many' but rarely 'all'. What is more, everyone is on a personal timetable of expectations. Six year olds know that they are ill but may expect to be well by Christmas. A mother may already have given her child up for dead, having begun a long process of mourning from the moment of diagnosis. A father may look forward grimly to years of harsh treatment which will culminate in cure. The doctor may not look beyond the results of the next blood test.

This chapter considers a model of psychosocial support for children and their families based on the principle that underlying all treatment is an expectation that families will be partners in the enterprise.

Recent literature reviews have been provided by Wass and Corr (1984), Carpenter and Onufrak (1985) and van Dongen-Melman and Sanders-Woudstra (1986). In this chapter we offer the viewpoint of a psychologist and a paediatrician, who work in the combined haematology/oncology department at the Great Ormond Street Hospital for Sick Children.

The key to the provision of care is the ability to call on a wide range of staff. Medical and nursing colleagues are acknowledged to be in the forefront of the work; they can be supplemented by play specialists, social workers, chaplains, teachers, psychologists and psychiatrists. A unique contribution to care in our hospital is the symptom care team, comprising a doctor and three nurses. With such numbers of staff concerned with support some coordination is vital. The use of a weekly psychosocial meeting is discussed to illustrate one way of doing this.

Support itself takes several forms in several locations. One area to be tapped is that already available in the community. As far as possible we share care with hospitals near the child's home and we try whenever possible to establish links with health visitors and other local colleagues. Educational problems, many of which are iatrogenic, are well-known in children being treated by conventional methods and liaison with teachers is of the utmost importance.

Siblings are not without their problems; in some cases they have more overt psychological difficulties than patients. Work with them is hampered by factors related to distance and the undesirability of missing school. The symptom care team, which is largely a domiciliary service, can often try to meet these needs.

Central to all the work is the need to communicate with the children themselves, about their illness, their treatment, their fears, their hopes, their fantasies and their thoughts about death. An understanding of child development and individual differences is vital for everyone working in this area.

As we try to include parents and patients into the treatment team so we feel it essential that all members of the support group, whatever their status or experience, should feel able to share thoughts and feelings and to ask for help when necessary. The greatest fear of the dying child is isolation; the greatest pitfall for the professional is imagining that one can work alone.

We have omitted any discussion of bereavement, not because we see this topic as unimportant, but for reasons of space. For a discussion of bereavement and care of the cancer patient's family see Bluglass, this volume.

Epidemiology

Fortunately cancer in children is rare: about 1,400 cases are diagnosed each year in the United Kingdom. The prognosis has improved remarkably so that 60 per cent of children can expect to reach long-term remission now (Morris Jones, 1987). This is a great source of strength and hope to the families during treatment. However, 40 per cent of patients do still die, some of these from complications of therapy and some from overwhelming disease. Cancer remains the most common illness causing death in children aged between 1 and 14 years.

Children from birth to adolescence may be affected and they suffer from a range of malignancies, of which leukaemia is the most common. Most tumours are responsive to some type of chemotherapy and this forms the mainstay of treatment, with surgery and radiotherapy as appropriate for some patients. Side-effects, both medical and psychological, are inevitable in cancer therapy. Most drugs and many investigations entail intravenous injections, so anxiety and needle phobia may develop. Alopecia, nausea and vomiting are common to many agents and periods of severe infection are not infrequent. Variable amounts of time in hospital and off school occur for all the children, and family life is disrupted (Zeltzer *et al.*, 1980).

The outlook for children with cancer is significantly better when they are treated at one of the recognized paediatric oncology centres which now exist around the country (Lennox *et al.*, 1979). In these centres multidisciplinary teams have the experience and facilities not only for intensive medical care but also for extensive psychosocial support.

APPROACHES TO PSYCHOLOGICAL SUPPORT

Overall Aims

It is easy to be woolly when talking of 'support for families': we rarely define this commodity. At a mundane level our contribution may mean providing fares to visit the hospital. At another level it will involve helping families to ask appropriate questions and giving appropriate answers so that they may feel more in command of what is happening. We try to give people an opportunity to feel that they are, in some way, contributing to the task on hand. At first this is a struggle against an illness, later it may become the need to ensure a peaceful death. Overall it means listening and opening possible avenues of thought and action.

The Provision of Support

The wide-ranging medical and psychological needs of the patient with cancer and his or her family require the expertise of a multidisciplinary team. There will be some situations where appropriate care can be given by any one of the team and other occasions when specialist skills are needed.

Medical and nursing staff are the people on the spot, available both day to day and at times of crisis. Their role in the psychological support of the children is essential. It is the medical staff who break the news to the family, explain the results of tests, determine therapy and above all understand the implications and prognosis. They and the nursing staff just by being there consistently provide much of the routine support and stability for families.

Formal explicit psychological support should ideally be available to all parents (Maguire *et al.*, 1979). Individual work should be as flexible as the system will allow. It is a good idea to introduce the key worker to all families as soon as possible after the diagnosis as a matter of routine. In this way there is no danger that families will feel they are being singled out; the onus is on them to maintain the contact if they wish.

People offering explicit support are usually social workers, psychologists or psychiatrists. Although there are distinctive contributions from each discipline – for example, psychologists have played a major role in investigating children's understanding of death and illness, and only social workers are legally able to undertake child care statutory work – there are ample opportunities for a blurring of boundaries. In many centres the type of work done depends more on personality and interest than professional label.

Group work takes several forms, on wards or in sessions quite separate from the main treatment areas (Gilder *et al.*, 1978). Parent groups have the advantage of allowing participants to realize that they are not alone in their fears and anxieties. It is probably better if groups are led by non-medical staff, because it allows parents a chance to be critical in a safe environment.

Play specialists do far more than occupy children. They can reduce uncertainty by providing play that is familiar, a welcome relief after all the strange sights, sounds and bodily discomfort that the children experience. They can also help prepare children for procedures and for events like hair loss. A set of photographs of the insertion of an indwelling catheter for long-term venous access (Hickman), plus a Hickman teddy (a teddy-bear with a Hickman catheter inserted in the appropriate place) in the hospital corner of the play room allow children to go through the event in anticipation and thus to have some sense of mastery over it.

In recent years a new development has been to extend the hospital's care to the home and community. This may be in the form of liaison nurses or a symptom care team who can maintain continuity of care from diagnosis through to cure or terminal care and have the chance to work with the families in their own homes.

The hospital chaplain plays a key role for some families and, indeed, for some staff, being prepared to approach people's spiritual needs, an area of which other staff are often shy. Neuberger (1987) has written helpfully about caring for people of different faiths.

The Co-ordination of Support

This topic receives little attention in the literature, yet it is easy for the right hand not to know that the left exists, let alone know what it does. Several hospitals now have weekly psychosocial ward rounds (Lansdown, 1986). These meetings, attended by medical, nursing and other staff, mirror a medical round, with emphasis on the psychosocial needs of the children and their families. They can also be a forum for discussion of staff feelings, especially when there has been a particularly distressing death.

'Who cares for the carers?' is a question increasingly asked. The last 25 years have seen a mushrooming growth of research on occupational stress. The relevant literature has been recently reviewed by Payne and Firth-Cozens (1987).

INVOLVING THE FAMILY IN TREATMENT

When a family is directly involved in the treatment of their child they have both a greater sense of control and also an opportunity to prepare themselves and their child appropriately for each stage of the disease. Parents need to go on learning about the disease, its manifestations, treatment and side-effects. In turn, they themselves then take the role and status of teacher and pass on the information to the rest of the family, the community and the child's school. They are the best people to prepare their child for chemotherapy, surgery or radiotherapy since they know their own child's strengths and fears and pattern of communication so much better then anyone else. Members of the oncology team can help parents by reassurance or by suggesting appropriate play techniques and approaches, but frequently we can stand back and learn from them.

Practical aspects of care, which used to be the exclusive province of nursing and medical staff, are now increasingly shared by parents. While a child is on treatment and in hospital, parents can help with day-to-day activities including filling in records of fluid intake and output and giving medicines. A number of children have indwelling catheters for long-term venous access which the parents maintain at home over many months, using sterile techniques. Many families looking after a terminally ill child at home take on all the care. Clearly not all families are comfortable drawing up drugs for infusions and re-sitting subcutaneous needles, but with good support, as their confidence grows, many manage well. This level of involvement in care can bring great satisfaction, particularly if it enables the child to stay at home, although it is also exhausting.

It is also important to be aware that what is appropriate for one family may be an unreasonable burden to another. Even within one family, parents frequently take unequal shares of responsibility, either by choice or force of circumstance, and may need help in coming to terms with this.

SHARED CARE

Because childhood cancer is so uncommon, the main centres are referred children from very wide geographical areas. Partly as a result of this but also because of the severe pressure on hospital beds and staffing, many centres have developed a system of shared care with the local referral hospital and the primary health-care teams. This tends to be presented to the patients as an advantage – they will not have to travel so far and will have a source of help locally. However, families frequently find it difficult to place the same confidence in their local hospital as they have in the centre, whose staff see so many more patients. They often miss the support of the other parents on the ward and feel more isolated and vulnerable. Misunderstandings or even small differences in approach between the hospitals can be worrying to a family already under stress.

There can be advantages for both the patients, the centre and the referral hospital in a shared care programme, but an active commitment by all members is needed for it to be effective. Shared care study days are one way of promoting education and communication, giving the local paediatricians the information and confidence they need to deal with these uncommon diseases and rapidly changing treatment protocols. It helps if members of the different centres can visit and see the problems facing each other. This may be by informal encouragement, by the consultant doing occasional outpatients locally or by giving some particular member of the centre's department a liaison role. Shared care cards, which hold details of treatment and current investigations and which can be carried by the patients, can be valuable. These avoid problems of delays with letters between centres. Also, when parents are party to the information on the cards and given the responsibility for carrying them, their role as part of the team and their sense of control are enhanced.

COMMUNITY SUPPORT NETWORKS

The extra stress of trying to look after other children and maintain a home often many hours' journey from the hospital should not be underestimated. An effective support network can make a great difference practically and emotionally to a family coping with childhood cancer. The lack of it can make bereavement worse (Worden, 1983).

Community 'carers' have rarely met the situation of childhood cancer. They frequently lack confidence, fear they will be unable to help and therefore do not try. Schools may be under- or overprotective or unwilling to take responsibility for the child. Primary health-care teams may feel superfluous in the wake of the specialist centre and wait to be called rather than actively offer support. Grandparents deserve a special mention. It is usually assumed that they will be a strength to parents. Often they are but many are not. Their distress and emotional needs can become an extra burden on the parents. They may offer false and unrealistic reassurance or undermine the parents' confidence in the medical centre by suggesting alternative opinions. Frequently, they are of a generation when frank discussion with children was not encouraged and so may feel uncomfortable with the current approach.

The hospital team should help the family find what support networks are available and appropriate to them and help establish links. Social workers and community liaison staff are in a good position to do this. Isolated families can be identified and extra support offered.

EDUCATIONAL PROBLEMS

Some children sail back into school after a period of illness with no apparent difficulties. Others face serious social and intellectual problems (Findley *et al.*, 1969; Kagen-Goodheart, 1977, Lansky *et al.*, 1975; Deasy-Spinetta, 1981; Wheeler *et al.*, 1988). The immunosuppresant nature of the drugs used in treatment can mean that children have to be shielded from contact with measles or chicken pox, either of which can be fatal. Some families deny illness to such an extent that they give no information to their child or the teachers – the resulting family secret is a threat to everyone's peace of mind. Older children may worry about the changes in their physical appearance – hair loss for example – and children of all ages may worry about falling behind with school work.

Problems can be pre-empted to some extent by encouraging contact between the child and school throughout the time of absence. Teachers can contact the hospital school and discuss work that might be done by the hospital teacher, and once a return is imminent they can ease the transition by telling other children that one of their number is about to come back looking a little different. Children can capitalize on their hard-won knowledge of a life-threatening illness by carrying out a project on it or by giving a talk to the rest of the class. In this context, it is important to note that teachers may have exaggerated ideas of the imminence of the child's death, they may have had unresolved experiences of bereavement themselves, they may be even more protective than the parents (van Eijs, 1977).

Some of these children have learning problems. In part this can be explained by frequent absences from school. But there is now convincing evidence that some of the difficulties are iatrogenic (Eiser, 1978; Moss *et al.*, 1981). The more recent study by Jannoun and Chessells (1987) found that nine out of 18 long-term survivors of leukaemia had both lowered IQs and specific auditory learning deficits. Children diagnosed under five years run the greatest risk of central nervous system damage.

SIBLINGS

The Nature of the Problem

Siblings suffer psychologically when a child has a long-threatening illness. Some authorities maintain that they exhibit greater problems than the patients (Cairns *et al.*, 1979; Spinetta, 1981). It takes time and commitment to be a good parent; when a child is first diagnosed even the best parents find that demands on both their time and commitment are excessive. The whole family system is upset: there is physical disruption because parents spend so much time in hospital or visiting, there is emotional disruption because the attention of parents – and, frequently, of the extended family – is focused on the sick child to the exclusion of others. Parents may also become disproportionately indulgent to the patient.

Observed Behaviour

There is however no consistent pattern to the behaviour problems that have been observed in siblings of children with a malignant disease. They include: irritability and social withdrawal (Lavigne and Ryan, 1979); jealousy; academic underachievement; enuresis; acting out behaviour (Kagen-Goodheart, 1977; Peck, 1979; Powazek, *et al.*, 1980). What is striking is the frequency with which there are similarities between the emotional distress of siblings and that of patients, especially in areas of anxiety, social isolation, vulnerability to illness and injury and self-esteem (Cairns *et al.*, 1979; Spinetta, 1981).

Lindsay and MacCarthy (1974) analyzed the needs of siblings within a developmental framework. Infants were found to be at the greatest risk because mothers were so preoccupied that they could not respond normally to cues given by their offspring. Pre-school children cannot understand what is going on (or perhaps adults think that they cannot understand and so tell them nothing) and so they interpret changes in family systems as rejection. The school child will understand more or less fully, depending on age, and will feel angry, resenting both illness and its consequences. Older siblings are likely to share the same emotions as those of school age but because their options are wider they are able to channel their feelings into providing support for the rest of the family, assuming the parental or caretaker role.

One particular at-risk group are those siblings who have been donors in bone marrow transplants. If the transplant goes well, the donor is likely to feel suitably satisfied with the part played; if not, there is a ready-made opportunity for the donor to feel guilty. A difficult dilemma for adults arises when the potential donor refuses to cooperate. Staff and parents are then put in the unenviable position of trying to persuade a child to undergo a painful and mildly dangerous procedure which is not primarily in that child's interest.

The effect of a death on siblings is a grossly under-researched topic. Pettle Michael and Lansdown (1986) found a noticeably higher incidence of disturbance than would be expected from the general population. They also found that the longer a child had to prepare for a brother's or sister's death, the better the subsequent adjustment.

Management

To a large extent the needs of siblings are not very different from those of the patient: to be told what is happening, why it is happening and as far as possible what is likely to happen in future. It is unwise to give siblings more information than is given to the patient, unless there is a great difference in age. The sibling who knows more may feel unable to enjoy a normal relationship with the patient, especially when they are rivals. As one boy said, sadly, 'I can't hit her now like I used to because I know that she might die and she doesn't know'.

It is of the utmost importance to get across to young children that they are not to blame for their brother's or sister's illness. Concepts of causality and illness develop slowly (Eiser, 1985) and children up to the age of seven or eight may remember a hasty word uttered during a quarrel ('I hate you and wish you were dead') and think that this caused the cancer. As well as giving information, it is essential also to allow the siblings opportunity to talk anxiety through and, perhaps, to mourn in anticipation. Parents are not always the best people to provide this support (although they may be) since they are so often preoccupied with the sick child. Teachers should be alerted to the possibility of a change in the child's work. This may be a falling off but there may also be a surge in activity, as though one child were working for two. Sometimes stress manifests itself in the development of physical symptoms.

The provision of support to siblings is easier to describe than to arrange. Most families have to travel long distances to a treatment centre and frequent family visits are not feasible. One answer is to link with community resources. Some centres have home visiting staff and it is likely that the work they do with the family is just as important as that carried out with the patients.

COMMUNICATING WITH CHILDREN

Why Communication is Necessary

Parents and children themselves may resist communication in order to protect each other. The phenomenon of mutual pretence is a well-established defence mechanism which leads parents and children to pretend to each other that neither is worried about the future (Bluebond-Langner, 1978). The result is that children may be denied the opportunity to express their fears. It is not suggested that mutual pretence is to be attacked – for many people it performs a valuable function – but it can be acknowledged, and both parties can allow the other space with a third person who can meet individual needs. Some parents go as far as lying, saying that the child has anaemia, or flu. Both parents and staff sometimes worry that they will not be able to answer questions adequately and so they avoid situations in which they might be asked. However, anxiety in children is commonly reduced, just as it is in adults, when they can anticipate events (Kelly, 1955). It follows that just as staff have a duty to be open with parents, so they should be with children, commensurate with the child's understanding of illness and possibly, of death.

Who Should Communicate

Many children gain much information, and a good deal of support, from other children. When there is a need to communicate with adults they often make their own choices. They may select a parent, a teacher, a student nurse. Often night staff receive more confidences than their colleagues who work during the day. Whoever it is, he or she is likely to need back-up support, partly so that communication can be monitored and partly because most people need support in their own right at such a stressful time.

How Children Communicate

Question and answer is the obvious mode of communication for adults and some children. Others prefer oblique approaches: 'I don't think I'll get any Christmas presents this year'. Some express themselves through play and/or drawings. Spinetta and Deasy-Spinetta (1981) discuss a number of studies in which projective tests and the scoring of children's drawings were used. A small portion of children express anxiety by changes in behaviour: moodiness, aggression or withdrawal.

Adults are often at a loss when they try to open communication with children. One good way in is to use a story involving serious illness or death. One of several sensitively written books on the topic of death, suitable for children, is *Badger's Parting Gifts* (Varley, 1984). Others are listed by Wass (1984) and Lamers (1986).

What Should be Communicated

It is wise to stay as close as possible to the truth in whatever one says. Throughout the illness, information about treatment, about the course of the disease and about anticipated side-effects should always be available to children.

As well as giving information, adults should also communicate the implicit message that they are treating children with respect. This is exemplified in the very difficult time when conventional treatment has failed and all that remains is symptom relief or experimental chemotherapy of unknown value. To what extent should we encourage children to make the choice or at least to join the decision making? There have been few studies in this area (Nitschke *et al.*, 1982; Kamps *et al.*, 1987), and no agreement on what is acceptable or desirable.

Equally important is the communication of an understanding of the child's emotions. Cheryl was four when her parents told her of her impending death. She refused then to be alone but was unable to put her fear into words. Her parents explained that it might be scary to think she would be alone when she died but this was not going to happen just yet and they would be sure to tell her when the time was near. They also promised not to leave her at this time. This calmed her, and the problem was resolved.

Telling Children That They May Die

Most children with a malignant disease learn, somehow, that their illness is potentially fatal. Parents may say that children will die if they do not cooperate with treatment; another patient in the ward may die; children may read something about their disease in a newspaper or see something on television.

Parents agonize about whether to tell a child when death is near. Judgements on this will depend on the conceptual development of the child, on the religious beliefs of the family, on the general communication style that has been adopted so far. Discussion with an experienced professional can often help parents. Children who are told that death may occur soon often seem to relax once the news is given and may need no more than the fact. Others need to ask more questions: 'Will you be able to visit me in heaven?'. The rule of thumb of always getting as close as possible to the truth is worth bearing in mind at this time.

THE CONCEPTS OF DEATH AND OF ILLNESS

Claire Mulholland, the mother of a child who died of leukaemia, published a collection of poems to her dead daughter (Mulholland, 1973). The shortest was:

> Worst of all was the agony
> Of not knowing
> What you knew.

Part of knowing what children know is understanding what they mean when they talk of death. The literature indicates that the concept is fully developed by the age of seven or eight, but this does not mean that a six year old can have no understanding of the subject. Five-year-old Matthew said to his mother: 'People do die, don't they. . .the doctors can't save everyone, can they. . .but Jesus can save me. He will cure me with love and kisses and send me back to you.'

That brief comment contains almost all the ingredients of this section. Children do not go to bed without a concept of death and wake up next morning with one; it develops gradually and various components fall into place over time. Kane (1979) put forward nine components, including the ideas that death is universal and irrevocable and that a dead person is immobile and without sensation. Matthew understood, at least in part, that death is not avoidable and that it means separation. He seems not fully to have grasped the notion of irrevocability.

Lansdown and Benjamin (1985) examined the development of the concept of death in healthy children, reporting that about two-thirds of the five year olds they questioned had a complete, or almost complete, understanding, using Kane's criteria. Children almost always seem to understand more than adults give them credit for – but one must always be wary of the child who partly understands, the one who says, for example, with confidence that 'everyone dies' but goes on to add 'when they are a hundred.'

Eiser (1985) has described attempts at delineating children's concepts of the nature and cause of illness. Bluebond-Langner (1978) and Lansdown (1987) have pointed to the importance of realizing that children's awareness proceeds in a series of distinct stages, from 'I am seriously ill' to 'I am dying'. There is no agreement on whether all children who die reach this last stage; but the possibility of them all coming to it, even when as young as three or four years, should, nevertheless, be considered.

AROUND THE TIME OF DEATH

After a family have been told that it is impossible to cure their child and have accepted, at least to some extent, that death is inevitable, they are faced not only with the immense emotional burden but also with numerous practical questions. How long will my child live? How long will he or she remain reasonably well? What shall we say to the child, to the siblings, to the rest of the family? Will there be pain or other symptoms? What can be done for them? Who will do it? Will it have to be in hospital? Where will our child die? What will the death be like? What do you do once someone has died? How do you know you've got the right ashes after a cremation? How can we possibly cope with any or all of this? Most of these questions and many more occur, at some point, to virtually every parent, although not everyone will acknowledge them unless encouraged. Often they are afraid they are peculiar or feel guilty for anticipating the child's death. Often they feel even more guilty for wanting, with part of their mind, the child to die, to be free of suffering.

Staff, at this time, need to reassure the family that they will not be abandoned just because active treatment has stopped. It is their responsibility to be sure that care will be available for the child and family, to answer questions, provide symptom relief and give emotional support. Parents can usually choose to have the child at home or in hospital and need to spend time talking over the advantages and difficulties each presents.

Most terminally ill children can expect a period of time after relapse during which they are either entirely or almost entirely symptom free. Although it can be difficult to predict how long this may last, most families want to take advantage of this time at home, together, in as normal an environment as possible for as long as they can. Treats can be arranged; short holidays, visits to relatives and friends and even premature celebrations for birthdays can be organized while the child is well enough to enjoy them.

During this period the family and the carers have some time to consider what they would like to do when the child develops symptoms and eventually when they are dying. Death at home is the first choice for many and the advantages for the child are clear; however, the responsibilities for the family are great. Most primary health-care teams have no experience of terminal care in children and feel uncomfortable with the situation. Sometimes community facilities for adult terminal care can be used but this means introducing new staff – who themselves have little paediatric experience – at a crucial time. Many centres are now increasingly aware of the needs of their terminally ill patients and are providing a home care service, which may be in the form of a symptom care team or a community liaison nurse. This has the advantage for the child and family of maintaining continuity and it provides the local health-care team with a resource of expertise and confidence (Lauer and Camitta, 1980; Corr and Corr, 1985).

Not all families choose to be at home – for some, the thought of living in the house where their child died is unbearable. The choices then are generally between the centre and the local paediatric ward. Both of these are more restricted than home and are geared to active treatment rather than terminal care, but usually, having known the family over some time, are able to accommodate to their needs. For some families the reassurance of being in hospital is important.

It is sometimes suggested that the child might go to a hospice, terminally. There are now two paediatric hospices open in the UK. Unlike adult facilities, their primary role has not been as a place for children to die but as a supportive facility for the families and child with progressive life-threatening diseases. Relatively few of their patients have had cancer (Burne *et al.*, 1984; Dominica, 1987). Unless the family have already established a relationship with a hospice, few will choose to make this new contact at a late stage.

SERVICE ORGANIZATION

At the risk of stating the obvious, the greatest practical need is financial. The National Health Service does not meet the cost of all our medical staff and pays for only a fraction of the psychosocial team. The social workers and symptom care team are paid by charitable organizations, teachers are funded by the local educational authority.

Next in order of importance is space on or near the ward, on or near the outpatients' department, so that parents and children can be seen with some privacy.

Time is not easily found in a very busy day. The organization of meetings at a regular time in a location that is easy to get to has been shown to be critical. After experimenting with several different locations the most successful so far has been the doctors' office on the ward.

There is the value of regular feedback to all staff on whatever psychosocial interventions have taken place. This can be formal, at the regular psychosocial meeting but it can be informally given.

Finally there is a need to be constantly self-critical, for each member of the team to feel free to make suggestions about how better to carry out the task.

Conclusion

In her novel *George Beneath a Paper Moon*, Nina Bawden wrote: 'The really unexpected happens so seldom that few of us know how to deal with it. We all move, for most of the time in a small circle of known possibilities to which we have learned the responses. Outside of this circle lies chaos; a dark land without guidelines.' Caring for children with malignant diseases involves helping them and their families to find some guidelines through the chaos.

Acknowledgements. The authors would like to thank Gillian Tindall and Tom Lissauer for their support and constructive criticism, and Juliet Grainger for typing the manuscript. Ann Goldman is grateful to the Rupert Foundation for Children with Life Threatening Disease who funded the symptom care team from 1986 to 1990.

References

BLUEBOND-LANGNER, M. (1978) *The Private Worlds of Dying Children.* Princeton, NJ: Princeton University Press.

BURNE, S.R., DOMINICA, F. and BAUM, J.D. (1984) Helen House – A hospice for children: Analysis of the first year. *British Medical Journal*, 289, 1665–1668.

CAIRNS, N.U., CLARK, G.M., SMITH, S.D. and LANSKY, S.B. (1979) Adaptation of siblings to childhood malignancy. *Journal of Pediatrics*, 95, 484–487.

CARPENTER, P.J. and ONUFRAK, B. (1984) Pediatric psychosocial oncology: A compendium of current professional literature. *Journal of Psychosocial Oncology*, 2, 119–136.

CORR, C.A. and CORR, D.M. (1985) Pediatric hospice care. *Pediatrics*, 76, 774–780.

DEASY-SPINETTA, P. (1981) The school and the child with cancer. In. J.J. Spinetta and P. Deasy-Spinetta (Eds) *Living With Childhood Cancer*. St. Louis: C.V. Mosby.

DOMINICA, F. (1987) The role of the hospice for the dying child. *British Journal of Hospice Medicine*, 38, 334–342.

EISER, C. (1978) Intellectual abilities among survivors of childhood leukaemia as a function of CNS irradiation. *Archives of Diseases in Childhood*, 53, 391–395.

EISER, C. (1985) *The psychology of childhood illness.* New York: Springer-Verlag.

FINDLEY, I.I., SMITH, P., GRAVES, P.J. and LINTON, M.L. (1969) Chronic disease in childhood: A study of family reactions. *British Journal of Medical Education,* 3, 66–99.

GILDER, R., BUSCHMAN, P.R., SITARZ, A.L. and WOLFF, J.A. (1978) Group therapy with parents of children with leukaemia. *American Journal of Psychotherapy,* 32, 276–287.

JANNOUN, L. and CHESSELLS, J. (1987) Long term psychological effects of childhood leukaemia and its treatment. *Paediatric Oncology and Haematology,* 4, 293–308.

KAGEN-GOODHEART, L. (1977) Re-entry: living with childhood cancer. *American Journal of Orthopsychiatry,* 47, 651–658.

KAMPS, W.A., AKKERBOOM, J.C., KINGMA, A. and HUMPHREY, G.B. (1987) Experimental chemotherapy in children with cancer – A parent's view. *Pediatric Hematology and Oncology,* 4, 117–124.

KANE, B. (1979) Children's concepts of death. *Journal of Genetic Psychology,* 134, 141–153.

KELLY, H. (1955) *The Psychology of Personal Constructs,* New York: W.W. Norton.

KOOCHER, G.P. and O'MALLEY, J.E. (1981) *The Damocles Syndrome.* New York: McGraw-Hill.

LAMERS, E. (1986) Books for adolescents. In C.A. Corr and J.N. McNeil (Eds) *Adolescence and Death.* New York: Springer-Verlag.

LANSDOWN, R. and BENJAMIN, G. (1985) The development of the concept of death in children aged 5–9 years. *Child: Care, health and development,* 11, 13–20.

LANSDOWN, R. (1986) The care of the child facing death. (Paper read at the 11th International Congress of the International Association of Child and Adolescent Psychiatry and Allied Professions, Paris.)

LANSDOWN, R. (1987) The development of the concept of death and its relationship to communicating with dying children. In E. Karas (Ed.) *Current Issues in Clinical Psychology.* London: Plenum Press.

LANSKY, S.B., LOWMAN, J.T., VATS, T. and GYULAY, J.E. (1975) School phobia in children with malignant neoplasms. *American Journal of Diseases of Children,* 129, 42–46.

LAVIGNE, J.V. and RYAN, M. (1979) Psychological adjustment of siblings of children with chronic illness. *Pediatrics,* 63, 616–627.

LAUER, M.E. and CAMITTA, B.M. (1980) Home care for dying children: A nursing model. *Journal of Pediatrics,* 97, 1032–1035.

LENNOX, E.L., STILLER, C.A., MORRIS JONES, P.H. and KINNIER WILSON, L.M. (1979) Nephroblastoma: treatment during 1970–3 and the effect on survival of inclusion in the first MRC trial. *British Medical Journal,* 2, 257–9.

LINDSAY, M. and MACCARTHY, D. (1974) Caring for the brothers and sisters of a dying child. In L. Butlin (Ed.) *Care of the Child Facing Death.* London: Routledge & Kegan Paul.

MAGUIRE, P., COMAROFF, J., RAMSELL, P.J. and MORRIS JONES, P.H. (1979) Psychological and social problems in families of children with leukemia. In P.H. Morris Jones (Ed.) *Topics in Paediatrics I. Haematology and oncology.* Tunbridge Wells: Pitman Medical.

MORRIS JONES, P.H. (1987) Advances in managing childhood cancer. *British Medical Journal,* 245, 4–6.

MOSS, H.A., NANNIS, E.D. and POPLACK, D.G. (1981) The effects of prophylactic treatment of the central nervous system on the intellectual functioning of

314 *Richard Lansdown and Ann Goldman*

children with acute lymphocytic leukaemia. *American Journal of Medicine,* 71, 47–52.

MULLHOLLAND, C. (1973) *I'll Dance With the Rainbows.* Glasgow: Patrick Press.

NEUBERGER, J. (1987) *Caring for Dying People of Different Faiths.* London: Austen Cornish Publishers, in association with the Lisa Sainsbury Foundation.

NITSCHKE, R., HUMPHREY, G.B., SEXAUER, C.L., CATRON, B., WUNDER, S. and JAY, S. (1982) Therapeutic choices made by patients with end-stage cancer. *Journal of Pediatrics, 101,* 471–476.

PAYNE, R. and FIRTH-COZENS, J. (1987) *Stress in Health Professionals.* Chichester: John Wiley.

PECK, B. (1979) Effects of childhood cancer on long-term survivors and their families. *British Medical Journal, 1,* 1327–1329.

PETTLE MICHAEL, S. and LANSDOWN, R. (1986) Adjustment to the death of a sibling. *Archives of Disease in Childhood, 61,* 278–283.

POWAZEK, M., SCHIJVING, J., GOFF, J.R., PAULSON, M.A. and STAGNER, S. (1980) Psychosocial ramifications of childhood leukaemia: One year post-diagnosis. In J.L. Schulman and M.J. Kupst (Eds) *The Child with Cancer.* Springfield, IL: Charles C. Thomas.

SPINETTA, J.J. (1981) The sibling of the child with cancer. In J.J. Spinetta and P. Deasy-Spinetta (Eds) *Living with Childhood Cancer.* St Louis: C.V. Mosby.

SPINETTA, J.J. and DEASY-SPINETTA, P. (Eds) (1981) *Living with Childhood Cancer.* St Louis: C.V. Mosby.

VAN DONGEN-MELMAN, J.E.W. and SANDERS-WOUDSTRA, J.A.R. (1986) Psychosocial aspects of childhood cancer: A review of the literature. *Journal of Child Psychology and Psychiatry, 27,* 145–180.

VAN EIJS, J. (1977) *The Truly Cured Child.* Baltimore: University Park Press.

VARLEY, S. (1984) *Badger's Parting Gifts.* London: Andersen Press.

WASS, H. (1984) Books for Children. In H. Wass and C.A. Corr (Eds) *Childhood Death.* London: Hemisphere.

WASS, H. and CORR, C.A. (Eds) (1984) *Childhood Death.* London: Hemisphere.

WHEELER, K., LEIPER, A.D., JANOUN, L. and CHESSELLS, J.M. (1988) Medical cost of curing childhood acute lymphoblastic leukaemia. *British Medical Journal, 296,* 162–166.

WORDEN, J.W. (1983) *Grief Counselling and Grief Therapy.* London: Tavistock Publications.

ZELTZER, L., KELLERMAN, J., ELLENBERG, L., DASH, J., and RIGLER, D. (1980) Psychological effects of illness in adolescence II. Impact of illness in adolescents – crucial issues and coping styles. *Journal of Pediatrics, 97,* 132–138.

INDEX